a LANGE medical book

# LANGE
## SMART CHARTS

# PATHOLOGY

**Robert Groysman, MD**

University of Medicine and Dentistry of New Jersey
Robert Wood Johnson Medical School
New Brunswick, New Jersey

**LANGE MEDICAL BOOKS / MCGRAW-HILL**
Medical Publishing Division

New York   St. Louis   San Francisco   Auckland   Bogotá   Caracas   Lisbon   London
Madrid   Mexico City   Milan   Montreal   New Delhi   San Juan
Singapore   Sydney   Tokyo   Toronto

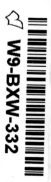

W9-BXW-332

*McGraw-Hill*

*A Division of The **McGraw·Hill** Companies*

**LANGE SMART CHARTS: PATHOLOGY**

Copyright © 2001 by The McGraw-Hill Companies, Inc.  All rights reserved.
Printed in the United States of America. Except as permitted under the United States
Copyright Act of 1976,  no part of this publication may be reproduced or distributed
in any form or by any means, or stored in a data base or retrieval system, without the
prior written permission of the publisher.

1 2 3 4 5 6 7 8 9 0 KGP KGP 0 9 8 7 6 5 4 3 2 1 0

ISBN 0-8385-8175-7
ISSN  1529-7780

This book was set in Goudy by Octal Publishing, Inc.
The editors were Janet Foltin, Harriet Lebowitz, and Nicky Panton.
The production supervisor was Rohnda Barnes.
The cover designer was Mary Skudlarek.
The index was prepared by Marilyn Rowland.

Quebecor World/Kingsport was printer and binder.

This book is printed on acid-free paper.

### Notice

Medicine is an ever-changing science. As new research and clinical experience broaden our knowledge, changes in treatment and drug therapy are required. The author and the publisher of this work have checked with sources believed to be reliable in their efforts to provide information that is complete and generally in accord with the standards accepted at the time of publication. However, in view of the possibility of human error or changes in medical sciences, neither the author  nor the publisher nor any other party who has been involved in the preparation or publication of this work warrants that the information contained herein is in every respect accurate or complete, and they are not responsible for any errors or omissions or for the results obtained from use of such information. Readers are encouraged to confirm the information contained herein with other sources. For example and in particular, readers are advised to check the product information sheet included in the package of each drug they plan to administer to be certain that the information contained in this book is accurate and that changes have not been made in the recommended dose or in the contraindications for administration. This recommendation is of particular importance in connection with new or infrequently used drugs.

This book is dedicated to my beautiful wife Jennifer and daughter Angelica for inspiring and believing in me and to my family, Sam, Minna, and Maya, and in-laws, Teresa, Victor, and Janene, for helping in their own way.

# CONTENTS

*Preface* . . . . . . . . . . . . . . . . . . . . . . . . . . . . . . . . . . . . . . . . . . . . . . . . . . . . . . . . . . . . . . . . . . . . . . . . . . . . . . . . . . vii

*How to Use This Book* . . . . . . . . . . . . . . . . . . . . . . . . . . . . . . . . . . . . . . . . . . . . . . . . . . . . . . . . . . . . . . ix

1. Basic Concepts of Pathology . . . . . . . . . . . . . . . . . . . . . . . . . . . . . . . . . . . . . . . . . . . . . . . . 1

2. Cardiovascular System . . . . . . . . . . . . . . . . . . . . . . . . . . . . . . . . . . . . . . . . . . . . . . . . . . . 25

3. Immunopathology and Autoimmune Diseases . . . . . . . . . . . . . . . . . . . . . . . . . . . . . . . . 45

4. Hematopoietic and Lymphoreticular Disorders . . . . . . . . . . . . . . . . . . . . . . . . . . . . . . . 57

5. Respiratory System . . . . . . . . . . . . . . . . . . . . . . . . . . . . . . . . . . . . . . . . . . . . . . . . . . . . . 93

6. Urinary System . . . . . . . . . . . . . . . . . . . . . . . . . . . . . . . . . . . . . . . . . . . . . . . . . . . . . . 109

7. Male and Female Reproductive Systems, the Breast, and Pregnancy . . . . . . . . . . . . . . 131

8. Endocrine System . . . . . . . . . . . . . . . . . . . . . . . . . . . . . . . . . . . . . . . . . . . . . . . . . . . . 163

9. Gastrointestinal Tract and the Oral Cavity . . . . . . . . . . . . . . . . . . . . . . . . . . . . . . . . . 189

10. Hepatobiliary System and the Exocrine Pancreas . . . . . . . . . . . . . . . . . . . . . . . . . . . . 213

11. The Skin . . . . . . . . . . . . . . . . . . . . . . . . . . . . . . . . . . . . . . . . . . . . . . . . . . . . . . . . . . . . 235

12. Musculoskeletal System and Soft Tissue Tumors . . . . . . . . . . . . . . . . . . . . . . . . . . . . 249

13. Nervous System . . . . . . . . . . . . . . . . . . . . . . . . . . . . . . . . . . . . . . . . . . . . . . . . . . . . . . 269

14. Nutritional and Environmental Diseases . . . . . . . . . . . . . . . . . . . . . . . . . . . . . . . . . . . 289

15. Diseases of Infancy to Childhood . . . . . . . . . . . . . . . . . . . . . . . . . . . . . . . . . . . . . . . . 299

Appendix A: Genetic Causes of Disease . . . . . . . . . . . . . . . . . . . . . . 317

Appendix B: Infectious Pathogens . . . . . . . . . . . . . . . . . . . . . . 319

INDEX . . . . . . . . . . . . . . . . . . . . . . . . . . . . . . . . 329

# PREFACE

*Lange Smart Charts: Pathology* was written and designed specifically for students in the field of medicine. It is geared towards how students study and learn, and what students need to know for course examinations and for the pathology component of the USMLE Step I boards.

The unique approach of this book is immediately apparent. Tables and diagrams are used exclusively to present the carefully selected information, clearly and concisely. This chart method gives an instant picture of how the various facts are connected, thereby making study time productive and successful. Special features include *Terms to Learn* and *Most Common Causes and Types*, which make the various topics quickly understandable and provide high-yield facts—those that are included on examinations and boards. A number of mnemonics that I have found to be particularly useful in remembering confusing details also appear throughout the book.

The material presented in *Pathology Smart Charts* is detailed enough for use in pathology class, yet concise enough for board review. This method is designed to reduce the amount of reading and re-reading required to master this subject area. The essence of this book is captured in the words of Albert Einstein, "Make everything as simple as possible, but not simpler."

I gratefully acknowledge Dr. Fred Skvara for the help that he gave me and David Barnes for his enthusiasm.

# HOW TO USE THIS BOOK

| | |
|---|---|
| **Layout of the book** | The book is composed entirely of tables and diagrams to facilitate comparison and clarify relationships between diseases and pathological processes. |
| **Using *Lange Smart Charts: Pathology* in conjunction with your medical pathology course** | Because learning pathology takes a considerable amount of time, it is generally not one of the areas in which cramming for examinations is possible. Therefore, start using this book early in the year as part of your pathology course. *Lange Smart Charts: Pathology* is designed to make the most of your studying time. Each chapter starts with an outline of diseases and conditions that will be the focus of study. This is followed by *Terms to Learn*, which provides an understanding of pathology concepts and the vocabulary with which to discuss them. The high-yield *Most Common Causes and Types* presents aspects of certain diseases that are heavily tested both on the boards and on pathology examinations. Mnemonics and other learning aids in each chapter facilitate learning some of the more confusing details. Use them, but also make up your own. Remember that the basic cellular and tissue processes and the histopathology (Chapter 1) has to be learned well since everything else builds on this. |
| **Using *Lange Smart Charts: Pathology* as a pathology review for the USMLE part I.** | Start by reviewing each of the chapter outlines, the *Terms to Learn*, and *Most Common* information. Use the mnemonics found in the book, and ones that you have made during your course. Then use a pathology question book to find your weaknesses and review these topics in the relevant chapters. With this approach, you should be able to review pathology in a matter of days. I recommend that you *actively* learn by adding your own notes to these *Lange Pathology Smart Charts*. |

# CHAPTER 1
# BASIC CONCEPTS OF PATHOLOGY

## I. CELLULAR AND TISSUE CHANGES
Granuloma
Steatosis (Fatty Change)
Hypoxic Cellular Injury
Storage Diseases

## II. TISSUE AND ORGAN INJURY
Types of Necrosis
Inflammatory Mediators
Causes of Edema
Mechanisms of Edema
Types of Thrombosis
Types of Embolism

## III. WOUND HEALING
Timing of Wound Healing

## IV. SHOCK
Types of Shock
Shock Stages

## V. NEOPLASTIC CHANGES
Malignant and Benign Tumor Nomenclature
Characteristics of Cancers
Tumor and Enzyme Markers
Oncogenes and Defective Tumor Suppressor Genes
Cancer Epidemiology
Infectious Causes of Tumors
Paraneoplastic Syndromes

**ABBREVIATIONS**
**ALT** (formerly SGPT) = alanine aminotransferase (serum glutamic-pyruvic transaminase)
**AST** (formerly SGOT) = aspartate aminotransferase (serum glutamic-oxaloacetic transaminase)
**ATP** = adenosine triphosphate
**CHF** = congestive heart failure
**CK-MB** = creatine kinase MB fraction
**LDH** = lactate dehydrogenase
**PMN** = polymorphonuclear leukocyte
**TB** = tuberculosis

# I. Cellular and Tissue Changes

## TERMS TO LEARN

| | |
|---|---|
| Agenesis | Absence of a tissue or organ anlage. In renal agenesis, kidneys fail to form from their mesodermal cell origins. |
| Anaplasia | Loss of cellular differentiation or orientation (cells no longer all face in the same direction). Increase in nuclear size (nuclear to cytoplasmic ratio) and change in cell shape. Mitotic figures or active cell division. Characteristic of malignant tumor cells. |
| Aplasia | Lack of organ or tissue development. In aplastic anemia, bone marrow cells fail to mature. Thymic aplasia (DiGeorge syndrome) also occurs. |
| Apoptosis | Programmed cell death without inflammation. Cytoplasm and the nucleus (nuclear karyorrhexis) break up into fragments that are enclosed by plasma membrane. Fragments are cleared by phagocytosis or karyolysis (nuclear fading). Normal process, unlike cellular necrosis. |
| Atrophy | Decrease in cell, tissue, or organ size or function. Seen in muscle after nerve injuries (denervation) or prolonged disuse. |
| Dysplasia | Disorganization of tissue or change in cell size or shape (not as severe as anaplasia). Can be seen in the cervix. Can progress to cervical anaplasia and cervical carcinoma. |
| Granuloma | Aggregation of inflammatory cells composed of modified macrophages (epithelioid), peripheral lymphocytes, and plasma cells. Granuloma surrounds or walls off a foreign body that is difficult for the body to eliminate, such as *Mycobacterium tuberculosis* or talc fragments. Giant cells may or may not be present within the granuloma (see Granuloma below). |
| Hyperplasia | Increase in cell number. |
| Hypertrophy | Increase in cell, tissue, or organ size. Seen in skeletal muscle with strength training and in cardiac muscle with hypertension. |
| Hypoplasia | Incomplete tissue development or decrease in tissue or cell size that is less severe than aplasia. |
| Metaplasia | Change of one mature tissue type into another. Squamous metaplasia (the most common type) occurs when columnar or pseudostratified ciliated columnar cells become stratified squamous epithelium. Associated with irritation (e.g., bronchi of smokers, the esophagus in chronic esophagitis, or the cervix). Also present in vitamin A deficiency. |
| Pyknosis | Chromatin clumping seen in cellular necrosis (compare with apoptosis above). Nucleus appears very dense. |

## GRANULOMA

Types of granulomas

- **Caseous:** Center undergoes liquefactive necrosis (looks like mush). Examples include **TB** and **histoplasmosis.**
- **Noncaseating:** Center does not undergo liquefactive necrosis and remains cellular. Examples include **berylliosis** and **sarcoidosis.**

Types of giant cells found within granulomas

- **Langhans-type giant cell:** Classically formed within the granuloma with **TB infection,** but can be seen in histoplasmosis and berylliosis. Nuclei form a horseshoe pattern within the giant cell.

- **Foreign-body giant cell:** Occurs within granulomas with foreign bodies such as **talc and silicone (silicosis).** Nuclei are scattered within the giant cell.

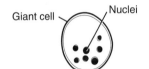

## STEATOSIS (FATTY CHANGE)

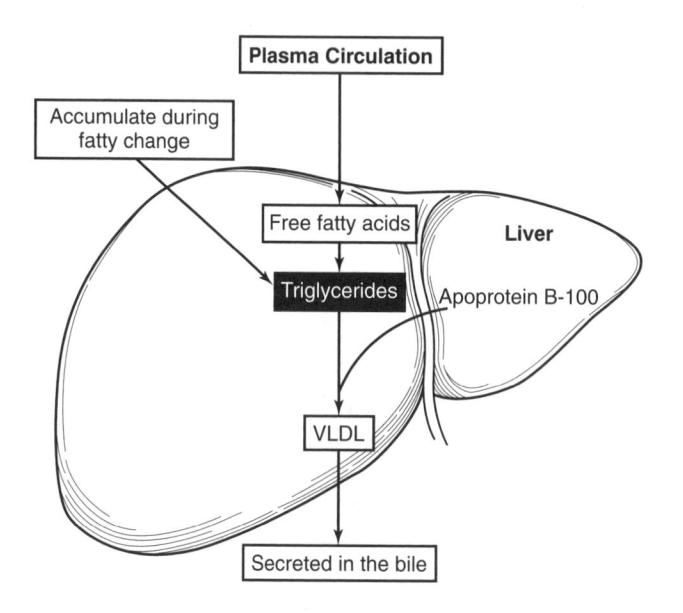

Seen primarily in alcohol abuse but also in diabetes mellitus and prolonged anemia. With Reye syndrome, acute fatty liver of pregnancy, tetracycline or acetaminophen overdose, and Wilson disease, there is associated liver failure. (See Chapter 10, Fatty Liver.) The sequence is as follows:

1. Increase in circulating free fatty acids.

2. Increase in fatty acid synthesis.

3. Decrease in apoprotein production.

4. Decrease in very low-density lipoprotein (VLDL) secretion.

# HYPOXIC CELLULAR INJURY

| Type | Histopathology |
|------|----------------|
| Reversible Injury | Initial cellular hypoxia → cellular (cloudy) swelling due to failure of the Na-K ATP pumps → swelling of organelles (mitochondria and endoplasmic reticulum) → failure of protein synthesis and mitochondrial ATP generation → increase in glycolysis in an attempt to generate more ATP, with resulting lactic acid generation. As pH declines, it causes chromatin to clump. Cell blebs (cell surface deformities) form because of cytoskeletal dysfunction. |
| Irreversible Injury (Cellular Necrosis) | With continued hypoxia, internal plasma membrane damage results in lysosomal content release. Damage to the external membrane results in myelin figures (whorls at the external membrane). Progresses to cell death. |
| Cell Death | Mitochondrial membrane damage allows $Ca^{2+}$ influx. Cells release proteins and enzymes as they die. Some proteins and enzymes are unique to a specific tissue or organ:<br><br>• Heart cells (myocytes) release AST (SGOT), $LDH_1$ (isozyme 1), creatine kinase, CK-MB, and troponin. Show early cell death with hypoxia.<br><br>• Liver cells (hepatocytes) release AST (SGOT) and ALT (SGPT). Show early cell death with hypoxia.<br><br>• Kidney tubular cells are the earliest to be damaged from hypoxia but do not release specific proteins or enzymes. Show early cell death with hypoxia.<br><br>• Pancreatic cells (acinar cells) release amylase (nonspecific) and lipase (specific to pancreatic cells). |

## STORAGE DISEASES

| Disease Category | Disease and Its Special Features | Substance That Accumulates | Organs, Systems, Areas of Body Involved |
|---|---|---|---|
| Glycogen Storage Diseases | Von Gierke disease (Type I)—autosomal recessive. Glycogen granules are evident on electron microscopy. Periodic acid Schiff stain is used for light microscopy. | Glycogen | Liver and kidneys |
| | McArdle syndrome (Type V)—autosomal recessive. Same as above. | Glycogen | Skeletal muscle |
| | Pompe disease (Type II)—autosomal recessive. Same as above. | Glycogen storage (resulting from acid maltase deficiency) | Heart, liver, and skeletal muscle ☞ Pompe = pump |
| Lipid or Lysosomal Storage Diseases | Tay-Sachs disease—autosomal recessive. Cells have "foamy" cytoplasm. | $GM_2$ ganglioside | Brain, retina (cherry red spot), autonomic nervous system, and others |
| | Gaucher disease—autosomal recessive. Cells have a "crinkly paper" appearance. | Glucocerebroside | Liver, spleen, bone marrow, brain, and the mononuclear phagocytic system (monocytes and macrophages) |
| | Niemann-Pick disease—autosomal recessive. Cells have "foamy" cytoplasm. | Sphingomyelin | Brain, liver, spleen, and the mononuclear phagocytic system |
| | Hurler syndrome—autosomal recessive. Cells have clear cytoplasm. | Mucopolysaccharides (heparan sulfate) | Liver, brain, skin, bone (deformities), and macrophages in different areas of the body |
| | Hunter syndrome—X-linked recessive. Cells have clear cytoplasm. | Mucopolysaccharides (heparan sulfate) | Liver, brain, and other organs |
| Other | Amyloidosis—deposition of a hyaline-like substance in tissue. Stains with Congo red (red) and hematoxylin and eosin (pink). Primary amyloidosis (AL type), multiple myeloma, and plasma cell dyscrasias can produce monoclonal light chains (Bence-Jones proteins). | Amyloid protein | Particularly damaging to the heart, pancreas, and kidneys |
| | Secondary amyloidosis—cellular protein generated by chronic diseases including rheumatoid arthritis, Hodgkin lymphoma, inflammatory bowel disease, diabetes mellitus, and Alzheimer disease. Also chronic infectious diseases (tuberculosis, leprosy, osteomyelitis, and bronchiectasis). | Depends on the disease or condition | Variable |

| | | |
|---|---|---|
| Metastatic calcification—hypercalcemia (increased serum calcium) and hyperphosphatemia (increased serum phosphate). | Calcium | Kidneys, blood vessels, and gastric mucosa. Calcification appears black on electron microscopy |
| Dystrophic calcification—calcium deposition on previously damaged tissue. | Calcium | Heart valves. ☞ Dystrophic and damaged both start with a "d" |
| Wilson disease can cause liver failure and a degenerative dementia. | Copper | Liver, basal ganglia of the brain, and cornea (Kayser-Fleischer ring) |
| Jaundice can be caused by direct (conjugated) or indirect (unconjugated) bilirubin. See Chapter 10. | Bilirubin | Liver, skin, sclera (icterus), and organs. Basal ganglia in neonates (kernicterus; with unconjugated bilirubin only) |
| Gout can cause arthritis and kidney stones. See Chapter 12. | Sodium urate crystals | Joints and subcutaneous tissue of the skin |
| Hemosiderosis is secondary to bleeding and breakdown of hemoglobin without cellular necrosis. | Iron as ferritin or hemosiderin | Connective tissue, bone marrow, liver, spleen, and macrophages in different areas of the body |
| Hemochromatosis is primary or secondary to iron overload. There is cellular necrosis. | Iron as ferritin or hemosiderin | Connective tissue, bone marrow, liver, spleen, and macrophages in different areas of the body |
| Atherosclerosis can lead to vascular disease. See Chapter 2. | Cholesterol | Blood vessels and skin (xanthomas) |

# II. Tissue and Organ Injury

## TERMS TO LEARN

| | |
|---|---|
| Edema | Fluid accumulation in intercellular tissue spaces or body cavities. Edema is categorized as local (ascites, pleural effusion, or pericarditis) or general (anasarca). Also categorized by location. |
| Embolism | Solid, liquid, or gaseous mass found in the circulation. Most emboli are thrombotic. Other types of emboli include air, amniotic fluid, fat, infectious, and neoplastic tissue. |
| Hyperemia (Congestion) | **Active** hyperemia involves dilatation of arterioles, resulting in an increase in blood flow and active distention of capillaries. |
| | **Passive** hyperemia is caused by impaired venous drainage and passive distention of capillaries due to backup of blood flow. Examples: Lung congestion results from left ventricular failure. Liver and spleen congestion results from right ventricular failure. |
| Infarct | **Ischemic** necrosis results from prolonged cellular hypoxia that can occur from arterial or venous blood flow interruption. Obstruction of venous drainage causes an infarction in tissues that lack an alternate drainage system. Necrotic area can remain bland (sterile) or become septic (infected). Dead, necrotic tissue is eventually replaced by a fibrous scar. |
| | **Hemorrhagic** (red)—occurs in loose tissue (lung), in occlusion of venous drainage (ovary and testis), and in tissues with a collateral blood supply (intestines). |
| | **White** (pale)—occurs in solid organs with end arteries (heart, kidneys, and spleen). |
| Inflammation | Rubor (redness), dolor (pain), calor (warmth), tumor (swelling), and loss of function. |
| Necrosis | Death or degeneration of cells or tissues as a result of an infarct or toxic injury. |
| Thrombosis | Formation of a thrombus (clot). Thrombus consists of blood factors, platelets, and interwoven fibrin and cellular fragments. There are venous and arterial thrombi. A thrombus may or may not occlude blood flow. Mural thrombus is an example of a nonoccluding thrombus. |

## TYPES OF NECROSIS

| Necrosis | Pathogenesis | Organs or Areas of Body Affected | Histopathology |
|---|---|---|---|
| Coagulative | Hypoxic injury secondary to a thrombus or embolus causing tissue infarction. | Heart, kidney, and spleen undergo pale infarcts. Lungs, intestine, and brain undergo hemorrhagic infarcts. | Architecture is preserved, but nuclei are pyknotic. Cells appear more acidophilic (pink). |
| Liquefactive | Destructive enzymes are released by PMNs, macrophages, and necrotic cells. See Hypoxic Cellular Injury—Irreversible Injury above. | Brain and within a bacterial abscess. | With autolysis, enzymes released from dead cells destroy those cells and surrounding cells. Tissue appears necrotic, soft, and liquefied, without preservation of architecture. |
| Caseous | TB and *Histoplasma* granulomas. | Any infected organ. | Findings are intermediate between the above two. Architecture is not preserved. Consistency resembles cottage cheese. Appreciated best on gross pathology. |
| Fat | Pancreatic enzyme digestion of fat, or trauma to a fat-abundant area. | Abdominal fat and the fatty tissue of the breasts. | Calcium soap formation (appears black on electron microscopy). Acutely, fatty macrophages and PMNs surround the area. |
| Gangrenous | Ischemic injury (dry necrosis), which is often followed by infection (wet necrosis). | Feet, fingers, or bowel. | When dry, looks like coagulative necrosis. When wet, looks like liquefactive necrosis. |
| Fibrinoid | Part of immune-mediated vasculitis, such as polyarteritis nodosa. Also due to hypertension. | Blood vessels. | Deposition of proteinaceous (amyloidlike) material in blood vessels. |

## INFLAMMATORY MEDIATORS

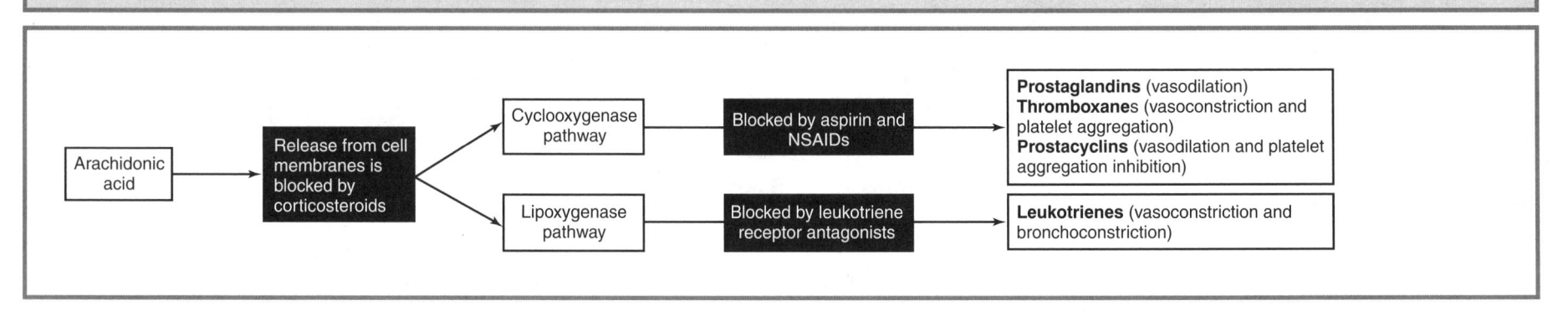

## CAUSES OF EDEMA

| Type | Underlying Conditions | Notes |
|---|---|---|
| Exudative Localized Edema | Cerebral edema—cerebral stroke, head trauma, meningitis, or encephalitis result in neural and glial necrosis and disruption of the blood-brain barrier. Brain may swell diffusely with larger injuries and cause increased intracranial pressure. | Caused by increased vascular permeability in capillaries due to inflammation. High protein content (> 3g/dl), specific gravity > 1.02, and high LDH. |
| | Joint effusion—associated with inflammatory joint diseases. | Pericardiocentesis (pericardial sac), arthrocentesis (joint spaces), paracentesis (peritoneal cavity), and thoracentesis (pleura) are procedures for withdrawing fluid from body cavities for analysis and diagnosis. |
| | Pericardial effusion—serous, fibroserous, or fibrinous fluid accumulation in the pericardial sac of the heart as a result of pericarditis. This is associated with inflammatory conditions, allergic reactions to drugs, and infections of the pericardium. | |

| | | |
|---|---|---|
| | Peritoneal effusion—associated with peritonitis (inflammation of the peritoneum). Exudate is rich in leukocytes and fibrin. | |
| | Pleural effusion—seen in pneumonia, malignancies, and some systemic diseases. | |
| | Subcutaneous or mucosal edema—found in localized burns, allergies (hives), trauma to the skin, inflammatory diseases, and localized infections. Angioneuritic edema is a hypersensitivity reaction localized to the face and neck. (Can be associated with an allergic reaction or an inherited complement deficiency.) | |
| **Exudative Generalized Edema** | Increased vascular permeability in capillaries in septic shock, widespread burns, and widespread allergies (including anaphylactic shock). | |
| **Transudative Localized Edema** | Subcutaneous edema—peripheral edema in the legs often results from local venous obstruction but can also be related to lymphatic obstruction (lymphedema). Varicose veins predispose to this kind of edema. Can also be the sole manifestation of CHF. | Can be caused by increased hydrostatic pressure, decreased plasma osmotic (oncotic) pressure, sodium retention, or blockade of venous drainage. Low protein content (< 3g/dl), specific gravity < 1.02, and low LDH. Similar to the ultrafiltrate formed by kidney nephrons. |
| | Pleural effusion, pulmonary edema (fluid in the alveoli or interstitium), ascites (fluid in the peritoneum), and hydropericardium (fluid in the pericardial sac)—can be associated with CHF, liver cirrhosis, renal disease (nephrotic syndrome), or starvation. | |
| **Transudative Generalized Edema** | May be seen in CHF, liver cirrhosis, and starvation. | |

## MECHANISMS OF EDEMA

| Pathogenesis | Description | Localization |
| --- | --- | --- |
| **Increased Hydrostatic Pressure** | Neoplasms or inflammatory lesions can cause leg edema or hydropericardium by venous obstruction. Interstitial lung edema can be due to CHF or pulmonary hypertension. | Generalized or local |
| **Reduced Oncotic Pressure** | Hypoproteinemia (hypoalbuminemia) can be caused by nephrotic syndrome, liver cirrhosis, malnutrition, and gastroenteropathy with protein loss. | Generalized |
| **Sodium Retention** | Excessive salt intake or increased resorption of sodium in the kidneys (excess aldosterone secretion) is seen in CHF. | Generalized |
| **Increased Capillary Permeability** | See Causes of Edema—Exudative Edema above. | Generalized or local |
| **Lymphatic Obstruction** | Local inflammation, neoplastic obstruction (*peau d'orange*), postsurgical inflammation, or postirradiation reaction. | Local |

## TYPES OF THROMBOSIS

| Type | Description | Pathology |
| --- | --- | --- |
| **Arterial Thrombosis** | Forms in areas of active blood flow. Occurs with vasculitis or more commonly after an atherosclerotic plaque rupture. | Lines of Zahn are light (platelets and fibrin) and dark (red blood cells, platelets, and fibrin) layers that can disappear or organize (recanalization and fibrosis). |
| **Venous Thrombosis** | Usually occurs in the deep leg veins where blood is more static. Venous stasis can occur with prolonged bed rest, varicose veins, surgery (particularly of the lower extremities), cancer, obesity, and fractures. | Complication is embolization to the lungs. Thrombophlebitis is an acute inflammation of veins that results in thrombus formation. |

## TYPES OF EMBOLISM

| Type | Description | Organs or Areas of Body Involved |
|------|-------------|----------------------------------|
| Thrombotic Embolus; | Pulmonary embolus—common in CHF and immobilized patients; a complication of venous thrombosis. See Venous Thrombosis above. | Pulmonary infarction (hemorrhagic) occurs if a small pulmonary artery branch is obstructed. Sudden death occurs if the pulmonary artery is obstructed. |
| | Systemic embolus—mural thrombosis (atrial) is associated with left atrial enlargement and subsequent atrial fibrillation (irregular atrial wall motion). Caused by CHF and mitral valve disease. | Embolus lodges in carotid artery branches including the middle cerebral artery (cerebral infarct), mesenteric artery (hemorrhagic intestinal infarct), or renal artery (pale infarct in renal cortex). Most emboli lodge in the legs (femoral artery or its branches). |
| | Systemic embolus—mural thrombosis (ventricular) is associated with poor ventricular wall motion as can be seen after a myocardial infarction, in dilated cardiomyopathies, and in CHF. | If embolus forms in the left ventricle, it can lodge in any organ that the aorta supplies (brain is the most concerning). Right ventricular thrombus can lodge in the pulmonary circulation. |
| | Paradoxical embolus—mural thrombus that has formed on the right side travels to the left side through a ventricular septal defect, atrial septal defect, or, more commonly, through a patent foramen ovale. | Embolization to the pulmonary artery can occur. |
| Septic Embolus | Embolization of infected tissue fragments from infected heart valves (endocarditis). | Systemic or pulmonary emboli, depending on the valve infected. Mitral valve emboli (the most common type) travel into the systemic circulation. |
| Fat Embolus | From bone marrow fragments following bone fractures. | Lung, liver, brain, or kidneys are possible lodging places. Can cause cutaneous petechiae, pulmonary infarcts, or cerebral infarctions. |
| Tumor Embolus | Originates from solid tumors. | Any area in the vascular system is a possible lodging place. |
| Amniotic Embolus | From amniotic fluid in the maternal circulation. | Disseminated intravascular coagulation or pulmonary embolism can result. |
| Air and Gas Embolus | Complication of central line placement. Also occurs in caisson disease, which can be seen in deep-sea divers who come to the surface too rapidly. | Any area in the vascular system is a possible lodging place. Of most concern is embolization to the brain. |

# III. Wound Healing

## TERMS TO LEARN

| | |
|---|---|
| Abrasion | Loss of superficial epidermal cells. Known as a scrape. |
| Avulsion | Tearing of a piece of tissue, such as tearing off skin, breaking a tooth, or ripping a tendon. Heals by second intention. |
| Contusion | Forms when surface capillaries rupture from a blunt hit. Known as a bruise. Can occur in any organ. Results in a hematoma or ecchymosis. Both are resorbed with time and change from black-blue (iron and hemoglobin deposits) to yellow (bilirubin from breakdown of hemoglobin). |
| First-Intention Healing | Healing in clean wounds when the edges are closely approximated. Granulation tissue appears without wound contraction and with minimal scarring. |
| Granulation Tissue | Normal component of tissue repair. Process consists of angiogenesis (new capillary formation), fibroblast cell proliferation, and stromal regeneration. Occurs in both first- and second-intention healing. Contrast with granuloma from previous section. |
| Healing (General) | Promoted by ultraviolet light, good nutrition, and youth. Inhibited by diabetes mellitus, corticosteroids, chronically infected area, vitamin C or zinc deficiency, and ionizing radiation. |
| Incision | Sharp cut made by a knife or a scalpel. If edges are apposed, the wound will heal by first intention. Otherwise, the gap will heal by second intention. |
| Laceration | Tear producing irregular or jagged wound edges. Heals like an incision. |
| Scarring | Normal tissue is replaced by fibrous connective tissue. Mainly seen with second intention. |
| Second-Intention Healing | Occurs in dirty, large, infarcted, or infected wounds. Different from first-intention healing in that it has more granulation tissue with wound contraction (myofibroblasts) and scarring. If on the skin, a small dimple remains. |
| Ulceration | Break in the skin or mucosa that does not heal. Examples include peptic ulcers, aphthous ulcers (edges of the lips), decubitus ulcers (bedsores), and lower extremity ulcers associated with arterial insufficiency or venous stasis. Ulcers are commonly seen overlying malignancy. Healing (second intention) occurs after the cause has been treated. |

## TIMING OF WOUND HEALING

| Time Elapsed | Histopathology | Strength of Original Skin |
|---|---|---|
| Initial | Clot forms with platelets and clotting factors. | |
| 1–3 days | PMNs infiltrate the clot. | |
| 1 week | Granulation tissue appears. | |
| 2 weeks | Granulation tissue becomes less cellular, then disappears. | 25% |
| 4 weeks | Same as above. | 30–40% |
| 2–3 months | Connective-tissue scar has formed. | 85% |

# IV. Shock

## TYPES OF SHOCK

| Condition | Cause(s) | Pathogenesis |
|---|---|---|
| Shock | Vital organs, including the brain, heart, and kidneys, do not receive adequate oxygen to supply their metabolic needs. | Hypoxia can occur when there is circulatory failure from damage to the heart, blood loss, or massive vasodilatation. |
| Cardiogenic Shock | Heart failure from myocardial infarction or arrhythmia (ventricular fibrillation). Also can occur with CHF because the heart is not pumping efficiently. | Shock occurs because there is pump failure and failure to circulate the blood. |
| Hypovolemic Shock | Loss of plasma from burns, severe fluid loss from vomiting or diarrhea, or blood loss (hemorrhagic shock). Also fluid sequestration from ascites in liver cirrhosis or pancreatitis. | Shock occurs because there is a low effective circulatory volume. |
| Septic Shock | Shock from bacterial infection (usually with gram-negative rods). Lipopolysaccharide endotoxin activates cytotoxic mediators (interleukin-1, tumor necrosis factor-$\alpha$, complement C5a and C3a). Mortality rate is 50%, even with treatment. | Shock occurs because peripheral vasculature vasodilates, shunting blood flow away from the heart and brain. |
| Neurogenic Shock | Spinal cord injury, severe trauma, pain, vasodilatory drugs, or a drug overdose. | Dysregulation of the autonomic nervous system mediates the vasodilatation. |
| Anaphylactic Shock | Severe and acute type I hypersensitivity reaction. Reaction is immediate (antibody mediated). | Inflammatory mediators interleukin-1 and tumor necrosis factor-$\alpha$ are released. Pathogenesis is similar to that of septic shock. |

## SHOCK STAGES

| Stage | Pathogenesis | Signs |
|---|---|---|
| Compensated (Nonprogressive) | Initial fall in cardiac output or a decrease in the delivery of that output results in a compensatory response:<br><br>• Heart rate increases (tachycardia) and respiratory rate increases (tachypnea).<br><br>• Peripheral vasoconstriction maintains blood flow to the brain, kidneys, and heart. | Mild hypotension, tachycardia, and colder extremities; otherwise normal. |
| Decompensated (Progressive) | Compensatory mechanisms can no longer maintain adequate oxygen supply to the vital organs. Some tissue hypoxia occurs. | Dyspnea (shortness of breath), metabolic acidosis (lactic acid excess), and acute renal failure (decreased urine production) can occur. |
| Irreversible Shock | Widespread hypoxia leads to endothelial and parenchymal cell damage, resulting in organ failure. | Coma or death. |

# V. Neoplastic Changes

## TERMS TO LEARN

| | |
|---|---|
| Choristoma | Normal tissue displaced to another organ, as seen in endometriosis. (See Chapter 7, Uterine Conditions.) |
| Desmoplasia | Tumor-induced proliferation of surrounding connective tissue. |
| Hamartoma | Benign tumor-like growth of cell types present in the organ. Examples include lipoma (fat tumor), fibroma, and hemangioma. |
| Initiation | Irreversible first step of carcinogenesis. Produces a mutation in the DNA. |
| Malignancy | Growth that shows metastasis (spread), invasiveness, and anaplasia. |
| Paraneoplastic Syndrome | Symptoms that are not directly due to a malignant tumor or its metastases. Mechanisms involve tumor, ectopic hormones, destruction of normal tissues, and unknown mechanisms. Provides an early warning sign that a cancer is present. Syndrome usually disappears once the tumor is treated or removed. Tumor recurrences are monitored by reemergence of the syndrome. |
| Primary Tumor | A tumor that originates in the organ, whether benign or malignant. |
| Promotion | Stimulation of cell proliferation. When it occurs with initiation, immortal cell lines can eventually arise. Can lead to dysplasia, anaplasia, and then malignancy. |
| Secondary Tumor | A tumor that originates in another organ but has metastasized to the organ in question |
| Tumor Grading | Degree of differentiation (aneuploidy or histology). What histopathologists describe after examining a tumor slice under the microscope. |
| Tumor Staging | Degree of spread, infiltration, or metastasis. What surgeons describe after exploring the body for a tumor and its metastases (i.e., clinical findings). |
| Tumor Suppressor Genes | Genes that suppress cancer formation by halting abnormal cell division or destroying cells with damaged DNA. (In contrast, oncogenes promote tumors). |

## MALIGNANT AND BENIGN TUMOR NOMENCLATURE

| Type | Tumors Ending in -oma | Tumors Ending in -carcinoma | Tumors Ending in -sarcoma |
|------|----------------------|-----------------------------|---------------------------|
| Benign | Adenoma (glands), lipoma (fat), fibroma (connective tissue), hemangioma (blood vessels), leiomyoma (smooth muscle), rhabdomyoma (skeletal muscle), osteoma, neuroma, others | None | None |
| Malignant | Hepatoma, lymphoma, seminoma, diffuse mesothelioma, melanoma, and immature teratoma | Squamous cell carcinoma, adenocarcinoma, hepatic carcinoma, bronchogenic carcinoma, renal cell carcinoma, and others | Fibrosarcoma, chondrosarcoma (cartilage), leiomyosarcoma (smooth muscle), rhabdomyosarcoma (striated muscle) |

## CHARACTERISTICS OF CANCERS

| Type | Origin | Preferential Metastasis |
|------|--------|-------------------------|
| Carcinoma | Epithelial origin. Carcinomas can differentiate into squamous cell carcinomas (contain keratin) and adenocarcinomas (produce mucin). | Spreads through the lymphatics (lymphatogenous). Exceptions are renal cell carcinoma (early venous invasion) and follicular thyroid carcinoma. |
| Sarcoma | Mesenchymal origin including bone, cartilage, lymphatics, fat, muscle, and fibrous tissue. | Spreads through the blood vessels (hematogenous). |
| Immature Teratoma | All 3 germ layers (epithelial, endothelial, and mesodermal). | Variable. |
| Carcinoid | Consists of amine precursor uptake and decarboxylation cells. | Depending on the site of origin, tumors can be locally infiltrating or have distant metastases. |

## TUMOR AND ENZYME MARKERS

| Enzyme | Associated Tumor |
| --- | --- |
| α-fetoprotein | Hepatocellular carcinoma, yolk sac tumor of the ovary |
| Carcinoembryonic antigen | Colon adenocarcinoma, pancreatic carcinoma |
| Prostate-specific antigen | Prostate adenocarcinoma (Prostate-specific antigen is present in small amounts in the normal prostate.) |
| Human chorionic gonadotropin | Choriocarcinoma; also elevated in hydatidiform moles and ectopic or normal pregnancy |

## ONCOGENES AND DEFECTIVE TUMOR SUPPRESSOR GENES

| Gene or Chromosome (Activity) | Associated Tumor |
| --- | --- |
| *rb* gene (defective) | Retinoblastoma, osteosarcoma |
| *BRCA-1* and *BRCA-2*, c-*ras*, erb B2/neu (HER-2) (presence) | Breast cancer |
| WT-1 (presence) | Wilms tumor |
| 8:14t (translocation causes increased *myc* expression) | Burkitt lymphoma |
| 14:18t (translocation) | Follicular lymphoma |
| 9:22t (translocation) | Chronic myeloid leukemia |
| 15:17t (translocation) | Acute myelocytic leukemia, M3 type promyelocytic leukemia |
| N-*myc* (amplification) | Neuroblastoma |

## CANCER EPIDEMIOLOGY: 1999 Estimated Cancer Rates and Deaths for All Adults per Year

| Cancer Rank | Incidence in Men (Number and %; 623,800 total cancers) | Mortality in Men (Number and %; 291,100 total deaths) | Incidence in Women (Number and %; 598,000 total cancers) | Mortality in Women (Number and %; 272,000 total deaths) | Overall Incidence (Number and %; 1,221,800 total cancers) | Overall Mortality (Number and %; 563,100 total deaths) |
|---|---|---|---|---|---|---|
| 1 | Prostate 179,300 (29%) | Lung and bronchus 90,900 (31%) | Breast 175,000 (29%) | Lung and bronchus 68,000 (26%) | Prostate 179,300 (15%) | Lung and bronchus 158,900 (28%) |
| 2 | Lung and bronchus 94,000 (15%) | Prostate 37,000 (13%) | Lung 77,600 (13%) | Breast 43,300 (16%) | Breast 176,300 (14%) | Colorectal 56,600 (10%) |
| 3 | Colorectal 62,400 (10%) | Colorectal 27,800 (10%) | Colorectal 67,000 (11%) | Colorectal 28,800 (11%) | Lung and bronchus 171,600 (14%) | Breast 43,700 (8%) |
| 4 | Urinary bladder 39,100 (6%) | Pancreas 13,900 (5%) | Uterine corpus 37,400 (6%) | Pancreas 14,700 (5%) | Colorectal 129,400 (11%) | Prostate 37,000 (7%) |
| 5 | Non-Hodgkin lymphoma 32,600 (5%) | Non-Hodgkin lymphoma 13,400 (5%) | Ovary 25,200 (4%) | Ovary 14,500 (5%) | Non-Hodgkin lymphoma 56,800 (5%) | Pancreas 28,600 (5%) |
| 6 | Skin melanoma 25,800 (4%) | Leukemia 12,400 (4%) | Non-Hodgkin lymphoma 24,200 (4%) | Non-Hodgkin lymphoma 12,300 (5%) | Urinary bladder and renal pelvis 54,200 (4%) | Non-Hodgkin lymphoma 25,700 (5%) |
| 7 | Oral cavity and pharynx 20,000 (3%) | Esophageal 9400 (3%) | Skin melanoma 18,400 (3%) | Leukemia 9700 (4%) | Skin melanoma 44,200 (4%) | Leukemia 22,100 (4%) |
| 8 | Kidney and renal pelvis 17,800 (3%) | Liver and biliary tree 8400 (3%) | Urinary bladder 15,100 (3%) | Uterine corpus 6400 (2%) | Uterine corpus 37,400 (3%) | Ovary 14,500 (3%) |
| 9 | Leukemia 16,800 (3%) | Urinary bladder 8100 (3%) | Pancreas 14,600 (2%) | Central nervous system 5900 (2%) | Leukemia 30,200 (2%) | Liver and biliary tree 13,600 (2%) |
| 10 | Pancreas 14,000 (2%) | Stomach 7900 (3%) | Thyroid 13,500 (2%) | Stomach 5600 and multiple myeloma 5600 (each 2%) | Pancreas 28,600 (2%) | Stomach 13,500 (2%) |
| Notes | Carcinomas represent 99% of all cancers, whereas sarcomas make up the other 1% in adults. Even though breast and prostate cancers are listed as #1 in the respective sexes in which they occur, basal cell carcinoma of the skin is considered the #1 occurring cancer (> 400,000 per year). However, because this cancer grows very slowly, almost never metastasizes, and has a cure rate of 98% or more, it is not listed with the above cancers. | | | | | |
| | For childhood cancers, see Chapter 15, Childhood Tumor Epidemiology. | | | | | |

Adapted from Landis, Murray, Bolden, Wingo. Cancer statistics, 1999. CA *Cancer J Clin* 1999;49:8–31.

## INFECTIOUS CAUSES OF TUMORS

| Infectious Agent or Toxin | Associated Tumor |
| --- | --- |
| *Aspergillus* (aflatoxin) | Hepatocellular carcinoma |
| Epstein-Barr virus | Burkitt lymphoma; nasopharyngeal carcinoma (in Asia) |
| Hepatitis B virus | Hepatocellular carcinoma |
| *Helicobacter pylori* | Gastric adenocarcinoma and gastric lymphoma |
| Human papillomavirus | Cervical and vaginal cancer |
| Human herpesvirus #8 | Kaposi sarcoma |
| Human T-cell lymphotropic virus type I | T-cell lymphoma or leukemia |
| *Schistosoma haematobium* | Transitional cell carcinoma of the bladder |

## PARANEOPLASTIC SYNDROMES

| Tumor | Paraneoplastic Syndrome(s) |
|---|---|
| Small Cell Carcinoma of the Lung | Adrenocorticotropic hormone (causes Cushing syndrome) and antidiuretic hormone–like hormone |
| Squamous Cell Bronchogenic Carcinoma of the Lung | Parathyroid hormone-like factor causing hypercalcemia |
| Breast Carcinoma | Hypercalcemia (from osteolytic bone metastases) |
| Renal Cell Carcinoma | Polycythemia and fever |
| Hepatoma | Hypoglycemia, polycythemia, and fever |
| Multiple Myeloma | Hypercalcemia (from osteolytic bone metastases) |
| Lymphoma | Fever and humoral immune deficits (B-cell malfunction) |
| Thymoma | Humoral immune deficits (B-cell malfunction), fever, and neuromyopathy |
| Prostatic Carcinoma | Coagulopathy and hypercalcemia |
| Pancreatic Adenocarcinoma | Migratory thrombophlebitis, known as Trousseau sign, and coagulopathy |
| Choriocarcinoma | Gonadotropin (see Tumor and Enzyme Markers above) |
| Carcinoid Tumors | Sterile plaque-like vegetations on the tricuspid and pulmonary valves |
| **Notes** | In general:<br>• Visceral malignancies can cause acanthosis nigricans and dermatomyositis.<br>• Metastatic tumors to bone can cause hypercalcemia.<br>• Many tumors can cause disseminated intravascular coagulopathy. |

# CHAPTER 2
# CARDIOVASCULAR SYSTEM

## I. VASCULAR DISEASES

Arteriosclerotic Disorders

Aneurysms

Other Vascular Diseases

Diseases by Vessel Size

Types of Vasculitides
(Vasculitis)

Primary Vascular Tumors or
Tumor-like Conditions

## II. CARDIAC DISEASES

Ischemic Heart Diseases

Myocardial Infarction
Timetable

Cardiomyopathies

Infective Endocarditis

Noninfective Endocarditis

Valvular Diseases

Pericarditis

Primary Heart Tumors

## III. HYPERTENSION

Types of Hypertension

**ABBREVIATIONS**

**AIDS** = acquired immunodeficiency syndrome
**CK, CK-MB** = creatine kinase, creatine kinase MB fraction
**CNS** = central nervous system
**ECG** = electrocardiogram
**HDL** = high-density lipoprotein
**LDH** = lactate dehydrogenase

**LDL** = low-density lipoprotein
**MI** = myocardial infarction
**PMN** = polymorphonuclear leukocyte
**SLE** = systemic lupus erythematosus
**TB** = tuberculosis

## MOST COMMON Causes and Types

| Disorder | Common Cause |
| --- | --- |
| Pulmonary embolism | Deep leg vein thrombosis |
| Early death after a myocardial infarction | Arrhythmias |
| Acute infective endocarditis | *Staphylococcus aureus* infection |
| Subacute infective endocarditis | *Streptococcus viridans* infection |
| Hypertension | Essential hypertension |
| Myocarditis | Rheumatic fever worldwide and Coxsackie B virus in the United States |

| Disorder | Common Type |
| --- | --- |
| Primary cardiac neoplasm | Myxoma |
| Valvular lesion | Aortic stenosis |
| Cardiomyopathy | Dilated cardiomyopathy |
| Congenital cardiac anomaly | Ventricular septal defect |

# I. Vascular Diseases

| | |
|---|---|
| Aneurysm | Balloon-like swelling in a wall of an artery or the heart. |
| Arteriosclerosis | Rigidity and thickening of arterial walls. Do not confuse with atherosclerosis. |
| HDL (High-Density Lipoprotein) | HDL's role is to exchange protein markers with the other lipoproteins, resulting in the transport of cholesterol esters back to the liver. Referred to as the "good cholesterol." |
| LDL (Low-Density Lipoprotein) | LDL's role is to transport cholesterol to peripheral tissues, but it tends to leave cholesterol "footprints" in blood vessel walls. Referred to as the "bad cholesterol." LDL forms from very low-density cholesterol (VLDL). |
| Vasculitis | An inflammatory and necrotizing vascular lesion (immune mediated) that results in vascular fragility and easy bruising. |

## ARTERIOSCLEROTIC DISORDERS

| Disease | Description | Risk Factors | Pathology |
|---|---|---|---|
| Mönckeberg Disease (Medial Calcific Sclerosis) | Patient develops stiff "pipe-stem arteries." Blood flow is normal | Age > 50 years | Media has ring-like calcifications in medium-sized muscular arteries. Often involves the radial and ulnar arteries. ☞ All start with M. |
| Arteriosclerosis | Hyaline deposition or hyperplastic changes within arterioles | Diabetes mellitus and hypertension | Hyaline deposition occurs with benign hypertension. In the kidneys, it is known as benign nephrosclerosis. |
| | | | Hyperplastic changes involve concentric "onion skin" thickening (fibrinoid deposition) of arteriolar walls and are associated with malignant hypertension. In the kidneys, this is known as malignant nephrosclerosis. |
| Atherosclerosis | Affects large elastic arteries such as the coronary arteries (heart), branches of the carotid arteries (brain), and renal arteries (kidneys) | Age > 45 years (most important), male gender, hypercholesterolemia, high levels of LDL, hypertension, diabetes, and smoking | Simple plaque (fibrous plaque or atheroma) is a lesion located within the intima of arteries. Contains a central lipid core covered by a fibrous cap containing smooth muscle cells, foam cells, and coagulative proteins. |
| | | | Complicated plaque is an ulcerated or calcified plaque. Plaque may rupture, causing a thrombus. Aneurysm also may occur because of structural weakness at the plaque. |

## ANEURYSMS

| Type | Description | Predisposing Factor(s) | Pathology |
|---|---|---|---|
| Atherosclerotic Aneurysm | Aneurysm of the descending (abdominal) aorta. | Risks associated with atherosclerosis | Aneurysm can grow and rupture, leading to death. |
| Syphilitic Aneurysm | Aneurysm of the ascending (thoracic) aorta. May cause aortic valvular insufficiency because of dilation at the base of the aortic valve. | Tertiary syphilis and Marfan syndrome | Media necrosis develops years after the initial infection and may cause sudden death from cardiac tamponade. |
| Berry Aneurysm | Aneurysm in the circle of Willis develops at arterial bifurcations and may cause hemorrhage into the subarachnoid space. Patients have sudden onset of the "worst headache of my life." This condition is fatal if not immediately treated. | Adult polycystic kidney disease and hypertension | Berry aneurysms can resemble berries when viewed on an arteriogram (X-ray with arterial contrast injected). |
| Dissecting Aneurysm | Not a true aneurysm. In an ascending aortic dissection a false lumen can dissect into the pericardial sac, resulting in cardiac tamponade. Can be fatal if the pericardium is not evacuated. | Hypertension (most common), cystic medial necrosis (destruction of elastic and muscular tissue), and Marfan syndrome | Intraluminal tear in the wall of the ascending aorta forms a second, false lumen in the media. |

## OTHER VASCULAR DISEASES

| Disease | Description | Risk Factors |
|---|---|---|
| Varicose Veins | Dilated and tortuous veins; affects the superficial veins in the legs. | Increased venous pressure. Seen in pregnant women, obese patients, in workers whose jobs require prolonged standing, or in those with superficial vein thrombophlebitis. |
| Raynaud Disease | Recurrent vasospasm of small arteries and arterioles, resulting in cyanosis of the fingers and toes. Raynaud phenomenon is similar to varicose veins. | Cold temperatures can initiate. Usually occurs in young women. Occurs secondary to SLE or scleroderma. |

# DISEASES BY VESSEL SIZE

| Small Vessels | Medium Vessels | Large Vessels |
|---|---|---|
| Wegener granulomatosis[1] | Polyarteritis nodosa[2] | Temporal arteritis |
| Hypersensitivity vasculitis[1,2] | Mönckeberg disease | Takayasu arteritis |
| Buerger disease (thromboangiitis obliterans) | Kawasaki disease | |
| Mixed cryoglobulinemia[2] | | Atherosclerosis |

[1] Associated with acute glomerulonephritis.
[2] Immune complex mediated.

# TYPES OF VASCULITIDES (VASCULITIS)

| Disease | Description | Associated Factors | Pathogenesis |
|---|---|---|---|
| Polyarteritis Nodosa | Acutely, can cause generalized symptoms of fever, weight loss, and headache. Multisystem disease:<br>• Hematologic (> 50%)—thrombocytopenia and anemia<br>• Kidneys (50%)—hypertension, glomerulonephritis, or hematuria<br>• Skin (30–50%)—nonspecific rashes<br>• Musculoskeletal (30–50%)—myalgias, arthralgias, or arthritis<br>• Heart (< 30%)—ischemic heart disease<br>• Gastrointestinal (< 30%)—nausea, vomiting, or abdominal pain secondary to hepatomegaly or bowel perforation | Hepatitis B and men | Necrotizing immune complex can form that destroys the media and internal elastic layer. Acutely, disease involves medial fibrinoid necrosis and inflammation. Both ruptured microaneurysms and thromboses result in tissue ischemia. Lesions occur at different times. Chronically, disease involves thickened, fibrosed, and narrowed arteries. |

| | | | |
|---|---|---|---|
| **Hypersensitivity Vasculitis** | Henoch-Schönlein purpura (anaphylactoid purpura) affects children. Patient presents with urticarial wheals that become petechial or purpuric. Fever, arthralgias, and gastrointestinal and renal disease (glomerulonephritis) may also occur. | Upper respiratory infections. Also certain drugs, foods, connective tissue disorders, and malignancies. | Immune complex mediated, but unlike polyarteritis nodosa, all the lesions occur at the same time. |
| | Serum sickness involves deposition of antibody–antigen complexes in joints, kidneys, and heart. | Reaction to blood products | Immune complex mediated. |
| **Mixed Cryoglobulinemia** | Arthralgias, diffuse weakness, and nephritis may result. | Hepatitis C and rheumatoid factor | Immune complex mediated. |
| **Wegener Granulomatosis** | Rapidly progressive vasculitis presents with lung signs (hemoptysis) and kidney signs (glomerulonephritis). | c-ANCA (cytoplasmic anti-neutrophil cytoplasmic antibody) | Necrotizing granulomatous vasculitis. Fibrinoid necrosis with early PMN infiltration. Granulomas form with giant cells. |
| **Buerger Disease** | Also known as thromboangiitis obliterans. Progressive, painful ischemic disease of the extremities found in smokers, involving intermittent claudication of the legs or fingers. May remit, but relapses with smoking. | Men aged 20–30 years of eastern European descent | Thrombosis with infiltration of PMNs leads to fibrosis. ☞ Think of eating burgers with your fingers. |
| **Giant Cell Arteritides** | Temporal arteritis is a disease of the temporal and intracranial arteries. Presents with fatigue, headache, absent temporal artery pulse, and palpable nodules over the temporal artery. Visual impairment may occur (ophthalmic artery = unilateral blindness). Associated with polymyalgia rheumatica—pain and stiffness in the shoulder or hip. | Age > 50 years | Granulomas form with giant cells; may cause infiltrates of eosinophils. |
| | Takayasu disease (pulseless disease and aortic arch syndrome) is a slowly progressive disease with aortic involvement (usually the aortic arch). Branching arteries are obstructed, causing absent pulses from the carotid, radial, or ulnar arteries. | Young women | Fibrosis of all layers of the aorta and branching arteries. Infiltration of the media and adventitia by PMNs and macrophages. Giant cells may be evident. |
| **Kawasaki Disease** | Also known as mucocutaneous lymph node syndrome. Acute, self-limited disease that affects the skin and mucous membranes of the mouth, nose, and conjunctiva. Attacks coronary arteries, causing aneurysms in 25%. (Also see Chapter 11, Desquamation Syndromes.) | Children | Acute necrotizing vasculitis. |

## PRIMARY VASCULAR TUMORS OR TUMORLIKE CONDITIONS

| Tumor | Description | Pathology |
|---|---|---|
| **Benign Tumors** | | |
| Hemangioma | Most common tumor of infancy. In capillary hemangioma, small capillarylike vessels in the skin, liver, pancreas, spleen, or kidneys are affected. Associated with von Hippel-Lindau disease. | Vascular spaces lined by endothelial cells are well defined except in cavernous hemangiomas. |
| | Cavernous hemangioma is a dilated, spongy, vascular mass in the dermis, mucosa, liver, pancreas, spleen, or brain. | |
| Telangiectasia | Also known as vascular ectasia. Not a true tumor. May occur in the skin or mucosa. Prone to bleeding. Associated with Sturge-Weber syndrome. | Prominent, distended, but otherwise normal capillary, venule, and arteriole structures. |
| | Spider telangiectasia is a pulsatile, red macule with small radiating channels. Associated with pregnancy and high estrogen levels. | |
| | Hereditary hemorrhagic telangiectasia is a progressive autosomal dominant disorder, also known as Osler-Weber-Rendu syndrome. Patients have multiple small vascular lesions in the skin and mucous membranes and are prone to epistaxis and gastrointestinal bleeding. | |
| Glomangioma (Glomus Tumor) | Small, purple, firm, painful nodule commonly occurring in a finger or toe. | Composed of vascular spaces. |
| **Malignant Tumors** | | |
| Angiosarcoma (Hemangiosarcoma) | Rare malignant vascular tumor occurring in the skin, musculoskeletal system, breast, or liver. Has widespread and early metastasis. | Composed of endothelial cells. Rapidly growing soft, hemorrhagic mass. Arsenic and thorium dioxide are causes. Polyvinyl chloride is associated with liver angiosarcoma. |
| Kaposi Sarcoma | Malignant vascular tumor now thought to be caused by human herpesvirus 8. Commonly involves the intestines, lung, lymph nodes, liver, and the skin. (See Chapter 11.) | Found frequently in patients with AIDS. |

# II. Cardiac Diseases

| | |
|---|---|
| **Cor Pulmonale** | Right-sided hypertension; hypertrophy and dilatation of the right ventricle from pulmonary hypertension. |
| **Creatine Kinase** | CK-MB is the myocardial fraction of creatine kinase, a mitochondrial enzyme. Serum CK levels rise with heart or skeletal muscle cell necrosis. |
| **Eisenmenger Syndrome** | Condition in which a left-to-right shunt reverses to a right-to-left shunt. Can happen with in patent ductus arteriosus, atrial septal defect, ventricular septal defect, and certain congenital heart diseases (tetralogy of Fallot, transposition of the great vessels, and truncus arteriosus). Mechanism: pulmonary volume overload → pulmonary hypertension → right ventricular hypertrophy → right ventricular pressure > left ventricular pressure → right-to-left heart shunting. |
| **Endocarditis** | Endocardial inflammation, particularly in the valves; infectious or noninfectious. |
| **Heart Failure** | Pumping action of one or both of the ventricles is inadequate, leading to low cardiac output or pulmonary congestion. Heart failure is left or right sided. Either can result in inadequate left-sided blood volume ejection. <ul><li>Left-sided failure presents with orthopnea (difficulty breathing while lying down) from pulmonary edema and lung congestion.</li><li>Right-sided failure causes an enlarged, congested liver and spleen. Liver resembles a "nutmeg" pattern. The most common cause is left-sided failure.</li><li>Systolic failure occurs acutely after an MI or chronically from dilated cardiomyopathy or mitral regurgitation. Dilated ventricle appears baggy with thin walls.</li><li>Diastolic failure causes stiff, hypertrophic ventricular walls from chronic hypertension (the major cause) or from restrictive cardiomyopathy.</li></ul> |
| **Hypertension** | Systemic hypertension is a sustained blood pressure greater than 140/90 mmHg. More than 50% of people in the United States have elevated blood pressure. Hypertension can be classified as: <ul><li>Essential: Age > 40 years, no known cause, and tends to run in families</li><li>Secondary: Age < 40 years and with a specific cause</li></ul> |

*Continued*

## TERMS TO LEARN (continued)

| | |
|---|---|
| **Ischemic Heart Disease** | Atherosclerotic narrowing or vasospasm of the coronary arteries. |
| **Lactate Dehydrogenase** | $LDH_1$ is a good measure of myocardial cell necrosis. Normally, $LDH_2 > LDH_1$ in the plasma. When this reverses, MI can be suspected. LDH peaks late. |
| **Myocarditis** | Inflammation of the myocardium. Rheumatic fever is the primary cause worldwide. Occurs during the acute stages in rheumatic fever. Coxsackie B virus is the most common cause in the United States. Complications include arrhythmias. |
| **Pericarditis** | Inflammation of the pericardium with pericardial effusion. Presents with fever and acute pleuritic chest pain, which is worse on inspiration and better while sitting and leaning forward. Pericardial friction rub and S-T elevation are seen on every ECG lead. Cardiac tamponade occurs with large effusion. |
| **Rheumatic Fever** | Immunologic reaction to group A β-hemolytic streptococci (after "strep throat"). Rheumatic heart disease: pancarditis (inflammation of endocardium, myocardium, and pericardium) and mitral stenosis. Patients may have fever, migratory polyarthritis (arthritis moves from one joint to another), erythema marginatum (small, painless subcutaneous swellings over bony prominences), and CNS involvement (Sydenham chorea-involuntary muscular movements). ☞ Remember the major Jones criteria of rheumatic fever with J = joints, ♡ = carditis, N = nodules, E = erythema marginatum, S = Sydenham chorea. |
| **Ventricular Hypertrophy** | Response to the increased pressure required to eject blood from the ventricles. Initially hypertrophy compensates, but eventually, the ventricles become too thick to pump effectively. Causes ventricular failure (see Heart Failure above). Increased muscle mass requires more oxygen to function, and accordingly the threshold for cardiac ischemia is lowered. |
| | Left ventricular hypertrophy: caused by hypertension or aortic valve stenosis. |
| | Right ventricular hypertrophy: caused by chronic lung disease, pulmonary hypertension, mitral valve stenosis, and any congenital heart disease with left-to-right shunting. |

# ISCHEMIC HEART DISEASES

| Disease | Description | Cause(s) | Complications |
|---------|-------------|----------|---------------|
| **Angina Pectoris** | Episodes of crushing chest pain from transient ischemia of the heart. | Narrowed coronary arteries secondary to atherosclerosis or vasospasm cannot meet oxygen demands of the heart. | Patients with unstable angina or Prinzmetal variant angina are at risk for developing an MI. |
| | Stable angina (most common)—pain caused by exertion and relieved by rest or vasodilators (nitroglycerin). | | |
| | Unstable angina—prolonged or recurrent pain at rest. Must check for possible MI. | | |
| | Prinzmetal angina—intermittent chest pain at rest. | Vasospasm of the coronary arteries creates a temporary shortage of blood flow and oxygen to the heart. | |
| **Myocardial Infarction** | Prolonged ischemia from thrombosis, probably due to atherosclerotic plaque rupture or ulceration. Presents with crushing chest pain. ECG changes and release of cardiac enzymes (CK, troponin, myoglobin, and LDH) are evident. (See Arteriosclerotic Disorders—Atherosclerosis above and Chapter 1, Types of Thrombosis.)<br><br>• Transmural infarction—Entire wall is involved.<br><br>• Subendothelial infarction—Necrosis is limited to the interior third of the left ventricular wall. | Hypercoagulability, collagen vascular diseases (SLE, scleroderma), smoking, hypertension, and hyperlipidemias. | Arrhythmias (main cause of death in the first several hours), left ventricular failure, ruptured papillary muscle, mural thrombosis, ventricular aneurysm, and pericarditis. |

## MYOCARDIAL INFARCTION TIMETABLE

| Time (After MI) | Gross Picture | Histopathology | Enzymes | Complications |
|---|---|---|---|---|
| Hours | No change | Myocyte edema | CK-MB, myoglobin, and troponin | Arrhythmias (most common complication) |
| 1–2 days | White (pale) infarct | Coagulative necrosis | CK-MB and troponin | Fibrinous pericarditis |
| 2–4 days | Pallor with some hyperemia | Acute inflammation (PMN infiltration), hyperemia, tissue changes due to phagocytosis of dead myocytes | $LDH_1 > LDH_2$ and troponin | None |
| 5–10 days (1 week) | Hyperemia with central necrotic yellow area | Granulation tissue | Troponin | Myocardial rupture (especially papillary muscle) |
| 6 weeks | Gray-white area with recanalized coronary artery | Acellular, fibrous, contracted scar | None | Dressler syndrome—autoimmune cause of pericarditis, but not clinically significant |

## CARDIOMYOPATHIES

| Disease | Description | Histopathology | Cause(s) or Predisposing Factors |
|---------|-------------|----------------|----------------------------------|
| Dilated Cardiomyopathy | Most common form of cardiomyopathy, involving dilation of both ventricles and heart failure. Baggy heart = $S_3$ extra heart sound. ☞ Say "bag-gy, $S_3$." | Poor contraction of muscle fibers is due to hypertrophy and possible necrosis with intermixed fibrous scars. | Alcoholism, thiamine ($B_1$) deficiency, and iron toxicity (hemochromatosis or intravascular hemolytic anemia). Also occurs peripartum (of unknown cause) during the last month of gestation. |
| Hypertrophic Obstructive Cardiomyopathy | Formerly known as idiopathic hypertrophic subaortic stenosis. Presents in adolescence with hypertrophy of the left ventricular wall, especially the septum (asymmetric hypertrophy). Left ventricular obstruction during systole can cause syncope and sudden death. Stiff heart = $S_4$ extra heart sound. | Disorganized muscle fibers; hypercontracted and poorly compliant myocardium. | Probable hereditary component. Associated with increased risk of atrial fibrillation, mural thrombosis, and sudden death. |
| Restrictive Cardiomyopathy | Rare. The stiff heart muscle interferes with pumping. Stiff heart = $S_4$ sound. | Infiltration of myocardium with amyloid. | Cardiac amyloidosis occurs in Alzheimer disease, systemic amyloidosis, or light chain disease. (See Chapter 1, Storage Diseases.) |

# INFECTIVE ENDOCARDITIS

| Disease | Description | Cause(s) or Predisposing Factors | Pathology |
|---|---|---|---|
| Bacterial Endocarditis | Bacterial endocarditis is the most common type. Both infective types of endocarditis are treated with antibiotics. Before the antibiotic era, the terms acute and subacute were used to denote death before 6 weeks and death after 6 weeks, respectively. | Transient bacteremia (bacteria in the blood). | Vegetations on valves occur downstream of the blood flow. Pressure past the valve is lower than the pressure before the valve. All manifestations are mediated by an immune type III hypersensitivity vasculitis. Septic emboli may complicate infective endocarditis.<br>• Osler node—painful, red, raised lesion on fingers and toes<br>• Janeway lesion—painless, red, flat lesion on proximal extremities<br>• Roth spots—petechiae in the retina |
| Acute (< 6 weeks) | Typically occurs in patients with a healthy heart and valves. The disease affects the aortic and tricuspid valves. Manifestations include fever, rigors, septic emboli, neurologic symptoms, and leukocytosis. New murmur from valve regurgitation. | The most common cause is S. aureus infection in IV drug users. In other patients, endocarditis can develop from bacteremia. | Positive blood culture. More aggressive than the subacute type and usually destroys the valve cusps. |

| Subacute (> 6 weeks) | Affects the mitral valve. Manifestations include fever, splenomegaly, petechiae, anemia, hematuria, and elevated rheumatoid factor. | • History of valve disease, ventricular septal defect, patent ductus arteriosus, or atrial septal defect<br>• *S. viridans* infection after oral or dental procedures<br>• *Staphylococcus epidermidis* infection of prosthetic heart valves<br>• *Enterococcus faecalis* (group D) in older men with genitourinary or gastrointestinal problems or surgery<br>• *Streptococcus bovis* (group D) associated with colon cancer<br>• Fungi (*Candida*, *Aspergillus*) and gram-negative rods (*Pseudomonas*, *Serratia*) in IV drug users | Less aggressive than the acute type. Usually thickens the cusp but leaves it intact. |

## NONINFECTIVE ENDOCARDITIS

| Disease | Description | Cause(s) or Predisposing Factors | Pathology |
|---|---|---|---|
| Nonbacterial Thrombotic Endocarditis | Affects mitral valve or aortic valves | Terminal stages of debilitating disorders (e.g., metastatic cancer, adenocarcinoma of the lung, or prostatic cancer) | Small fibrin deposits arranged along the line of closure on valve leaflets; usually involve only one side of the valve leaflet. No inflammation (should be called endocardiosis) or valve damage. |
| Libman-Sacks Endocarditis | Affects any cardiac valve(s) (See Chapter 3, Systemic Autoimmune Disorders—SLE.) | Associated with SLE | Small vegetations on one or both surfaces of valve leaflets. Wartlike lesions found at the angles of the mitral or tricuspid valves. |
| Endocarditis of Carcinoid Syndrome | Affects tricuspid and pulmonary valves | Products of carcinoid tumors (vasoactive amines and peptides such as serotonin) cause these plaques. Plaques are not part of tumor or its metastases | Thick plaques in the endocardium and valves of the right side of the heart. Smooth muscle cells are embedded in a stroma of collagen and other components. Presumably, the responsible compound is detoxified in the liver and lungs. |
| Rheumatic Fever Endocarditis | Affects mitral and aortic valves | Rheumatic fever | Wartlike vegetations on valve (do not embolize), fibrosis and thickening, and deformation of valves with calcification. |

# VALVULAR DISEASES

| Condition | Description | Predisposing Factors | Pathology |
|---|---|---|---|
| **Regurgitation or Insufficiency** | Mitral valve regurgitation occurs because the leaflets do not close normally. Patients can be asymptomatic for years, but can present with exertional dyspnea. Predisposes to atrial fibrillation and subacute infective endocarditis. | Rheumatic heart disease, coronary artery disease, acute infective endocarditis, myxoid degeneration, and Marfan syndrome | Myxoid degeneration causes valve prolapse by destruction of the valve ground substance. Produces a floppy cusp that rises too far into the atrium during systole. Similar action occurs in Marfan syndrome. See Cardiomyopathies above. |
| | Aortic valve regurgitation is usually asymptomatic until middle age, when it presents with exertional dyspnea, angina, or fatigue. Predisposes to subacute infective endocarditis and atrial arrhythmias. | Rheumatic heart disease, syphilitic aortitis with aortic valve ring dilatation, nondissecting aortic aneurysm from cystic medial necrosis, acute infective endocarditis, and Marfan syndrome | Both mitral and aortic valve regurgitation increase the volume load for the left ventricle and cause ventricular dilatation over time. See Cardiomyopathies above. |
| **Stenosis** | Aortic valve stenosis (most common valve lesion) is usually asymptomatic except in severe stenosis. Symptoms are angina pectoris, CHF, or syncope. When symptomatic, surgery should be considered. | Congenital bicuspid valve or calcification in the elderly. Valve degeneration is more common with smoking and hypertension | Calcific aortic stenosis is secondary to calcium deposits over time. Ventricular hypertrophy occurs. |
| | Mitral valve stenosis may be asymptomatic with mild disease. With severe disease, dyspnea and fatigue occur. Atrial fibrillation is common. | Rheumatic heart disease | Pulmonary edema. See Noninfective Endocarditis—Rheumatic Fever above. |
| **Prosthetic Valves** | Tricuspid or mitral valves are replaced if regurgitation or stenosis is present. Pulmonary valve may be replaced if stenosis is present. Replacement requires antibiotic prophylaxis against infective endocarditis. Biologic valves deteriorate faster but do not require anticoagulation. Mechanical valves last longer but require anticoagulation treatment. | Nature of foreign valve | Foreign valve material may facilitate bacterial adhesion to valve surfaces. Irregular surfaces of the valve can trigger the clotting cascade. |

## PERICARDITIS

| Type | Description | Cause(s) | Associated Findings |
|---|---|---|---|
| Fibrinous, Serous, or Serofibrinous Pericarditis | Fibrinous exudate with or without a serous effusion (higher in protein content than transudative effusion). | Uremia, SLE, acute rheumatic fever, Coxsackie B, echoviruses, Dressler syndrome, and Mycobacterium tuberculosis | Inflammatory exudate on the pericardium is fibrin rich and presents with a friction rub |
| Purulent Pericarditis | Pericardium is covered with yellow-gray exudate. Purulent pericardial effusion. | S. aureus, Streptococcus pneumoniae, M. tuberculosis, and fungi | Inflammatory cells (PMNs) and the organism found in the effusion; friction rub |
| Hemorrhagic Pericarditis | Inflammatory exudate—serous, serofibrinous, or purulent. | Uremia, M. tuberculosis, severe acute infections, and neoplasms (lung, renal cell, and lymphomas) | Hemorrhagic effusion. Can result in tamponade |
| Chronic Constrictive Pericarditis | Destruction of the pericardial cavity. Scarring → stiff pericardial sac → tamponade. | S. aureus, M. tuberculosis (now rare), radiation therapy, and histoplasmosis | Interferes with venous return and can result in cardiac tamponade |

## PRIMARY HEART TUMORS

| Tumor | Pathology |
|---|---|
| Myxoma | Most common primary heart tumor. (Note: The most common neoplasms of the heart are metastases to the pericardium.) Most myxomas form in the left atrium and may cause obstruction or embolization. This is a benign tumor and also a hamartoma. (See Chapter 1, Neoplastic Changes—Terms to Learn.) |
| Lipoma | Poorly encapsulated, benign tumor of adipose tissue, also called a hamartoma. Occurs in the left ventricle, right atrium, or septum. |

# III. Hypertension

## TYPES OF HYPERTENSION

| Disease | Description | Cause(s) or Predisposing Factors | Pathology |
|---|---|---|---|
| Essential Hypertension (Benign) | Most common type of adult hypertension. Initially asymptomatic. Chronic disease may cause heart hypertrophy, renal ischemia, hypertensive encephalopathy, or hypertensive retinopathy. | Idiopathic. Tends toward familial aggregation. More common in blacks. | Medial thickening from muscular hypertrophy may progress to intimal hyalinization and fibrosis. Benign renal nephrosclerosis in kidneys. (For cerebral encephalopathy, see Chapter 13, Cerebrovascular Diseases. For renal disease, see Chapter 6.) |
| Secondary Hypertension (Benign) | Most common type of hypertension in children. See Essential Hypertension above for complications and pathology. | Renin-angiotensin-aldosterone activation, hyperaldosteronism, acromegaly, Cushing syndrome, steroid use, pheochromocytoma, hyperthyroidism, pregnancy toxemia, CNS tumors, and use of drugs, chemicals, amphetamines, or cocaine. | Unilateral kidney involvement: Renal artery stenosis leads to renin-dependent hypertension (high renin levels). Unilateral hydronephrosis. Most common causes are fibromuscular dysplasia (females) and renal artery atherosclerosis (males). Bilateral kidney involvement: caused by diabetic nephropathy, chronic glomerulonephritis, chronic pyelonephritis, adult polycystic kidney disease, interstitial nephritis, and coarctation of the aorta. Leads to renin-independent hypertension (intrinsic renal failure is responsible rather than the increased renin). Hyperaldosteronism: results from a kidney renin-secreting tumor or Conn syndrome (aldosterone-secreting adenoma in the adrenals). Pheochromocytoma: secretes epinephrine and norepinephrine. |
| Malignant Hypertension | Characterized by papilledema, retinal hemorrhages and exudates, and blood pressures of 200/140 mmHg or greater. (See Chapter 6, Vascular Kidney Disorders.) | Progressive condition that results from long-standing hypertension (either of the above two, but more common with essential hypertension). | Fibrinoid necrosis (onion skinning) is seen in arteries and arterioles. Extreme thickening of the intima leads to narrow arterioles, tissue ischemia, and hemorrhage. Malignant nephrosclerosis causes renal insufficiency, further fueling the hypertension. |

# CHAPTER 3
# IMMUNOPATHOLOGY AND AUTOIMMUNE DISEASES

## I. BASIC IMMUNOLOGY

Immune Complement Cascade System

Important Cytokines

MHC Antigen Type and Associated Diseases

Complications of Tissue Transplants

## II. AUTOIMMUNE DISORDERS

Hypersensitivity Diseases

Systemic Autoimmune Disorders

Autoimmune Disease Summary

## III. GENERAL IMMUNODEFICIENCIES

Inflammatory Response Failure

Immunodeficiency by Immune Component

Immunodeficiency Conditions

**ABBREVIATIONS**

**ADP** = adenosine diphosphate
**CMV** = cytomegalovirus
**CNS** = central nervous system
**EBV** = Epstein-Barr virus
**HLA** = human leukocyte antigen
**H$_2$O$_2$** = hydrogen peroxide
**HIV** = human immunodeficiency virus

**Ig** = immunoglobulin
**MHC** = major histocompatibility complex
**NADPH** = reduced nicotinamide adenine dinucleotide phosphate
**PMN** = polymorphonuclear leukocyte
**SCID** = severe combined immunodeficiency disease
**VDRL** = Venereal Disease Research Laboratory (test for syphilis)

## TERMS TO LEARN

|  |  |
|---|---|
| Arthus Reaction | Type III hypersensitivity. Injection of allergen into skin causes local tissue vasculitis and necrosis. |
| Congenital Condition | A condition that is present at the time of birth, whether genetic or not. |
| Coombs' Test | Identifies type II hypersensitivity.<br><br>• Direct Coombs' test is for antibodies attached to red blood cells. Used to diagnose hemolytic disease of the newborn, acquired hemolytic anemias (due to methyldopa, penicillin), and transfusion hemolytic anemias.<br><br>• Indirect Coombs' test of serum is for free antibodies reactive to red blood cells. Used to diagnose cold agglutinin-type anemia (IgM) and some drug-induced hemolytic anemias. |
| Enzyme-Linked Immunosorbent Assay (ELISA) | Enzyme immunoassay used for quantification of an antibody or antigen. Used as a screening test in HIV. |
| Opsonin | Serum component that attaches to bacteria. The combination facilitates phagocytosis by macrophages and other phagocytes. |
| Perinatal Period | Occurs shortly before birth, during delivery, or some time after. |
| Radioallergosorbent Test (RIA) | Immunologic test that helps identify reactive IgEs to allergens. Allergens can be tested by radioallergosorbent test or enzyme-linked immunosorbent assay. |
| Sequestered Tissue | Immunologically privileged tissues (sperm, cornea, lens, and CNS) that develop after the immune system is competent. For example, no rejection problems occur with lens and corneal transplants. |
| Tuberculin Reaction | Type IV hypersensitivity. Indurated, erythematous plaque forms at the site of subcutaneous tuberculin antigen injection. |
| Tzanck Preparation | Staining of skin scrapings from a lesion. Test helps identify herpes and varicella viruses. |
| Western Blot | Electrophoresis detection of antibodies to viral proteins. Useful as a confirmatory test in HIV. |

# I. Basic Immunology

## IMMUNE COMPLEMENT CASCADE SYSTEM

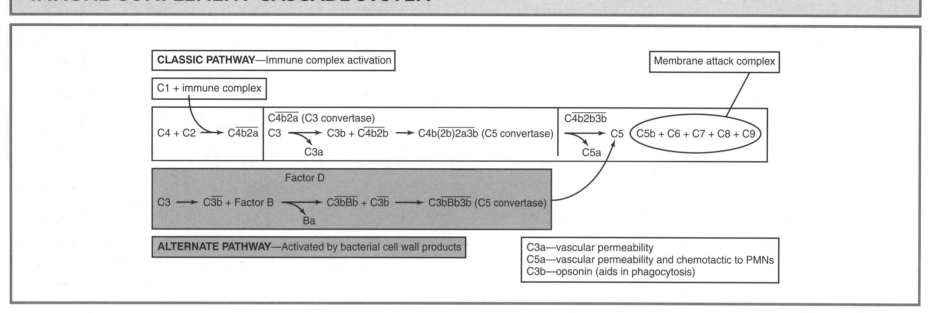

## IMPORTANT CYTOKINES

| Cytokine | Manufactured in | Functions |
|---|---|---|
| Interleukin-1 | Macrophages | Causes T-cell proliferation and interleukin-2 production |
| Interleukin-2 | T cells | Causes T-cell proliferation and B-cell stimulation |
| Interleukin-3 | T cells | Causes proliferation of bone marrow stem cells |
| Tumor Necrosis Factor-α | Macrophages | Causes T-cell proliferation and interleukin-2 production |
| Bradykinin | Plasma protein; high-molecular-weight kininogen | Mediates pain; increases vascular permeability and PMN chemotaxis |

## MHC ANTIGEN TYPE AND ASSOCIATED DISEASES

| MHC Type | HLA Types | Expression Site | MHC Restriction | Associated Diseases |
|---|---|---|---|---|
| I (diseases more common in men) | HLA-A, HLA-B, and HLA-C are located on chromosome 6 and consist of up to 6 different MHC type I antigens. | On all nucleated cells | Expresses endogenous antigen (from virus or tumor) to CD8 T cells, which lyse the cell | • HLA-B27—ankylosing spondylitis and Reiter syndrome<br>• HLA-A3—primary hemochromatosis |
| II (diseases more common in women) | HLA-DP, HLA-DQ, and HLA-DR consist of up to 10 different MHC type II antigens. | Only on immunocompetent cells or antigen-presenting cells, macrophages, PMNs, lymphocytes, natural killer cells, and histiocytes | Expresses exogenous antigens to CD4 helper T cells | • HLA-DR4—rheumatoid arthritis<br>• HLA-DR3—Graves disease and myasthenia gravis |

## COMPLICATIONS OF TISSUE TRANSPLANTS

| Condition | Time From Transplantation | Pathogenesis | Histopathology |
|---|---|---|---|
| Solid Organ: Hyperacute Rejection | Minutes to a day | Antibody mediated. Need previous exposure to same donor antigen to cause this reaction. | Vasculitis. |
| Solid Organ: Acute Rejection | 1 week to months | Cell or antibody mediated. | Lymphocyte and macrophage infiltration. Arteritis is antibody mediated. |
| Solid Organ: Chronic Rejection | Months to years | Cell or antibody mediated. | Vascular damage with organ scarring and atrophy. |
| Bone Marrow Transplant | Short- or long-term | Immunocompetent donor T cells attack host tissue, such as in graft-versus-host disease. T-cell depletion can reduce graft-versus-host disease. | T-cell mediated. Donated organ's rejection of host cells. Liver, skin, and gastrointestinal tract are most affected. |

## II. Autoimmune Disorders

### HYPERSENSITIVITY DISEASES

| Hypersensitivity Type | Pathogenesis | Associated Diseases | Reaction or Test |
|---|---|---|---|
| I (Immediate) | Mast cells and basophils degranulate when presented with an allergen. Immediate, IgE-mediated, preformed histamine release and slower leukotriene synthesis and release (slow reacting substance). | Most allergies and atopic conditions, including allergic asthma, allergic rhinitis, atopic dermatitis, and anaphylaxis | Localized pruritic skin wheal and erythema within 15–20 minutes. Severe reaction can cause bronchoconstriction and vasodilatation (anaphylactic shock). |
| II (Cytotoxic or Antibody Mediated) | Antibodies react with cell-membrane components. Complement may be involved in the cell lysis. | Hemolytic disease of the newborn (Rh or ABO incompatibility), Goodpasture disease, Graves disease, systemic lupus erythematosus, Addison disease, myasthenia gravis, pernicious anemia, Hashimoto disease, and diabetes mellitus type I | Coombs' test is used for detection. Damage results from direct binding and complement fixation. |
| III (Immune Complex) | Antibody–antigen complexes are deposited in various sites (mostly in joints and kidneys), and complement-mediated lysis occurs. These complexes act as chemotactic agents for inflammation. | Serum sickness, polyarteritis nodosa, poststreptococcal glomerulonephritis, rheumatoid arthritis, acute hypersensitivity pneumonitis, and primary (lupoid) biliary cirrhosis | Arthus reaction occurs—localized cutaneous and subcutaneous response to an injected allergen. |
| IV (Cell Mediated) | CD4-specific memory T cells are responsible for the reaction. | Contact dermatitis and chronic hypersensitivity pneumonitis | Tuberculin reaction occurs with a non-pruritic, erythematous, raised skin lesion. This slow reaction takes 48–72 hours to develop. |

## SYSTEMIC AUTOIMMUNE DISORDERS

| Syndrome | Description | Population Commonly Affected | Pathologic Findings |
|---|---|---|---|
| Systemic Lupus Erythematosus | Disease of body-cavity linings, kidneys, skin, joints, and lungs. Causes fever, lymphadenopathy, weight loss, and photosensitive butterfly rash over the base of nose. Other features include Raynaud phenomenon, diffuse pneumonitis, Libman-Sacks endocarditis, vasculitis, glomerulonephritis, and CNS symptoms. | Women | Markers include antinuclear antibodies, anti-Smith antigen antibody (antiribonucleoproteins), antibody against double-stranded DNA, and false-positive VDRL test (cardiolipin released). Findings include fibrinoid change, dermal-epidermal junction complex deposition, basement membrane thickening, and hematoxylin bodies (nucleoprotein and antinuclear antibody complexes). |
| Systemic Sclerosis (Scleroderma) | Progressive disease of the gastrointestinal tract, heart, lungs, muscle, skin, and joints. Causes tight, contracted skin, esophageal sclerosis (dysphagia), glomerular disease (renal failure), and pulmonary sclerosis (pulmonary failure). Variant syndrome is CREST: Calcinosis, Raynaud phenomenon, Esophageal dysfunction (dysphagia), Sclerodactyly (finger clawing), and Telangiectasia. | Young women, but peak is 50–60 years | Vasculitis with fibrosis and degenerative changes. Subcutaneous fibrosis of the facial skin can produce a masklike appearance. Anticentromere antibody activity. |
| Sjögren Syndrome | Produces the triad of xerostomia (dry mouth), keratoconjunctivitis sicca (dry eyes with corneal abrasion), and rheumatoid arthritis. May cause bilateral enlargement of the parotids. | Middle-aged women | 75% have rheumatoid factor and 70% have antinuclear antibodies. Antiribonucleoproteins anti-Ro (ss-a) and anti-La (ss-b) are present 60% of the time. |
| Rheumatoid Arthritis | Chronic inflammatory disorder of the synovial joints. Presents with fatigue, weight loss, fever, and myalgias. (See Chapter 12, Types of Joint Diseases—Arthritis.) | Young to middle-aged persons | Main characteristic is proliferation of a pannus (synovium) into the joint. Rheumatoid factor (autoantibody against IgG) is seen with immune complex deposition. |

## AUTOIMMUNE DISEASE SUMMARY

| Disease | Type of Hypersensitivity | Antibodies Involved |
|---|---|---|
| Addison Disease | II | Antibody to adrenocortical microsomes and plasma membranes |
| Diabetes Mellitus | II | Antibody to β (insulin-secreting) pancreatic islet cells and insulin-associated antibody |
| Goodpasture Syndrome | II | Antibody against glomerular and lung basement membrane |
| Graves Disease | II | Anti–thyroid-stimulating hormone receptor antibody (stimulates the receptor) |
| Hashimoto Thyroiditis | II | Antibody to thyroglobulin and thyroid peroxidases |
| Lupoid Autoimmune Cirrhosis | III | High antimitochondrial antibodies, antinuclear antibodies, and anti–smooth-muscle antibodies |
| Myasthenia Gravis | II | Antibody to the acetylcholine receptor |
| Pernicious Anemia | II | Antibody to parietal cells |
| Polyarteritis Nodosa | III | Immune complexes in blood vessels (may have antibody to hepatitis B antigen) |
| Primary Biliary Cirrhosis | III | Antimitochondrial antibody |
| Rheumatoid Arthritis | III | Autoantibody to synovium, called rheumatoid factor |

# III. General Immunodeficiencies

| INFLAMMATORY RESPONSE FAILURE |
|---|

| Disease or Syndrome | Dysfunction | Cause(s) | Associated Problems |
|---|---|---|---|
| Chédiak-Higashi Syndrome | Migration and chemotaxis of PMNs due to a microtubular problem | Autosomal recessive | Bacterial and fungal infections. PMNs have characteristic cytoplasmic inclusions called the Chédiak-Higashi anomaly (many large lysosomes containing undigested bacterial particles). |
| Chronic Granulomatous Disease | Absence of NADPH oxidase, which catalyzes the respiratory burst (abnormal nitrogen blue tetrazolium test, which checks the oxidative burst) | X-linked or autosomal recessive | Infection with pyogenic catalase-producing organisms (do not generate $H_2O_2$), including *S. aureus*, *Klebsiella*, *E. Coli*, *Shigella*, *Salmonella*, *Pseudomonas*, *Serratia*, *Candida*, and *Aspergillus*. *Streptococcus* and *Haemophilus influenzae* pose no problem. Infectious organism persists within phagocytes, causing a chronic inflammatory reaction which leads to granulomas. |
| Asplenia | Macrophages in the spleen | Acquired or congenital | Infection with encapsulated bacteria—*Streptococcus pneumoniae*, *Neisseria meningitidis*, *Haemophilus influenzae*. |
| Diabetes Mellitus | PMNs and macrophage phagocytosis | Inheritable | Increased incidence of bacterial respiratory infections. |

# IMMUNODEFICIENCY BY IMMUNE COMPONENT

| Immune Component | Cause of Deficiency | Likely Infections as a Result of Deficiency |
|---|---|---|
| Pancytopenia (B and T cells, Neutrophils) | Aplastic anemia due to bone marrow–infiltrating tumors (lymphomas, metastatic carcinomas Such as breast, lung, colorectal, and prostate), fibrosis, cancer, cytotoxic therapy, radiation, several viruses (parvovirus B19, CMV, and EBV), SCID. | May involve any of the pathogens listed below. NOTE: Pancytopenia involves RBC and Platelets as well. |
| Neutropenia (Neutrophils) | Absolute neutrophil count is < 1000. Chédiak-Higashi syndrome and chronic granulomatous disease can cause this. | Systemic infection with gram-negative rods (*Pseudomonas aeruginosa, Enterobacteriaceae*, and *Legionella*) or fungi (*Candida* and *Aspergillus*). Fever in a neutropenic patient indicates infection and needs immediate attention. |
| Lymphopenia (T Cells) | For all T cells, causes are corticosteroids, sarcoidosis, and lymphomas. For CD4 T cells only, causes are HIV and hyper-IgM syndrome. | Infection with intracellular pathogens (*Toxoplasma, Strongyloides, Mycobacterium*), DNA viruses (CMV, varicella zoster virus), fungi (*Cryptococcus, Coccidioides, Pneumocystis carinii*), *Listeria*, and *Nocardia*. |
| Lymphopenia (B Cells) | Multiple myeloma, IgA deficiency, and infections with EBV or CMV | Infection with encapsulated bacteria (*S. pneumoniae, N. meningitidis*, and *H. influenzae*); sinobronchial infections. |
| Complement | C2 deficiency is the most common (asymptomatic). Also liver damage or failure, hypoproteinemia (nephrotic syndrome), and congenital complement deficiencies. | Pyogenic bacterial infections; recurrent *Neisseria* infections (especially with terminal complement deficiencies of C5, C6, C7, C8, and C9). |

## IMMUNODEFICIENCY CONDITIONS

| Disease or Syndrome | Dysfunction | Cause(s) or Risk Factors | Associated Problems |
|---|---|---|---|
| X-Linked Agammaglobulinemia of Bruton | Mature B cells: maturation stops at the pre-B stage. No plasma cells (no antibodies) or germinal centers. | X-linked (males only); appears after 6 months of life (after maternal antibodies disappear) | Recurrent infections with encapsulated bacteria (*Staphylococcus aureus*, *H. influenzae*, *S. pneumoniae*) early in life. |
| DiGeorge Syndrome | T cells | Thymic aplasia (malformation of the third and fourth pharyngeal pouches) | Infection with intracellular pathogens (viruses, some bacteria, and fungi). Because the parathyroid gland (forms from the same pouches) is missing, hypocalcemia and tetany will result. |
| Severe Combined Immunodeficiency Disease | B and T cells (lymphopenia); thymic hypoplasia and lymph organ hypoplasia. | Autosomal recessive (adenosine deaminase deficiency with toxic ADP accumulation in lymphocytes) | Viral, bacterial, and fungal infections. Higher risk of malignancy. May require a bone marrow transplant. ☞ Say "Let's SCIDADA here" to remember which enzyme is deficient (ADA is adenosine deaminase). |
| IgA Deficiency | Most common B-cell defect. IgA-secreting B cells do not mature to plasma cells. | Inherited | Anaphylactic reactions to blood products (due to IgA autoantibody). |
| Wiskott-Aldrich Syndrome | T cells | X-linked recessive | Poor response to bacterial polysaccharide antigen. Also causes eczema and thrombocytopenia. ☞ "Wisk" to get out the tea (T) stain. |

*Continued*

## IMMUNODEFICIENCY CONDITIONS (Continued)

| Disease or Syndrome | Dysfunction | Cause(s) or Risk Factors | Associated Problems |
|---|---|---|---|
| AIDS

*Acute Stage:* HIV positive, flu or infectious mononucleosis like symptoms, general lymphadenopathy
*End Stage:* wasting from tuberculosis, CMV, or *Cryptosporidium* | Depletion of CD4 cells, Langerhan's cells, dendritic cells, microglia (CNS), and neural cells. Monocytes and macrophages are reservoirs. | Homosexual activity in men, IV drug use, multiple blood transfusions (hemophilia, thalassemia major), and vertical transmission to infants of infected mothers at delivery (25%). Now, heterosexual activity may also lead to transmission of the virus. | Failure of humoral immunity (no CD4 T cells to stimulate) and cell-mediated immunity. Paradoxical hypergammaglobulinemia (polyclonal but nonfunctional). Opportunistic infections: *P. carinii, Mycobacterium tuberculosis*, CMV, *Mucor* (fungus), *Mycobacterium avium-intracellulare, Cryptosporidium, Coccidioides, Cryptococcus, Toxoplasma, Histoplasma,* and *Giardia.* Opportunistic malignancies: Kaposi sarcoma, non-Hodgkin B-cell lymphoma (immunoblastic), and CNS tumors (primary lymphoma). |
| Leukemias and Solid Tumors | T-cell malfunction or bone marrow infiltration with resulting pancytopenia. | Metastases to bone or leukemia. | Infection with intracellular pathogens (viruses, certain bacteria, and fungi). If leukemia or solid tumors infiltrate into bone marrow, presentation is similar to SCID. |
| Chemotherapy Toxicity | Bone marrow failure with resulting pancytopenia. | Chemotherapy destroys dividing blood cell precursors in bone marrow. | Similar to SCID. |

# CHAPTER 4
# HEMATOPOIETIC AND LYMPHORETICULAR DISORDERS

**I. GENERAL HEMATOLOGY**

Hematopoiesis

**II. ANEMIAS AND POLYCYTHEMIA**

Iron-Carrying Proteins

RBC Morphology in Anemias

Abnormal Blood Indices in Anemias

Pathogenesis of Microcytic Anemias

Types of Microcytic Anemias

**II. ANEMIAS AND POLYCYTHEMIA** *(Continued)*

Types of Hemoglobin

Globin-Chain Genes: Pathogenesis of Thalassemias

Macrocytic Anemias

Schilling Test

Normochromic Anemias

Hemolytic Anemias

Polycythemia

**III. LEUKOCYTIC DISORDERS**

Myeloproliferative Syndromes

Hodgkin Lymphomas

Non-Hodgkin Lymphomas

Myelodysplastic Syndromes

Leukemias

Plasma Cell Dyscrasias

Langerhans Cell Histiocytosis

**IV. HEMOSTATIC DISORDERS**

Summary of Bleeding Disorders

Comparison of von Willebrand Disease and Hemophilia

Thrombocytopenia

Clotting Cascade

Hemostasis System Modifiers

Disseminated Intravascular Coagulation

**ABBREVIATIONS**

**ADP** = adenosine diphosphate
**G6PD** = glucose-6-phosphate dehydrogenase
**Hct** = hematocrit
**Hgb** = hemoglobin
**MCV** = mean corpuscular volume
**NSAID** = nonsteroidal anti-inflammatory drug
**PT** = prothrombin time

**PTT** = partial thromboplastin time
**RBC** = red blood cell
**TdT** = terminal deoxynucleotidyltransferase
**TT** = thrombin time
**vWF** = von Willebrand factor
**WBC** = white blood cell

## MOST COMMON Causes and Types

| Disorder | Common Cause |
| --- | --- |
| Microcytic anemia | Iron-deficiency anemia |
| Macrocytic anemia | Megaloblastic anemia |
| Thrombocytopenia | Aplastic anemia |

| Disorder | Common Type |
| --- | --- |
| Hodgkin lymphoma | Nodular sclerosis |
| Childhood leukemia | Acute lymphocytic leukemia |
| Plasma cell dyscrasias | Multiple myeloma |
| Childhood thrombocytopenia | Acute idiopathic thrombocytopenic purpura |

# I. General Hematology

| | |
|---|---|
| Acanthocytosis | Cells with thorny projections (burr cells). |
| Anemia | Deficiency of RBCs. Hct is low. Normal response is an increase in reticulocyte production unless the anemia is caused by bone marrow failure. Anemia is classified based on RBC diameter: microcytic, normocytic, or macrocytic. Also classified by the cause of anemia: hypoproliferative, bone marrow failure, delayed nuclear maturation, and hemolytic. (See Abnormal Blood Indices in Anemias below.) |
| Anisocytosis | Variation in size among RBCs. |
| Aplastic Anemias | Group of disorders that includes at least 2 cytopenias caused by bone marrow failure. Can be any combination of anemia, thrombocytopenia, or leukopenia. |
| Erythropoiesis | Formation of the RBC line. |
| Extramedullary Erythropoiesis | Production of RBCs by hematopoietic tissue found outside the bone marrow, most commonly in the spleen and liver. Compensation for bone marrow failure. |
| Heinz Body | Round inclusions seen with new methylene blue stain (shows the oxidized, precipitated Hgb). Seen in G6PD deficiency. |
| Hematocrit (Het) | Ratio of total RBC volume to the total blood volume. Dilution decreases Hct; dehydration increases it. Used together with Hgb to diagnose anemia or polycythemia. |
| Hematopoiesis | Formation of new blood cells including WBCs, RBCs, and platelets. Includes erythropoiesis and leukopoiesis. |
| Howell-Jolly Body | Round blue bodies in RBCs representing nuclear debris. Seen in pernicious anemia, hemolytic anemia, or asplenia. |
| Ineffective Erythropoiesis | Failure to generate mature RBCs even though precursors exist. Caused by iron deficiency and defective heme or hemoglobin synthesis. Also caused by chronic diseases (liver and kidney), chronic inflammatory states, and infiltrative diseases (bone marrow failure). |

*Continued*

## TERMS TO LEARN (Continued)

| | |
|---|---|
| Leukopoiesis | Formation of the WBC line, including granulocytes (PMNs, eosinophils, and basophils) and agranulocytes (mononuclear cells—lymphocytes, monocytes, and macrophages). |
| Macrocyte | Larger than normal RBC diameter, with MCV > 100 $\mu m^3$. Most common causes are vitamin $B_{12}$ and folate deficiency. |
| Microcyte | Smaller than normal RBC diameter, with MCV < 80 $\mu m^3$. Iron studies including serum iron, total iron-binding capacity, and serum ferritin are used to differentiate among the causes of microcytic anemias. Most common cause of microcytic anemia is iron deficiency. |
| Myeloid Cells | Immature bone marrow cells of the granulocyte cell line. Found in the circulation in myelocytic stem cell disorders (myeloproliferative disorders) and myelocytic leukemias. |
| Myelophthisic Anemia | Normocytic, normochromic anemia. Results from bone marrow infiltration by cells of leukemia, lymphoma, myeloma, fibrosis, or granulomas. Can cause extramedullary erythropoiesis, pancytopenia, many nucleated RBC precursors, and formation of abnormally shaped RBCs called teardrop cells (poikilocytosis). |
| Pappenheimer Bodies | Siderotic granules (excess precipitated iron) in RBCs. |
| Poikilocytosis | Irregularities in RBC shape. |
| Polycythemia | Increase in circulating RBCs. |
| Reactive Erythropoiesis | Appropriate reaction (reticulocytosis and erythrocytosis) to subacute or chronic loss of RBCs. Seen in hemolytic anemias. |
| Rouleaux Formation | Stacked RBCs (resembling a stack of cards), seen in multiple myeloma and Waldenström macroglobulinemia. |
| Schistocyte | Severe poikilocytosis with cell fragmentation. |
| Sickle Cell | RBC that resembles a quarter moon. Seen in sickle cell anemia and in sickle cell trait. |
| Spherocyte | Sphere-shaped RBC without the pale center. Seen with spherocytosis. |
| Target Cell | RBC that resembles a bull's-eye target (dark circle within the pale center area). Seen in liver disease. |

# HEMATOPOIESIS

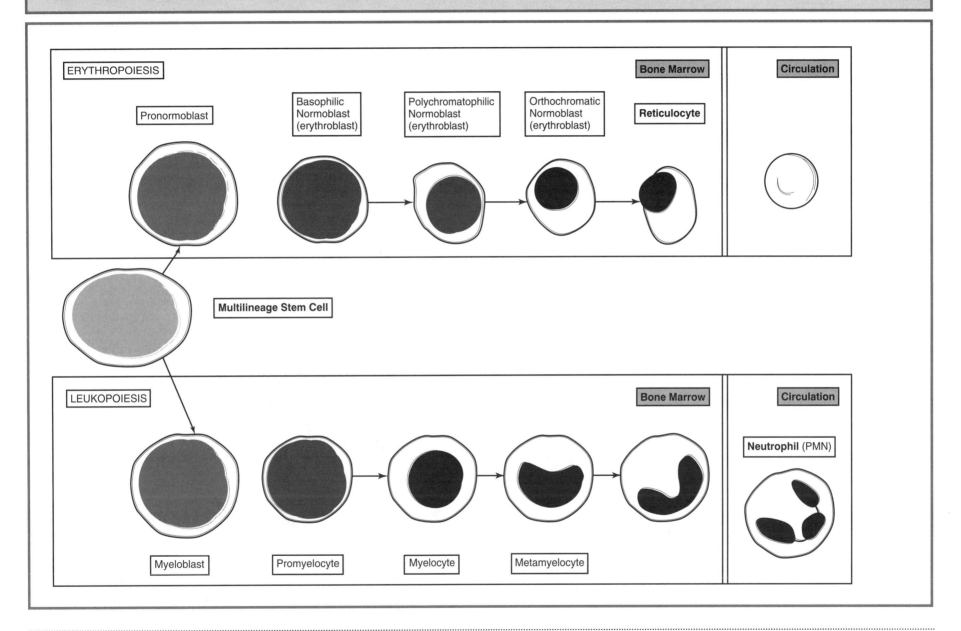

ERYTHROPOIESIS

Pronormoblast

Basophilic Normoblast (erythroblast)

Polychromatophilic Normoblast (erythroblast)

Orthochromatic Normoblast (erythroblast)

**Reticulocyte**

**Bone Marrow**

**Circulation**

**Multilineage Stem Cell**

LEUKOPOIESIS

**Bone Marrow**

**Circulation**

**Neutrophil** (PMN)

Myeloblast

Promyelocyte

Myelocyte

Metamyelocyte

# II. Anemias and Polycythemia

## IRON-CARRYING PROTEINS

| Protein | Function |
| --- | --- |
| Ferritin | Major storage in an iron–protein complex. |
| Hemosiderin | Minor storage form. |
| Transferrin | Binds iron in plasma. Total iron-binding capacity measures the percentage of transferrin saturation with iron. The greater the iron-binding capacity, the less iron is available (assuming the transferrin is constant). |
| Myoglobin | Iron–protein complex in myocytes of the heart and skeletal and smooth muscle; used to store and transport oxygen |
| Hemoglobin | Iron–protein complex in RBCs; used to store and transport oxygen. |
| Haptoglobin | Transports loose Hgb (from intravascularly lysed RBCs). |

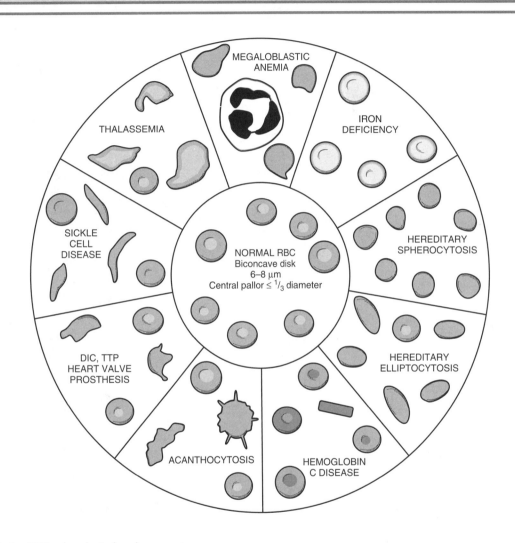

DIC = disseminated intravascular coagulation; TTP = thrombotic thrombocytopenic purpura.

Adapted from Rubin E, Farber J (editors): *Pathology,* 3rd ed. Philadelphia: Lippincott-Raven, 1999:1068.

## ABNORMAL BLOOD INDICES IN ANEMIAS

| Measurement | Normocytic Normochromic Anemias | Microcytic Hypochromic Anemias | Macrocytic Hyperchromic Anemias |
|---|---|---|---|
| **Mean Corpuscular Volume (MCV)** The average volume occupied by an RBC. MCV = Hct × 10/RBC ($10^{12}$/L). | 80–100 $\mu m^3$ | < 80 $\mu m^3$ | > 100 $\mu m^3$ |
| **Mean Corpuscular Hemoglobin (MCH)** The average weight of Hgb in an RBC. MCH = Hgb (g/dL) × 10/RBC ($10^{12}$/L). | 27–33 pg | < 27 pg | > 33 pg |
| **Mean Corpuscular Hemoglobin Concentration (MCHC)** Ratio of the weight of Hgb to the volume of the RBC. MCHC = Hgb (g/dL) × 100/Hct, or MCH/MCV. (Normal: 31–37 g/dL) | ≤ 30 g/dL | ≤ 30 g/dL (except in spherocytosis, where MCHC is up to 37 g/dL) | ≤ 30 g/dL |
| Representative Anemias | **Bone marrow failure with ineffective erythropoiesis:** aplastic anemia, myelodysplastic syndromes (refractory anemias), and myelophthisic anemia. **Hypoproliferative anemias:** renal disease (low erythropoietin). **Blood loss or hemolysis:** acute hemorrhage and hemolytic anemias (except thalassemias). **Other:** Chronic inflammation and iron deficiency in early stages. Hemolysis is compensated by reticulocytosis (increased reticulocyte formation) or effective erythropoiesis. Reticulocytes are larger than mature RBCs. | **Ineffective or decreased erythropoiesis without bone marrow failure:** iron-deficiency anemia (most common cause), thalassemias, hereditary sideroblastic anemia, and anemia of chronic disease. **Cytoskeletal membrane abnormality:** hereditary spherocytosis. | **Delayed nuclear maturation:** $B_{12}$ or folic acid deficiency—megaloblastic anemia (most common cause), Lesch-Nyhan syndrome, antimetabolite drugs, or DNA synthesis inhibitors. **Abnormal plasma protein incorporation:** liver disease (spur cell anemia) and chronic alcoholism. |

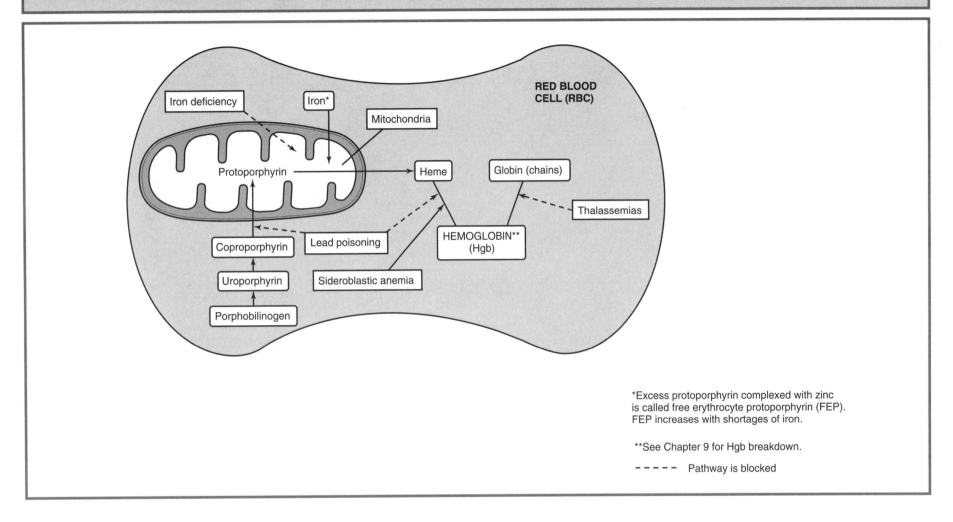

RED BLOOD CELL (RBC)

Iron deficiency

Iron*

Mitochondria

Protoporphyrin → Heme

Globin (chains)

Thalassemias

Coproporphyrin

Lead poisoning

HEMOGLOBIN** (Hgb)

Uroporphyrin

Sideroblastic anemia

Porphobilinogen

*Excess protoporphyrin complexed with zinc
is called free erythrocyte protoporphyrin (FEP).
FEP increases with shortages of iron.

**See Chapter 9 for Hgb breakdown.

– – – – – Pathway is blocked

## TYPES OF MICROCYTIC ANEMIAS

| Anemia | Pathogenesis | Associated Findings | Serum Iron | Total Iron-Binding Capacity | Serum Ferritin | Bone Marrow Iron | Findings on Peripheral Smear |
|---|---|---|---|---|---|---|---|
| Iron-Deficiency Anemia | Inadequate iron stores to incorporate into Hgb. Caused by menses in women or gastrointestinal bleeding in men. Dietary deficiency is seen only in neonates. | Low LDH and indirect bilirubin. Severe anemia causes brittle nails and nail spooning, smooth tongue, mucosal ulcerations, cheliosis, and ice craving. | ↓ | ↑ | ↓ | ↓ | Microcytic RBCs with large (> 1/3 diameter) pale area in centers |
| Anemia of Chronic Disease | Iron-release blockade from reticuloendothelial stores. Bone marrow cannot compensate (no available iron). Seen in chronic infections, cancer, or chronic liver disease. | High LDH and indirect bilirubin. Can cause fever, jaundice, and leukocytosis. | ↓ | ↓ | ↑ | ↑ | Normocytic normochromic cells (early); microcytic cells (later) |
| Sideroblastic Anemia | X-linked or acquired. Defective heme synthase halts heme synthesis. | Iron accumulates in tissues. | ↑ | ↑ | ↑ | ↑ | Dimorphic microcytic ring sideroblasts (with Prussian blue stain) and normal RBCs |
| Thalassemia | Deficiency of globin chain synthesis (Hgb A cannot form). Hgb $A_2$ and Hgb F form to compensate. | High LDH and indirect bilirubin. Can cause jaundice. | Normal | Normal | Normal | Normal-↑ | Increased RBCs from compensatory increase in other forms of Hgb. Unique for a microcytic anemia |
| Lead Poisoning | Heme and globin production are halted because of lead-mediated enzyme inhibition. | High urine coproporphyrin III. | Normal-↑ | Normal | ↑ | Normal | RBC basophilic stippling |
| Hereditary Spherocytosis | Autosomal dominant. Irregularity of the RBC membrane cytoskeleton results in hemolysis in the spleen (extravascular hemolysis). Osmotic fragility test is positive (hypotonic solution lyses cells). | High LDH and indirect bilirubin. MCHC is the highest it can be, 37 g/dL. Can cause jaundice, splenomegaly, and severe anemia. | Normal | Normal | Normal | Normal | Spherocytes (no pale region in center of RBCs) |

## TYPES OF HEMOGLOBIN

| Hemoglobin | Chains | α (Alpha) Chain(s) | β (Beta) Chain(s) | γ (Gamma) Chain(s) | δ (Delta) Chain(s) | Description or Pathogenesis |
|---|---|---|---|---|---|---|
| Hgb A (Adult) | $\alpha_2\beta_2$ | 2 | 2 | | | Normal Hgb. |
| Hgb A$_2$ (Adult) | $\alpha_2\delta_2$ | 2 | | | 2 | Minor increase occurs in thalassemias and sickle cell anemia. Normal variant of Hgb. |
| Hgb F (Fetal) | $\alpha_2\gamma_2$ | 2 | | 2 | | Hgb F does not bind 2,3-bisphosphoglycerate well. It holds on to oxygen better than the adult form. Increase in Hgb F in persistent disease and thalassemia major (all β chains defective). |
| Hgb H | $\beta_4$ | (1) | 4 | | | Hgb H cannot release oxygen. Alpha chain may be present but not in sufficient quantity to form Hgb F. |
| Hgb Lepore | $\alpha_2(\beta\delta)_2$ | 2 | 1 | | 1 | Hybrid βδ chain forms a normal variant of adult Hgb; carriers are asymptomatic. |
| Hgb S | $\alpha_2\beta_2{}^s$ | 2 | 2 (modified) | | | Seen in sickle cell disease. Amino-acid substitution in the β chain sequence causes it to form polymers with other Hgb S molecules in the RBC when the cell is desaturated in oxygen. |

## GLOBIN-CHAIN GENES: PATHOGENESIS OF THALASSEMIAS

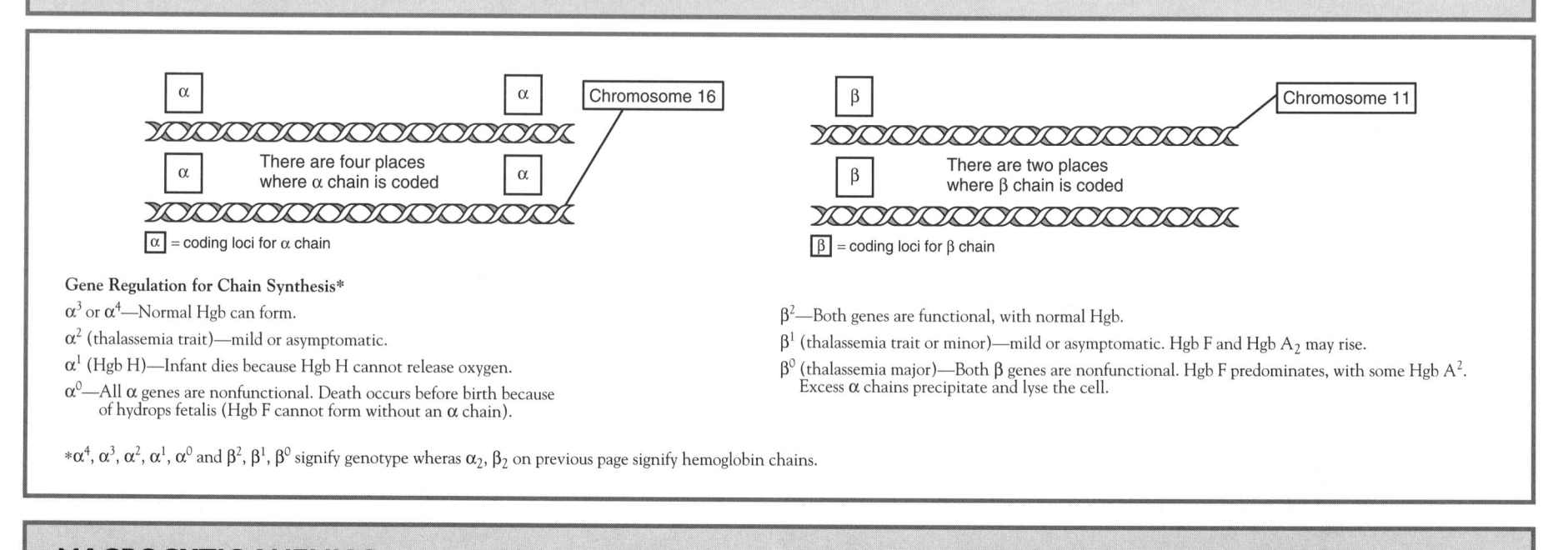

Gene Regulation for Chain Synthesis*

$\alpha^3$ or $\alpha^4$—Normal Hgb can form.

$\alpha^2$ (thalassemia trait)—mild or asymptomatic.

$\alpha^1$ (Hgb H)—Infant dies because Hgb H cannot release oxygen.

$\alpha^0$—All $\alpha$ genes are nonfunctional. Death occurs before birth because of hydrops fetalis (Hgb F cannot form without an $\alpha$ chain).

$\beta^2$—Both genes are functional, with normal Hgb.

$\beta^1$ (thalassemia trait or minor)—mild or asymptomatic. Hgb F and Hgb $A_2$ may rise.

$\beta^0$ (thalassemia major)—Both $\beta$ genes are nonfunctional. Hgb F predominates, with some Hgb $A^2$. Excess $\alpha$ chains precipitate and lyse the cell.

*$\alpha^4$, $\alpha^3$, $\alpha^2$, $\alpha^1$, $\alpha^0$ and $\beta^2$, $\beta^1$, $\beta^0$ signify genotype wheras $\alpha_2$, $\beta_2$ on previous page signify hemoglobin chains.

## MACROCYTIC ANEMIAS

| Cause of Anemia | Serum $B_{12}$ | Serum Folate | RBC Folate | Findings on Peripheral Smear | Findings in Bone Marrow | Signs and Symptoms | Pathogenesis and Treatment |
|---|---|---|---|---|---|---|---|
| $B_{12}$ Deficiency | ↓ | Normal | Normal | Macrocytes and ovalocytes. PMNs may be multilobed. | Immature WBC and RBC precursors. | Peripheral neuropathy and demyelination of the posterolateral spinal cord tracts, leading to a sensory and vibratory sense loss. | Delayed nuclear maturation. $B_{12}$ is insufficient with vegetarian diet, in neonates, and with pernicious anemia (autoimmune), tapeworm, and malabsorption (chronic diarrhea). Treatable with parenteral $B_{12}$. |

| | | | | | | | |
|---|---|---|---|---|---|---|---|
| **Folic Acid Deficiency** | Normal | ↓ | ↓ | Similar to above | Similar to above | Anemia | Delayed nuclear maturation. Dietary deficiency is the primary cause. Can occur if demands for folate increase (pregnancy or alcoholism). Never treat with folate alone. Folate will treat only the anemia and not the neurologic symptoms that may be caused by $B_{12}$ deficiency. |
| **Spur Cell Anemia** | Normal | ↓ | ↓ | Target cells and poikilocytosis | Normal | Hemolytic anemia; elevations of liver enzymes | Anemia from viral or alcoholic hepatitis or cirrhosis of the liver. Increased serum lipoproteins transfer cholesterol into RBC membranes, increasing their surface area. Treatment is unclear. |
| **Alcoholism** | ↓ | ↓ | ↓ | Macrocytes | Immature precursors | Anemia; elevated liver enzymes. (See Chapter 14.) | Direct interruption of Hgb synthesis in bone marrow. Unrelated to liver cirrhosis. Reverses with cessation of alcohol use. |
| **Antimetabolite Drugs** | Normal | Normal | Normal | Macrocytes | Hypercellular or immature precursors | Anemia | Toxicity from drugs such as 5-fluorouracil. Treatable by discontinuing the drug. |
| **Hereditary G6PD Deficiency** | Normal | Normal | Normal | Reticulocytes and hemolysis | Hypercellularity, with Heinz bodies seen with methylene blue | Asymptomatic until exposure to oxidizing agent, then hemolytic anemia occurs | X-linked. Oxidizing agents cause RBC lysis. Treatment is prevention: Avoid fava beans and oxidizing drugs. |
| **Autoimmune Hemolytic Anemia** | Normal | Normal | Normal | Reticulocytes, spherocytes, and hemolysis | Hypercellularity | Anemia, positive osmotic fragility test, and positive direct Coombs' test | Drugs such as chloramphenicol, methyldopa, or sulfonamides; 50% of cases are idiopathic. Treatable with prednisone. |

## SCHILLING TEST

The Schilling test identifies the defect, if any, that may interfere with the natural absorption of vitamin $B_{12}$. The test helps to differentiate a $B_{12}$-deficient diet from intrinsic factor (IF) shortage (pernicious anemia), ileal malabsorption, pancreatic insufficiency, and bacterial overgrowth.

**Step I:** Give oral radioactive $B_{12}$ (*$B_{12}$) followed by a large flushing parenteral (injected) dose of regular $B_{12}$ and record the amount of *$B_{12}$ in the urine. A functional system of IF and $B_{12}$ will cause more than 7% of the radioactive $B_{12}$ to be excreted. If $B_{12}$ is the only dietary deficiency, then this step will identify it.

**Step II:** Perform this test only if step I caused less than 7% excretion (not a dietary cause). Perform the steps below, giving oral $B_{12}$ first, then doing each modification until the condition is corrected and the cause is found.

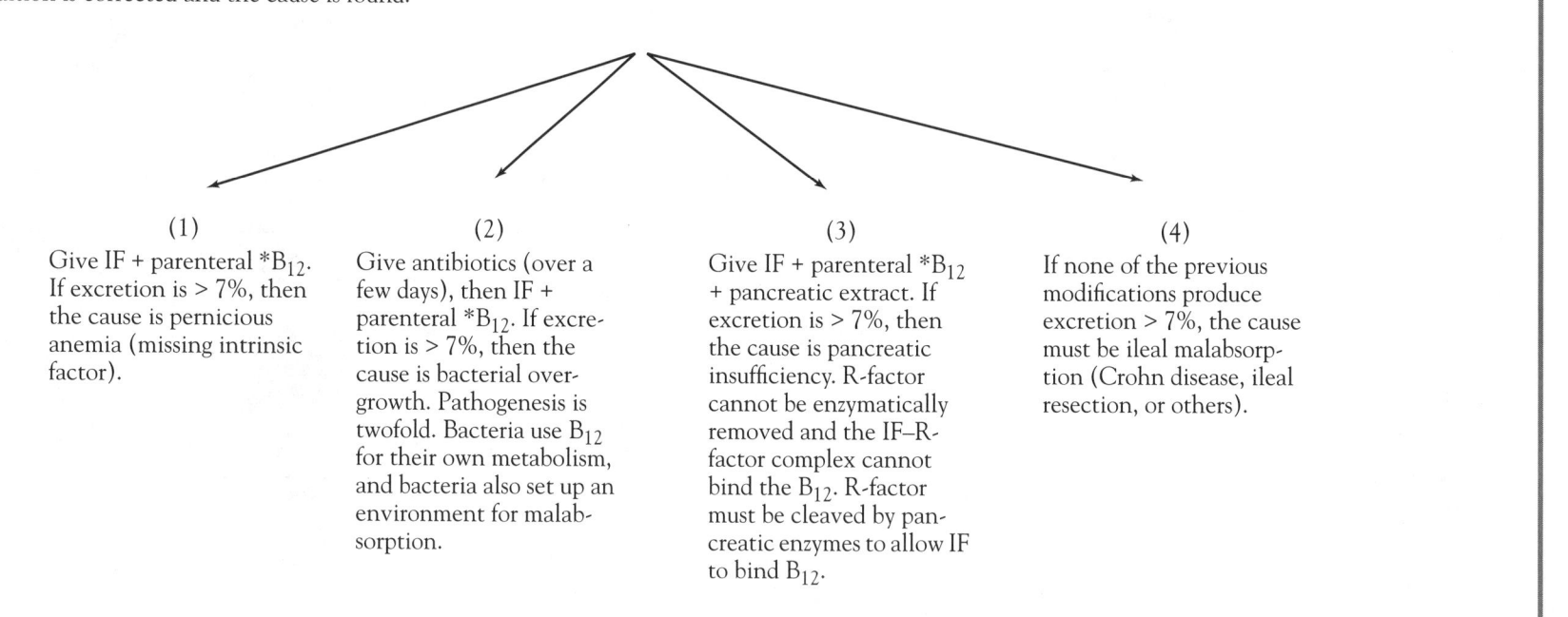

(1)
Give IF + parenteral *$B_{12}$. If excretion is > 7%, then the cause is pernicious anemia (missing intrinsic factor).

(2)
Give antibiotics (over a few days), then IF + parenteral *$B_{12}$. If excretion is > 7%, then the cause is bacterial overgrowth. Pathogenesis is twofold. Bacteria use $B_{12}$ for their own metabolism, and bacteria also set up an environment for malabsorption.

(3)
Give IF + parenteral *$B_{12}$ + pancreatic extract. If excretion is > 7%, then the cause is pancreatic insufficiency. R-factor cannot be enzymatically removed and the IF–R-factor complex cannot bind the $B_{12}$. R-factor must be cleaved by pancreatic enzymes to allow IF to bind $B_{12}$.

(4)
If none of the previous modifications produce excretion > 7%, the cause must be ileal malabsorption (Crohn disease, ileal resection, or others).

## NORMOCHROMIC ANEMIAS

| Anemia | Description and Cause(s) | Pathologic Findings |
|---|---|---|
| Acute Hemorrhagic Anemia | Rapid, moderate to severe bleeding. Normocytic rather than microcytic even though there is iron loss (in RBCs). No time for formation of microcytic cells, so RBCs retain their original size. | Can lead to hypovolemic shock if there is sufficient volume loss. |
| Hemolytic Anemia | See Hemolytic Anemias below. | Anemia with high LDH and indirect bilirubin. |
| Hypoproliferative Anemia | Chronic renal disease (decreased production of erythropoietin) or endocrine deficiency (low testosterone, high estrogen, or low thyroid hormone). | Anemia with low LDH and indirect bilirubin. |
| Myelophthisic Anemia | Caused by myelofibrosis, idiopathic fibrosis, or tumor infiltration (multiple myeloma, metastases to bone, or lysosomal storage diseases). | Extramedullary erythropoiesis. Teardrop cells are found on peripheral smear. |
| Red Cell Aplasia | Caused by an autoimmune reaction or infection with parvovirus B19. | Only the red cell line is suppressed. |
| Aplastic Anemia | Drug related—arsenic poisoning or chemotherapy.<br><br>Infiltrative—lymphomas, chronic lymphocytic leukemia, metastases from solid tumors, granulomas, or multiple myeloma. | Pancytopenia with no hematopoiesis. |

## HEMOLYTIC ANEMIAS

| Category | Intravascular Hemolysis | | Extravascular Hemolysis | |
| --- | --- | --- | --- | --- |
| | Intrinsic (Internal Defect) | Extrinsic (Acquired) | Intrinsic (Internal Defect) | Extrinsic (Acquired) |
| Diseases | Paroxysmal nocturnal hemoglobinuria and pyruvate kinase deficiency | Cold-type hemolytic anemia (IgM), microangiopathic anemias,[1] autoimmune hemolytic anemia, and malaria | Hereditary spherocytosis, thalassemias, and sickle cell anemia | Warm-type hemolytic anemia (IgG) |
| Laboratory Findings | Hemoglobinemia, hemoglobinuria, ↓ free haptoglobin (complexes with Hgb), ↑ indirect bilirubin (jaundice), and reticulocytosis | | Reticulocytosis | |
| Pathogenesis | Mechanical injury or complement-mediated lysis. Because the hemolysis occurs in the circulation, Hgb is partly broken down into bilirubin. | | Engulfed RBCs with membrane damage, reduced RBC flexibility, or opsonized RBCs by the reticuloendothelial system of the spleen. Because the cells are lysed by phagocytosis, the Hgb and iron are recycled. | |

[1]Microangiopathic anemias are caused by RBC fragmentation by small inflamed vessels or by prosthetic valves. Seen with vasculitis, disseminated intravascular coagulopathy, march hemoglobinuria, thrombotic thrombocytopenic purpura, and hemolytic-uremic syndrome.

## POLYCYTHEMIA

| Type | Description | Pathogenesis | Representative Diseases |
|------|-------------|--------------|------------------------|
| Relative | Plasma volume decreases while RBC mass is the same. Hct increases (RBC mass increases relative to total blood volume). Condition is transient. Dehydration is the primary cause. | | |
| Absolute | RBC mass increases. Hct increases. | | |
| | Appropriate polycythemia (secondary)—RBC mass increases in an appropriate response to increase oxygen-carrying capacity. Normal process (stress erythrocytosis). Process reverses when hypoxia no longer exists. | Chronic hypoxemia | Chronic lung disease, congenital cyanotic heart disease, smoking, and prolonged exposure to high altitudes |
| | Inappropriate polycythemia (primary)—RBC mass increases even though there is no requirement for extra oxygen-carrying capacity. | Uncontrolled or abnormal erythropoietin secretion | Thalassemias, polycythemia vera, erythropoietin-secreting renal adenocarcinoma, hepatocellular carcinoma (hepatoma), and myeloproliferative disorders |

# III. Leukocytic Disorders

## TERMS TO LEARN

| | |
|---|---|
| **Acute Inflammatory Response** | Includes the PMNs. |
| **Auer Bodies** | Rodlike inclusions in PMNs. |
| **Chédiak-Higashi Anomaly** | Large cytoplasmic inclusions found in leukocytes. |
| **Chronic Inflammatory Response** | Includes macrophages and lymphocytes, which replace the PMNs present during the acute response. |
| **Döhle Bodies** | Blue inclusions in PMNs. Remnants of rough endoplasmic reticulum. |
| **Eosinophilia** | Increased eosinophils. ☞ Remember the causes by NAACP, where N = neoplasms, A = allergies, A = asthma, C = connective tissue disorders, and P = parasites. |
| **Leukemia** | Excessive growth of abnormal leukocytes. Separated into lymphocytic and nonlymphocytic (myelocytic). Further subdivided into acute and chronic forms. All are primary bone marrow tumors. Patients present with fever, fatigue, bleeding (except for chronic myeloid leukemia), increased incidence of infections, or bone pain. <br> Hairy cell leukemia (rare B-cell leukemia) is identified by hairlike projections from the cell membrane. Cells infiltrate the bone marrow, spleen, and liver. No lymphadenopathy is present; diagnosed by the presence of tartrate-resistant acid phosphatase. |
| **Leukemoid Reaction** | Increase in reactive leukocytes because of inflammation. Consists of mostly mature PMNs. Leukocyte alkaline phosphatase score is used to differentiate between leukemia (low score) and a leukemoid reaction (high score). |
| **Leukocytosis** | Increase of WBCs. Analogous to absolute polycythemia. |
| **Lymphoma** | Neoplasm of lymphocytes that is generally confined to lymph nodes in the initial stages. Two general types are Hodgkin and non-Hodgkin lymphoma. Hodgkin lymphoma tends to present with nontender lymphadenopathy, fever, night sweats, and weight loss. |

| | |
|---|---|
| **May-Hegglin Anomaly** | Basophilic (purple) inclusions in leukocytes. |
| **Myelodysplastic Syndromes** | Group of related disorders with ineffective erythropoiesis, cytopenias, and hypercellular marrow. Some cases progress to acute nonlymphoblastic leukemia. Some secondary causes are chemotherapy, irradiation, or acquired stem cell disorders. Presents as a refractory anemia with many circulating precursors but few mature cells. |
| **Myeloproliferative Syndromes** | Hyperproliferation of the myeloid stem cell line. Includes clonal neoplastic proliferation of the erythroid (RBCs), megakaryocytic (platelets), or granulocytic cell line, depending on the disorder. See Myeloproliferative Syndromes below. |
| **Pelger-Huët Abnormality** | Bilobed nucleus in PMNs. Seen in myelodysplastic syndromes. |
| **Plasmacytosis** | Plasma cells present in the circulation (abnormal). |
| **Reactive Thrombocytosis** | Increased number of circulating platelets. Seen after splenectomy and in patients with malignancies, infections, or trauma. |
| **Smudge Cell** | Partially disintegrated cell, most often seen in acute leukemia. |
| **Toxic Granulation** | Coarse dark granules in PMNs. |

## MYELOPROLIFERATIVE SYNDROMES

| Disorder | Cells Involved | Description | Laboratory Tests or Smear |
|---|---|---|---|
| Polycythemia Vera | Predominantly erythroid differentiation, but can cause increased platelets and WBCs | Also known as essential polycythemia. With the exception of pruritus (itching of the skin), it is indistinguishable from normal erythrocytosis. Presents with massive splenomegaly, hypertension, neurologic symptoms, or thrombosis. Some cases can progress to chronic myelogenous leukemia (5% can become acute). Median survival is 11–15 years. | Increased Hgb, Hct > 60%, thrombocytosis, leukocytosis, high leukocyte alkaline phosphatase score, and elevated serum uric acid and serum $B_{12}$. |
| Essential Thrombocytosis | Platelet excess due to overactive megakaryocytes | Also known as essential thrombocythemia (idiopathic thrombocytosis). Average age at diagnosis is 50–60 years. Causes mild splenomegaly and hemorrhage or thrombosis. Small percentage of cases convert to an acute leukemia. | Thrombocytosis with large platelets and megakaryocyte fragments. Leukocyte alkaline phosphatase score can be high or normal. RBC mass is normal. |
| Myelofibrosis | Multilineage differentiation and extramedullary hematopoiesis | Patients are > 50 years old. Causes progressive anemia and thrombocytopenia, massive splenomegaly, and fatigue. Extramedullary hematopoiesis in the liver causes portal hypertension and eventual liver failure. Median survival is 5 years. | Teardrop cells, giant abnormal platelets, and megakaryocyte fragments. WBC count is variable. |

# HODGKIN LYMPHOMAS

7100 new cases and 1300 deaths from Hodgkin lymphoma were predicted for 1999 in the United States. Hodgkin disease is responsible for 15% of all lymphomas in adults. All types have Reed-Sternberg cells.

| Type (listed by declining prognosis) | Histopathology |
| --- | --- |
| Lymphocyte Predominant | Most cells are mature B cells. Note that only the Reed-Sternberg cells are neoplastic, not the lymphocytes. |
| Nodular Sclerosis | The most common type. Abnormal lymphoid nodules are separated by broad collagen bands. |
| Mixed Cellularity | Mixed cellular infiltration |
| Lymphocyte Depletion | Hypocellular (few lymphocytes) and fibrotic tissue |
| Classification | <ul><li>I—single lymph node region</li><li>II—two or more lymph node regions on one side of the diaphragm</li><li>III—lymph nodes involved on both sides of the diaphragm</li><li>IV—dissemination into organs</li></ul> Subscripts <ul><li>A—asymptomatic</li><li>B—sweats, fever, and 10% weight loss in 6 months</li></ul> |

Reed-Sternberg cell

# NON-HODGKIN LYMPHOMAS

Non-Hodgkin lymphoma is the fifth most common type of cancer. It is responsible for 25,700 deaths per year in the United States, placing it as the sixth most common cause of cancer mortality.

| Grade | Types | Markers | Description and Prognosis |
|---|---|---|---|
| Low Grade (Best Prognosis) | Follicular, small cell, and cleaved (most common; 35% of all lymphomas in adults). | B cell | Presents with painless peripheral lymphadenopathy. Fewer than 20% present with systemic symptoms of fever, weight loss, or night sweats. Can cause mediastinal adenopathy (mediastinal enlargement). |
| | Diffuse lymphocytic lymphoma, small lymphocytic type represents 10% of all lymphomas. May resemble chronic lymphocytic leukemia. | B cell | Untreated patients survive for years. Disease follows an indolent course. |
| Intermediate Grade (Intermediate Prognosis) | Follicular, mixed small and large cell, and cleaved. Represents a portion of the follicular type. | B cell | Untreated patients survive only for months. Disease is more aggressive than low-grade type. |
| | Follicular, large cell represents a portion of the follicular type. | B cell | |
| | Diffuse, mixed large and small cell. | B cell | |
| High Grade (Worst Prognosis) | Large cell (immunoblastic) lymphoma represents 10% of all lymphomas in adults. In children, it is the second most common lymphoma. | B cell | Highly aggressive lymphomas present similarly to above except that they cause more extralymphatic disease, such as skin lesions, liver infiltration, spinal cord compression, or solitary bone lesions. Untreated patients survive only for weeks. |
| | Lymphoblastic lymphoma represents 10% of all lymphomas. | T cell | |
| | Burkitt lymphoma, small cell, noncleaved represents a portion of the follicular type. | B cell Translocation t(8;14) | Childhood disease that presents with a jaw or abdominal tumor that spreads to extranodal sites, to bone (lytic lesions), and to bone marrow. There is little or no lymph node involvement. |

| T-Cell Lymphomas | Mycosis fungoides or cutaneous T-cell lymphoma. | T cell | Lymphoma of middle-aged adults, with a male predominance. Follows an indolent course and can present with lymphadenopathy. Involves mostly skin lesions. |
| --- | --- | --- | --- |
| | Sézary syndrome, a variant of cutaneous T-cell lymphoma. | T cell | Similar to above except with more peripheral blood involvement. Cells can infiltrate the bone marrow. Also follows an indolent course. |
| | Cutaneous T-cell lymphoma caused by human T-cell lymphotropic virus, adult T-cell leukemia, or lymphoma virus. | T cell | Human T-cell lymphotropic virus is a retrovirus similar to human immunodeficiency virus. Often presents with hepatosplenomegaly and skin lesions. |

# MYELODYSPLASTIC SYNDROMES

| Syndrome | Findings on Peripheral Smear | Findings in Bone Marrow | Description | Survival and Leukemic Conversion Rates |
|---|---|---|---|---|
| Refractory Anemia | < 1% blasts | Erythroid hyperplasia; < 5% blasts | Most patients present in their 60s with fatigue, infections, or bleeding. Anemia is due to bone marrow failure. Reticulocyte count is reduced. PMNs may have Pelger-Huët abnormality. | Best prognosis for long-term survival. Risk of conversion to acute leukemia is 0–20%. Survival is approximately 37 months. |
| Refractory Anemia With Ringed Sideroblasts | < 1% blasts | > 15% ringed sideroblasts (with Prussian blue stain); < 5% blasts | | Mean survival is 49 months. Risk of conversion to acute leukemia is 0–15%. |
| Refractory Anemia With Excess Blasts | < 5% blasts | 5–20% blasts | | Mean survival is 9 months. Risk of converting to acute leukemia is 20–50%. |
| Refractory Anemia With Excess Blasts in Transformation | > 5% blasts; blast cells have Auer rods | 20–30% blasts | | Mean survival is 6 months. Risk of leukemic transformation is 11–75%. |
| Chronic Myelomonocytic Leukemia | < 5% blasts and monocytosis | < 20% blasts; elevated numbers of promyelocytes | | Mean survival is 22 months. Risk of leukemic transformation is 3–55%. |

# LEUKEMIAS

Leukemia is the ninth most common cancer and ranks seventh in mortality due to cancer. There are a total of 30,200 cases and 22,100 deaths per year in the United States.

| Leukemia | Lymphocytic Leukemias<br>Have smudge cells | Myelocytic Leukemias<br>Have a specific esterase marker |
|---|---|---|
| **Acute Leukemias**<br><br>• Pancytopenia<br><br>• > 30% blasts in bone marrow<br><br>• Bone marrow failure | **Acute Lymphocytic Leukemia**<br><br>• Immature B cells<br><br>• Common in children<br><br>• TdT marker | **Acute Myeloid Leukemia**<br><br>• Common in adults<br><br>• No TdT marker<br><br>• Has several subdivisions, $M_0$–$M_7$. Most important is $M_3$ (promyelocytic leukemia), which is associated with disseminated intravascular coagulation and Auer bodies. |
| **Chronic Leukemias**<br><br>• Found in the elderly | **Chronic Lymphocytic Leukemia**<br><br>• Mature B cells<br><br>• CD19/CD5 marker (same as small lymphocytic lymphoma B-cell markers)<br><br>• Can cause an autoimmune anemia<br><br>• Hypoglobulinemia (no Ig production)<br><br>• No pancytopenia | **Chronic Myeloid Leukemia**<br><br>• Blast crisis (acceleration of bone marrow infiltration)<br><br>• High leukocytosis<br><br>• t(9;22)—Philadelphia chromosome<br><br>• Extreme splenomegaly (white pulp infiltration)<br><br>• Thrombocytosis (unique to this leukemia) |

## PLASMA CELL DYSCRASIAS

| Disease | Description | Bone Erosion(s) | Bence Jones Protein in Urine (Light Chain of Ig) | Histopathologic Findings |
|---|---|---|---|---|
| Multiple Myeloma | Responsible for 13,700 new cases and 11,400 deaths per year in the Unites States. Causes hypercalcemia, myeloma nephrosis (protein casts in collecting ducts), amyloid nephropathy, hyper-gammaglobulinemia, rouleaux formation, and high blood viscosity. Dissemination to the spleen, liver, and lymph nodes. | Yes | Yes | Plasma cells. Eccentrically placed nuclei and perinuclear clear areas. AL type amyloidosis. (See Chapter 1, Storage Diseases.) |
| Solitary Plasmacytoma | Can present with a solitary bone lesion or with extraosseous lesions. | Yes with bone lesion; no with extraosseous lesions | No | Plasma cells. Possible AL type amyloidosis. |
| Waldenström Macroglobulinemia | Causes splenomegaly, weight loss, fatigue, anemia, and a bleeding tendency; IgM (macroglobulin)-diffuse plasma cell infiltration; hyperviscosity syndrome (IgM binds RBCs together); Raynaud phenomenon. | No | Yes | Bone marrow is infiltrated with lymphocytes and plasma cells. Possible AL type amyloidosis. |
| Heavy-Chain Disease (AL amyloid type) | IgA heavy-chain producer. Intestinal infiltration causes atrophy of the villi and intestinal malabsorption. | No | No | Leads to amyloidosis of the AL type. |
| Monoclonal Gammopathy of Undetermined Significance | Diagnosed when all other causes of hypergammaglobulinemia have been ruled out. No bone marrow infiltration. Ig levels are elevated. | No | No | Bone marrow has < 10% plasma cells, normally and abnormally shaped. More than 25% of cases progress to multiple myeloma. Possible AL-type amyloidosis. |

## LANGERHANS CELL HISTIOCYTOSIS

| Disease | Description | Population Affected | Pathologic Findings and Prognosis |
|---|---|---|---|
| **Letterer-Siwe Disease** (Acutely Disseminated) | Aggressive and fatal. Presents with a rash, bone lesions, hepatosplenomegaly, lymphadenopathy, pancytopenia, or pulmonary involvement. | Infants | Can see tennis-racket–shaped Birbeck granules on electron microscopy. Histiocytes have the CD1 marker. Prognosis of Letterer-Siwe disease is the worst of the 3 diseases given here and the most likely to be fatal. |
| **Hand-Schüller-Christian Disease** (Multifocal) | Can affect bones, particularly the skull. Triad of skull lesions, diabetes insipidus, and exophthalmos due to orbit erosion. | Children < 5 years old | Prognosis is intermediate between eosinophilic granuloma and Letterer-Siwe disease. |
| **Eosinophilic Granuloma** (Unifocal) | Usually presents with a solitary bone lesion, but can also attack the lungs. | | Has the best prognosis of the 2 diseases above. |

# IV. Hemostatic Disorders

## TERMS TO LEARN

| | |
|---|---|
| Ecchymosis | Large hemorrhage into the skin. "Black and blue" mark of a bruise seen with blunt trauma. |
| Epistaxis | Bleeding from the nose. Can occur with trauma, irritation, and bleeding disorders. |
| Fibrinolysis | Normal process of dissolving a thrombus in the circulation. Helps to balance the coagulation system. See Thrombolysis below. |
| Hemarthrosis | Bleeding into the joint space. Can be seen after trauma to the joint, especially in patients who have hemophilia. |
| Hematemesis | Bloody vomitus. |
| Hematochezia | Extensive bright red bleeding from the rectum. |
| Hematoma | Blood that has collected within tissue. Can be seen in trauma and bleeding disorders. |
| Hematuria | Blood in the urine. |
| Hemoptysis | Coughed-up blood in the sputum originating from the lungs or bronchi. |
| Hemostasis | Normal control of bleeding. Platelets are responsible for primary hemostasis by forming the initial hemostatic plug. Clotting cascade is responsible for secondary hemostasis by layering fibrin polymers on top of the platelets and stabilizing the clot. Process can go awry from lack of platelets, dysfunctional platelets, or a dysfunctional clotting system. |
| Melena | Black, tarry stools from upper gastrointestinal bleeding. The stool is black rather than red because the blood oxidizes in the stomach. Stool must be guaiac test–positive for it to be considered melena. Other substances can turn the stool black, such as iron and certain medications. |
| Petechia | Small hemorrhage into the skin or mucous membrane from capillary leakage. A pinpoint, black-blue macule (flat) that does not blanch when pressed. |

| | |
|---|---|
| **Purpura** | Black-purple patches (flat) or plaques (raised) from hemorrhage or extravasation of blood into the skin. Caused by thrombocytopenia or vasculitis. |
| **Thrombolysis** | The process of dissolving a thrombus with a thrombolytic agent, such as streptokinase. |
| **Transfusion** | When blood replacement is needed, packed RBCs are used. Platelets, fresh frozen plasma, and cryoprecipitate (clotting factor VIII) can be administered as needed. Transfusions can induce a hemolytic transfusion reaction (extrinsic hemolysis mediated by an ABO or Rh incompatibility). Nonhemolytic febrile reaction (leukoagglutinin reaction) occurs if the recipient has formed antibodies against donor's WBCs or platelets from previous transfusions. |

## SUMMARY OF BLEEDING DISORDERS

| Category | Description | Representative Diseases |
|---|---|---|
| Fragile Blood Vessels | Palpable purpuric rash, easy bruising, and spontaneous bleeding. Normal platelet count and normal hemostatic tests. Normal coagulation times (PT and PTT). | Rickettsial and meningococcal infections |
| | | Any vasculitis |
| | | Poor vascular support due to connective tissue diseases such as Ehlers-Danlos syndrome, Cushing syndrome, or scurvy |
| | | Hereditary hemorrhagic telangiectasia |
| Reduced Platelet Count | Nonpalpable purpuric rash, ecchymoses, and hematomas. Spontaneous mucosal bleeding. Normal coagulation times (PT and PTT). | Thrombocytopenias |
| Qualitative Platelet Disorders | Nonpalpable purpuric rash, ecchymoses, and hematomas. Spontaneous mucosal bleeding. Prolonged bleeding time (TT) but normal coagulation time (PT). Can have prolonged PTT. Platelet count is normal. but platelets are dysfunctional. | von Willebrand disease—dysfunctional von Willebrand factor (vWF) protein, which is responsible for platelet adhesion. Most common hereditary disorder of hemostasis. |
| | | Bernard-Soulier syndrome—defective adhesion due to deficiency of Ib/IX (platelet receptor for vWF) |
| | | Glanzmann thrombasthenia—defective aggregation due to deficiency of IIb/IIIa (platelet receptor for binding fibrinogen) |
| | | Storage pool disease—defective secretion of platelet granule contents, especially ADP, preventing aggregation |
| | | Acquired disease from myeloproliferative disorders, drugs such as aspirin and other NSAIDs, heparin, or corticosteroids |
| Clotting Factor Deficiencies | Hemarthrosis and bleeding into muscles from minor trauma. Repeated hemarthroses cause disabling arthropathy. Prolonged bleeding after surgery. Prolonged coagulation times (PT or PTT). | Hemophilia A and B—normal bleeding time (TT) and PT. Prolonged PTT. Most common hereditary coagulopathy. |

## COMPARISON OF VON WILLEBRAND DISEASE AND HEMOPHILIA

| Disorder | Inheritance Pattern | Hemorrhage Site | Bleeding Time (TT) | PTT (Intrinsic) | PT (Extrinsic) | Pathogenesis |
|---|---|---|---|---|---|---|
| von Willebrand Disease | Autosomal dominant | Skin and mucous membranes | Long | Normal or long | Normal | Low factor VIII activity<br>• Type I—decrease in circulating vWF due to inhibited release<br>• Type II—no multimer assembly (active vWF is composed of large multimers) |
| Hemophilia A | X-linked | Muscles and joints | Normal | Long | Normal | Reduced circulating factor VIII |
| Hemophilia B (Christmas Disease) | X-linked | Muscles and joints | Normal | Long | Normal | Reduced circulating factor IX |

## THROMBOCYTOPENIA

| Type | Pathogenesis | Clinical Findings | Pathologic Findings |
|---|---|---|---|
| Idiopathic Thrombocytopenic Purpura | Platelet destruction in the spleen by complement against platelet glycoproteins. | Presents with spontaneous skin or mucosal bleeding. Nonpalpable purpuric rash, ecchymoses, and hematomas. No splenomegaly. | Isolated thrombocytopenia. Most commonly seen as a self-limited illness in children after a viral infection such as rubella, cytomegalovirus, hepatitis B, or Epstein-Barr virus. In adults, disease is chronic and more common in women. |
| Isoimmune Thrombocytopenia (Post-Transfusion Purpura) | Occurs after platelet transfusion. Antibodies to foreign donor platelets destroy the platelets. | Fever and bleeding. | Can cause neonatal hematologic problems if the mother is sensitized by previous platelet transfusions. Anti-platelet antibody (IgG) can cross the placenta. |
| Thrombotic Thrombocytopenic Purpura | Antibodies to endothelial cells cause microthrombi in capillaries and small arteries. No inflammation. | Microangiopathic hemolytic anemia, bleeding secondary to thrombocytopenia, transient neurologic changes, kidney failure, and fever. | Causes reticulocytosis. Coagulation tests (PT and PTT) are normal. |
| Hemolytic-Uremic Syndrome | Autoimmune mechanism. | Similar to thrombotic thrombocytopenic purpura, but without the neurologic problems. | In children, can occur after gastroenteritis with *Escherichia coli* O:157, *Shigella, Salmonella*, or viruses. In adults, can be precipitated by pregnancy. Coagulation tests (PT and PTT) are normal. |

# CLOTTING CASCADE

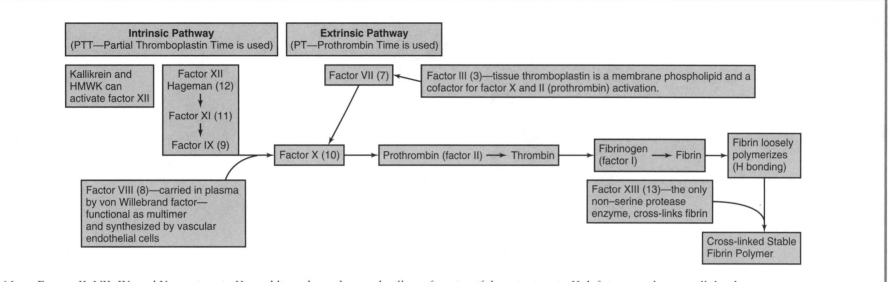

**Intrinsic Pathway**
(PTT—Partial Thromboplastin Time is used)

**Extrinsic Pathway**
(PT—Prothrombin Time is used)

Kallikrein and HMWK can activate factor XII

Factor XII Hageman (12)
↓
Factor XI (11)
↓
Factor IX (9)

Factor VII (7)

Factor III (3)—tissue thromboplastin is a membrane phospholipid and a cofactor for factor X and II (prothrombin) activation.

Factor X (10) → Prothrombin (factor II) → Thrombin

Fibrinogen (factor I) → Fibrin

Fibrin loosely polymerizes (H bonding)

Factor VIII (8)—carried in plasma by von Willebrand factor—functional as multimer and synthesized by vascular endothelial cells

Factor XIII (13)—the only non–serine protease enzyme, cross-links fibrin

Cross-linked Stable Fibrin Polymer

Note: Factors II, VII, IX, and X are vitamin K– and liver-dependent and will not function if there is vitamin K deficiency or hepatocellular damage.

Hemostasis promotors:

Thromboxane $A_2$ reduces blood flow by vasoconstriction.

ADP promotes platelet aggregation.

Factor III—tissue thromboplastin—promotes the clotting cascade.

HMWK = high-molecular-weight kininogen.

# HEMOSTASIS SYSTEM MODIFIERS

| Category | Agent(s) and Function(s) |
|---|---|
| **Natural Hemostasis Modification** | |
| **Anticoagulators (Clotting System)** | Antithrombin III—deactivates all the active serine proteases (all active factors except XIII). Heparin potentiates this factor and also irreversibly inactivates factors II, IX, X, and XI. May see an acquired antithrombin III deficiency with oral contraceptive pills. |
| | Thrombomodulin—protein on endothelial surfaces that sequesters active thrombin. It is vitamin K dependent. It activates protein C. Along with protein S, it destroys several factors. |
| **Platelet Down-Regulators** | Prostacyclin—inhibits platelet aggregation. |
| **Fibrinolysis** | Plasminogen—an endogenous agent that is proteolytically converted to plasmin and dissolves thrombi. |
| **Manufactured Hemostasis Modification** | |
| **Antiplatelet Medications** | Aspirin—irreversibly inhibits the cyclooxygenase pathway, causing irreversible platelet dysfunction, and reduces thromboxane $A_2$ (vaso-constrictor). NSAIDs reversibly cause platelet dysfunction. |
| | Ticlopidine, clopidogrel—inhibits ADP release from platelets. ADP is responsible for platelet aggregation. |
| | Abciximab, tirofiban, and eptifibatide are a newer class of intravenous drugs that inhibit platelet aggregation. They block von Wille-brand factor and fibrinogen from binding to glycoprotein IIb/IIIa receptors on platelets. |
| **Anticoagulation Medications** | Heparin—parenteral drug, safe for pregnant women (does not cross the placenta), is used to prevent further clot propagation in throm-bophlebitis, stroke, myocardial infarction, and pulmonary embolism. PTT is used to monitor it. Can cause osteoporosis with prolonged use. |
| | Warfarin—oral vitamin K antagonist (reversible deactivation of factors II, VII, IX, and X) is teratogenic to pregnant women. Active only in the liver (where it is not bound to albumin). Initially, warfarin acts as a weak procoagulant. Takes several days before the antico-agulant properties begin to work. For this reason, warfarin is started together with heparin, then heparin is slowly reduced. PT is used to monitor warfarin. Warfarin is often used on a long-term basis. |
| **Thrombolytic Medications** | Used to dissolve thrombi in cerebral strokes and myocardial infarctions. |
| | Streptokinase (isolated from *Streptococcus*)—forms a complex with plasminogen and indirectly activates it. |
| | Tissue plasminogen activator—directly activates plasminogen. |

## DISSEMINATED INTRAVASCULAR COAGULATION

| Causes | Pathogenesis |
| --- | --- |
| General | Caused by secondary problems such as obstetric complications (amniotic fluid embolism), infections (*Rickettsia* and *Meningococcus*), or massive tissue injuries. Involves platelet, fibrin, and coagulation factor consumption. Abnormal PT, PTT, and TT. Formation of fibrin split products (inhibit further clot formation). |
| Release of Tissue Factor | Tissue factor (thromboplastin) is expressed when interleukin-1 or tumor necrosis factor-$\alpha$ is present (mucus or degranulation of leukemic cells). |
| Endothelial Injury | Exposes collagen, initiating the intrinsic clotting pathway. |
| Organ Pathology | Bleeding and hemorrhage in the kidneys, lungs (adult respiratory distress syndrome), brain, adrenal glands, and placenta (separation). |

# CHAPTER 5
# RESPIRATORY SYSTEM

## I. OBSTRUCTIVE PULMONARY DISEASES

Normal Lung Morphology and Emphysema

Types of Obstructive Pulmonary Diseases

## II. RESTRICTIVE PULMONARY DISEASES

Types of Restrictive Lung Diseases

Pneumoconioses

Disease Distribution in the Lungs

Infiltrative Diseases

## III. PULMONARY INFECTIONS

Pathologic Classification of Pneumonias

Clinical Classification of Pneumonias

Tuberculosis

## IV. VASCULAR DISEASE AND TUMORS

Vascular Lung Diseases

Primary Lung Cancers

**ABBREVIATIONS**

**APUD** = amine precursor uptake and decarboxylation
**ARDS** = adult respiratory distress syndrome
**COPD** = chronic obstructive pulmonary disease
**TB** = tuberculosis

## MOST COMMON Causes and Types

| Disorder | Common Cause |
|---|---|
| Pulmonary hypertension | Acute pulmonary embolism |
| Lobar pneumonia | *Streptococcus pneumoniae* (pneumococcus) |
| Pulmonary hemorrhage | Pulmonary embolism |

| Disorder | Common Type |
|---|---|
| Pneumoconiosis | Silicosis |
| Bronchogenic carcinoma | Squamous cell carcinoma and adenocarcinoma of the lung |
| Atypical pneumonia | Mycoplasma |

# I. Obstructive Pulmonary Diseases

## TERMS TO LEARN

| | |
|---|---|
| Alveolitis | Inflammation of the respiratory alveoli due to hypersensitivity to inhaled antigens. Over time, may lead to chronic fibrosis, alveolar wall destruction, and a honeycombed lung appearance on X-ray (overlapping white circles). |
| Bronchogenic Tumors | May produce cough, hemoptysis, obstruction of the airways, atelectasis, or pneumonitis. |
| Consolidation | Lung alveoli become filled with exudative fluid, often because of pneumonia. Diagnosed by dull sound on percussion or by chest X-ray. |
| Empyema | Pus collection in the pleural cavity from pneumonia. Must be surgically drained. Do not confuse this term with emphysema. See Obstructive Pulmonary Diseases below. |
| Lung Abscess | A walled-off collection of pus that consists of polymicrobial anaerobes and inflammatory cells. |
| Obstructive Pulmonary Diseases | Increased resistance to air flow (expiratory phase) anywhere along the air-conducting system. Causes dyspnea, wheezing, or stridor. Seen in asthma, chronic bronchitis, emphysema, and with obstruction by foreign bodies (e.g., food chunks, small toys). Chronic obstructive pulmonary disease includes emphysema and chronic bronchitis. |
| Pneumoconioses | Collection of occupationally related diseases caused by chronic inhalation of organic or inorganic substances. Clinically important diseases include coal worker's pneumoconiosis, asbestosis, and silicosis. |
| Pneumonia | Inflammatory lung reaction involving the alveolar spaces. During pulmonary bacterial infection, the alveoli fill with pus. |
| Pneumonitis | Inflammatory lung reaction involving only the walls of the alveoli. Compare with pneumonia. |
| Pores of Kohn | Tiny openings between alveoli that can allow the spread of infections and exudate. |

*Continued*

## TERMS TO LEARN (Continued)

| | |
|---|---|
| **Restrictive Pulmonary Diseases** | Decreased capacity to expand the lung parenchyma; difficulty with the inspiratory phase. Causes dyspnea and tachycardia without wheezing. |
| | Chest-wall disorders or wall deformity (kyphoscoliosis), severe obesity, or pleural disease. |
| | Diaphragm weakness—Guillain-Barré syndrome, myasthenia gravis, phrenic nerve damage, muscular dystrophy, or *Clostridium botulinum* poisoning. |
| | Infiltrative diseases—interstitial pneumonias, pneumoconioses, or ARDS. |
| | Decreased lung volume—atelectasis, pneumothorax, or hemothorax. |
| **Tuberculosis** | *Mycobacterium tuberculosis* is an acid-fast bacillus responsible for TB. Can remain dormant for many years. A resurgence of TB is occurring in persons with human immunodeficiency virus infection. Others at risk include those in crowded living environments, homeless people, drug abusers, and those in poor health. TB is screened with a tuberculin skin test (see Chapter 3). A positive result confirms only TB exposure, not active TB. Definitive diagnosis is made with sputum stain and culture. Vaccination with BCG (bacille Calmette-Guérin) is available but is not widely used in the United States. |

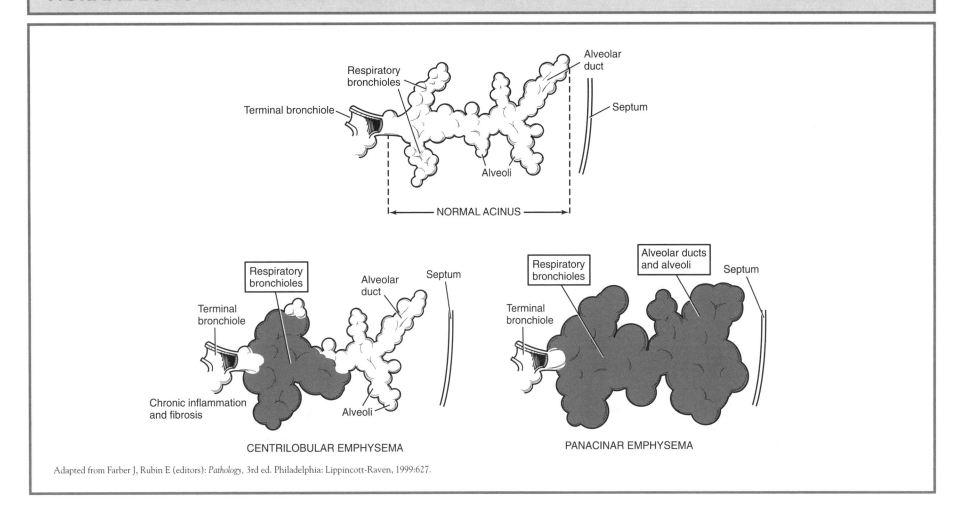

Adapted from Farber J, Rubin E (editors): *Pathology,* 3rd ed. Philadelphia: Lippincott-Raven, 1999:627.

## TYPES OF OBSTRUCTIVE PULMONARY DISEASES

| Disease | Description and Types | Pathogenesis | Findings and Prognosis |
|---|---|---|---|
| Bronchial Asthma | Presents with wheezing on expiration, dyspnea, and cough. Bronchial occlusion occurs with mucus plugs. Eosinophilia is seen in the lungs. | Hyperreactivity of the bronchi and bronchioles. | • Acute attacks of bronchoconstriction are reversible. |
| | Extrinsic (atopic or allergic)—presents in children with bronchoconstriction and mucus secretion. Associated with urticaria (hives) and allergic rhinitis. Precipitated by pet or plant allergens. | | • Status asthmaticus—prolonged asthmatic attack that does not respond well to treatment and may result in death. |
| | Intrinsic (nonatopic)—presents in adults with exacerbations secondary to viruses, cold temperature, irritants, stress, or exercise. | | • Cardiac asthma—bronchospasm induced by congestive heart failure. |
| | Intrinsic (drug-induced)—aspirin is the most common cause. Involves increased leukotriene production with blockade of the cyclooxygenase pathway. | | |
| | Occupationally induced—fumes, organic dusts, and chemicals may induce an attack. | | |
| Chronic Bronchitis (COPD) | Productive cough for 3 consecutive months over at least a consecutive 2-year period. Divided into asthmatic and obstructive types. Patients present in their 60s with wheezing, episodic dyspnea, and weight gain. Precipitating events include pneumonia, surgery, or trauma. | Hypersecretion of mucus because of increased goblet cells in small airways. Smoking can predispose. | Whereas acute bronchitis is reversible, chronic bronchitis is permanent. Patients are characterized as "blue bloaters." Squamous metaplasia is found in the bronchial endothelium. |

| | | | |
|---|---|---|---|
| **Emphysema (COPD)** | Causes wheezing, hunched-over breathing, progressive exertional dyspnea, and weight loss. Unlike chronic bronchitis, it produces little or no coughing. Symptoms classically present earlier than in chronic bronchitis. | Dilatation of distal air spaces. Can be caused by smoking or hereditary $\alpha_1$-antitrypsin deficiency. | Permanent condition from chronic destruction of alveolar walls without fibrosis and dilatation of air spaces. Patients are characterized as "pink puffers." |
| | Centrilobular—affects the respiratory bronchioles and occurs with smoking and chronic bronchitis. | | |
| | Panacinar—affects the entire acinus and occurs at the base of the lungs. Caused by $\alpha_1$-antitrypsin deficiency and smoking. | | |
| | Paraseptal—affects the pleura and septa. Can become a spontaneous pneumothorax if a bulla (enlarged, air filled bubble at the surface of the lung) ruptures into the pleura. | | |
| | Irregular—causes scarring and increase in alveolar size (inflammatory but usually asymptomatic). | | |
| **Bronchiectasis** | Most common cause is bacterial pneumonia. Presents with fever, persistent cough with purulent sputum, recurrent lung infections, hemoptysis, and pleuritic pain. Progressive dyspnea and cyanosis occur. Children are particularly susceptible because their bronchi are smaller in diameter and become obstructed more easily. | Bronchial obstruction by a tumor, foreign body, mucus impaction, or infection. Congenital from cystic fibrosis. | Permanent condition. Affects the lower lobes bilaterally. Pertussis toxin can cause bronchiectasis without the obstruction. |

# II. Restrictive Pulmonary Diseases

## TYPES OF RESTRICTIVE LUNG DISEASES

| Condition | Description | Pathogenesis | Pathologic Findings |
|---|---|---|---|
| **Adult Respiratory Distress Syndrome** | Also known as diffuse alveolar damage. Acute onset of respiratory insufficiency and noncardiogenic pulmonary edema. Presents with progressive tachypnea, then dyspnea, cyanosis, and bilateral crackles (rales). | Toxins, trauma, irritants, viral infections, oxygen toxicity, septic shock, or pancreatitis | Hyaline membranes demonstrate vascular congestion, interstitial and intra-alveolar edema, and subsequent fibrosis. Condition results in diffuse damage to alveolar capillary walls. |
| **Neonatal Respiratory Distress Syndrome** | Onset is at birth. Condition causes dyspnea and cyanosis resulting from the lack of pulmonary surfactant. | Prematurity, maternal diabetes, and cesarean section | |
| Atelectasis | In neonates, due to incomplete lung expansion. In adults, an area of lung can collapse on itself. Symptoms depend on the rapidity of onset and the extent of lung involvement, ranging from no symptoms to acute dyspnea and hypoxemia. | Complete obstruction of an airway<br><br>Compressive type—compression by fluid, tumors, blood (hemothorax), or air in the pleural cavity (pneumothorax)<br><br>Contractive type—tissue scarring<br><br>Patchy type—loss of surfactant (looks like ARDS) | Reversible condition if the obstruction or compression is temporary. Secondary infections may occur, leading to residual pathology of the lungs. |

## PNEUMOCONIOSES

| Condition | Description | Cause(s) or Population Affected | Pathogenesis |
|---|---|---|---|
| Anthracosis | Usually benign and asymptomatic | Air pollution, smoking, coal mining, and urban living | Macrophages become filled with carbon particles. |
| Coal Worker's Pneumoconiosis | Simple (benign) or appears as a chronic, progressive, massive fibrosis (results in respiratory failure) | Coal miners | Pathology occurs in the upper lobes. Macrophages contain carbon particles in nodules with collagen fibers. In progressive coal worker's pneumoconiosis, the nodules are larger. Increased risk of TB, chronic bronchitis, and emphysema (centrilobular). |
| Silicosis | Most common occupational pulmonary disease. Causes dyspnea with obstructive and restrictive lung dysfunction. | Sandblasters and miners | Pathology occurs in the upper lobes. Macrophages die after ingesting silicon particles. Eventual nodule formation can block airways. Greater incidence of TB in people with chronic silicosis. |
| Asbestosis | Causes dyspnea and inspiratory crackles. Increased risk of bronchogenic carcinoma and mesothelioma. Risk of bronchogenic carcinoma is magnified by smoking. | Mining, insulation, and ship building | Pathology occurs in the lower lobes. Ferruginous bodies (asbestos bodies) are yellow and rod shaped. Causes diffuse pulmonary interstitial fibrosis. |
| Berylliosis | Acute type involves pneumonitis with edema and exudate.<br><br>Chronic type involves dyspnea with cough and arthralgias. | Aerospace workers | In the chronic form, noncaseating granulomas form in the lungs. Increased risk of bronchogenic carcinoma. |

## DISEASE DISTRIBUTION IN THE LUNGS

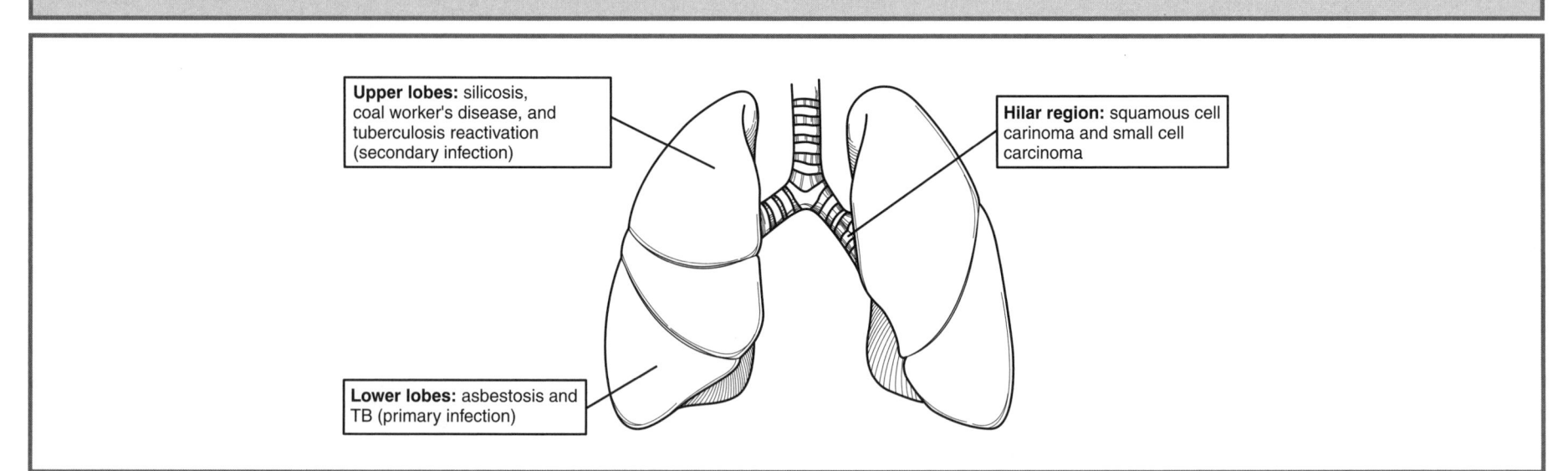

**Upper lobes:** silicosis, coal worker's disease, and tuberculosis reactivation (secondary infection)

**Hilar region:** squamous cell carinoma and small cell carcinoma

**Lower lobes:** asbestosis and TB (primary infection)

# INFILTRATIVE DISEASES

| Disease | Description and Symptoms | Causes and Pathologic Findings |
|---|---|---|
| Collagen Vascular Disease | Respiratory difficulty and cyanosis. | Can be caused by rheumatoid arthritis, systemic lupus erythematosus, or Wegener granulomatosis. |
| Hypersensitivity Pneumonitis | Symptoms result from an immune reaction to prolonged exposure to an antigen. Acute disease causes fever, chills, dyspnea, recurrent cough, and leukocytosis. Symptoms occur as soon as a few hours after exposure. Continuous exposure leads to respiratory failure and cyanosis. | Hyperreactivity of the alveoli. Acutely, lymphocytic and plasma-cell lung infiltrates and noncaseating granulomas occupy the alveoli and interstitial spaces. Chronically, diffuse pulmonary fibrosis occurs. Causes include thermophilic actinomycetes in air conditioners and humidifiers (humidifier's lung) and in moldy hay (farmer's lung), and bird feces (pigeon breeder's disease). Condition is reversible early on. |
| Idiopathic Pulmonary Fibrosis | Also known as cryptogenic fibrosing alveolitis. Patients present in their 60s to 70s with chronic cough and dyspnea. Progressive respiratory difficulty and cyanosis occur. Median survival is 4 years from symptom onset. | Interstitial lung disease. Involves chronic alveolitis and destruction of the wall architecture, hyperplasia of type II pneumocytes and fibrosis, and the development of cystic spaces. |
| Idiopathic Pulmonary Hemosiderosis | Presents with hemoptysis and recurrent pulmonary hemorrhages. | Resembles the lung component of Goodpasture syndrome. However, the alveolar wall necrosis is not prominent. |
| Sarcoidosis | Systemic disease of unknown etiology. Patients present in their 30s to 40s; 90% with bilateral lung involvement. Dyspnea, malaise, and fever occur. Can affect any other organ. Angiotensin-converting enzyme levels are elevated in 40–80% of patients. | Noncaseating granulomas with asteroid bodies (look like stars) and Schaumann bodies (laminated concretions). Diagnosed when biopsy shows noncaseating granulomas and all other granulomatous conditions are excluded. Increased incidence in black women. |
| Pulmonary Eosinophilia | Also known as extrinsic allergic alveolitis. | No vasculitic fibrosis or necrosis. Eosinophilic infiltrates in the alveoli and eosinophilia in peripheral blood can be found. |
| | Histiocytosis—eosinophilic granuloma. (See Chapter 4, Langerhans Cell Histiocytosis.) | |
| | Löffler syndrome—pulmonary lesions with eosinophilia. Can present with cough, fever, and serum eosinophilia. Associated with exposure to *Ascaris* (roundworm) or *Strongyloides*. | |
| | Other causes include drug allergies, asthma, polyarteritis nodosa, and idiopathic causes. | |

# III. Pulmonary Infections

## PATHOLOGIC CLASSIFICATION OF PNEUMONIAS

| Condition | Description | Pathologic Findings |
| --- | --- | --- |
| **Bronchopneumonias** | Most common pneumonia presentation. Caused by *Staphylococcus aureus* (most common), *Staphylococcus pyogenes*, *Haemophilus influenzae*, *Pseudomonas*, the coliform bacteria (*Klebsiella pneumoniae*, *Enterobacter*, and *Escherichia coli*), and TB. | Focal patches of intra-alveolar suppurative exudate surrounding bronchi and bronchioles. |
| | In patients with acquired immunodeficiency syndrome, premature infants, and people on immunosuppressive therapy, *Pneumocystis carinii* can cause pneumonia. Condition presents with fever, dyspnea, and a nonproductive cough. Patients are at risk when the CD4 count falls below 200 cells/μL. Lactate dehydrogenase is elevated. Without treatment, patients rapidly deteriorate and die. | Interstitial involvement and diffuse or focal intra-alveolar exudates, nodules, and cavitations within the nodules. Wright-Giemsa or silver stain may show round cysts. |
| **Lobar Pneumonias** | Caused by *S. pneumoniae* (pneumococcus; the most common cause), *K. pneumoniae*, *Staphylococcus*, and *H. influenzae*. Presents with fever, chills, productive cough with rusty sputum, and pleuritic chest pain. Radiopaque densities may be seen on chest X-ray. | Intra-alveolar suppurative exudate consolidates the entire lobe or only sections. Stages of untreated pneumonia: congestion → red hepatization (red blood cells, neutrophils, and fibrin) → gray hepatization (fibrosuppurative exudate) → resolution (granular debris and macrophages). |
| **Anaerobic Pneumonias (Aspiration Pneumonia)** | Caused by multiple anaerobic species, including *Prevotella* (*Bacteroides*) and *Fusobacterium*, and gram-negative rods. Presents with weight loss, fever, and a foul-smelling, productive cough. Caused by aspiration of oropharyngeal secretions. Patients at risk include neonates, the elderly, those with poor dental hygiene, debilitated persons, drug addicts, alcoholics, or those with seizures. | Necrosis or abscess. Infection is usually polymicrobial. |
| **Atypical Pneumonias** | *Mycoplasma pneumoniae* is the most common cause; also *Chlamydia psittaci* (ornithosis), *Legionella*, *Coxiella* (Q fever), and viruses such as influenza, parainfluenza, adenovirus, and respiratory syncytial virus. Presents with mild fever, muscle aches, a nonproductive cough, dyspnea, and headaches. | Alveolar architecture is preserved, with diffuse lymphocyte infiltration of the interstitium. No exudate in the alveoli. Technically, a viral pneumonia should be called viral pneumonitis (only the alveolar walls are involved). |

# CLINICAL CLASSIFICATION OF PNEUMONIAS

| Patient Group | Community-Acquired Pneumonias (in decreasing order of incidence) | Hospital-Acquired Pneumonias (in decreasing order of incidence) |
|---|---|---|
| Adults (< 60 years) | S. pneumoniae, M. pneumoniae, viruses, Chlamydia pneumoniae, and H. influenzae | Pneumonia is considered hospital-acquired (nosocomial) if it occurs 48 hours after the patient has been admitted to the hospital. The most common hospital-acquired pneumonias are: Pseudomonas aeruginosa, S. aureus, Enterobacter, K. pneumoniae, E. coli, Proteus, Serratia, and anaerobes such as Bacteroides. (For pneumonia in the pediatric population, see Chapter 15, Neonatal Infections.) |
| Adults (> 60 years) | S. pneumoniae, viruses, H. influenzae, gram-negative bacilli, S. aureus, Legionella, and Moraxella catarrhalis | |
| Hospitalized Adults | S. pneumoniae, H. influenzae, gram-negative bacilli, Legionella, S. aureus, C. pneumoniae, viruses, M. pneumoniae, and M. catarrhalis | |

# TUBERCULOSIS

| Condition | Description | Location in Lungs | Pathologic Process |
|---|---|---|---|
| Primary TB | Usually asymptomatic. | Lower lobes and hilar lymph nodes | Calcified granuloma called the Ghon complex forms. May or may not produce giant cells and caseation. Can disseminate and cause meningitis. |
| Secondary TB (Reactivated) | Most patients present with this type. Causes mild fever, night sweats, cough, hemoptysis (coughing up blood), weakness, and weight loss. | Lung apex or upper portions of the lower lobes | Spreads via the lymphatics. If cavitation occurs in an airway, it can then be spread by coughing. Cavitating lesions eventually become fibrinocalcific scars. |
| Miliary TB | Disease spreads throughout the lungs and to other organs via the lymphatics from the primary lesion. | Small patchy foci throughout the lungs | Spreads to the bone marrow, liver, and spleen. |
| Bronchopneumonia | Similar to other bronchopneumonias. See Pathologic Classification of Pneumonias above. | Surrounds bronchi and bronchioles | No tubercle formation. Mycobacterium is found in exudate. Usually associated with an immunocompromised state. |

# IV. Vascular Disease and Tumors

## VASCULAR LUNG DISEASES

| Condition | Description | Complications | Pathologic Findings |
|---|---|---|---|
| Pulmonary Edema | Acute onset of cardiogenic pulmonary edema presents with dyspnea at rest, productive frothy pink sputum, tachycardia, diaphoresis, and cyanosis. Rales, wheezing, or rhonchi may be heard. Condition is due to mitral stenosis, exacerbation of congestive heart failure, or acute myocardial infarction. (See Chapter 1, Causes of Edema.) | Pulmonary infection | Transudative fluid, containing macrophages filled with hemosiderin. Accumulates in the lower lobes of the lungs. |
| | Noncardiogenic pulmonary edema presents in an identical manner but lacks the cardiac history. Causes include ARDS, bacterial pneumonias, disseminated intravascular coagulation, sepsis, shock, malignancies, pulmonary embolism, and connective tissue diseases. | Pulmonary infection | Protein exudate fills first the interstitium, then the alveoli. |
| Pulmonary Embolism | Most often results from deep venous thrombosis in the legs. Risk factors include cancer, oral contraceptive use, and fractures. Emboli may be small and asymptomatic in young adults with good bronchial circulation. Pulmonary infarcts occur with compromised bronchial circulation (e.g., with congestive heart failure or lung disease), often in older adults. (See Chapter 1, Types of Embolism.) | May be fatal with a massive pulmonary infarct | From none to hemorrhagic infarct with eventual scar. |
| Pulmonary Hypertension | Presents with progressive dyspnea, fatigue, or dull chest pain (resembling angina). <br> Primary—idiopathic and rare, occurring in young women. Presents with a progressively worsening course, ending in death. <br> Secondary—Mechanisms include decreased cross-sectional area of the pulmonary vasculature, usually due to hypoxia. Acute pulmonary embolism is the primary cause. A left- to right-shunt, pulmonary stenosis, polycythemia, or systemic hypertension are other causes. | In advanced stages, tricuspid and pulmonary valve insufficiency | Endothelial cell dysfunction with decreased prostacyclin and nitrous oxide results in vasoconstriction. Pulmonary vessel smooth muscle hypertrophy and intimal proliferation occur. |

## PRIMARY LUNG CANCERS

Responsible for 171,600 new cases and 158,900 deaths per year in the United States, placing this cancer as the third most common in incidence and the most common cause of death due to cancer. Tumors secondary to metastases from the breast, colon, kidney, or melanoma are a more common cause of lung tumors than any primary lung tumor. Metastases are usually bilateral.

| Type | Disease Description | Pathologic Process |
|------|---------------------|--------------------|
| Bronchogenic Carcinomas | Represent 90% of all primary lung cancers. Patients present in their 50s to 70s with cough, dyspnea, chest pain, hemoptysis, anorexia, and weight loss. | • If the tumor involves the lung apex, it can present as Pancoast syndrome, causing compressive neurovascular complications.<br><br>• Superior vena cava syndrome (mediastinal tumor compression of the superior vena cava and recurrent laryngeal nerve) causes hoarseness and decreased drainage from the head and neck.<br><br>• Horner syndrome (sympathetic chains are compressed) causes ipsilateral miosis, anhydrosis, and ptosis.<br><br>• Bronchial obstruction predisposes to an obstructive pneumonia.<br><br>• Symptomatic lung cancer is generally unresectable because of the advanced stage at the time of presentation. Smoking is the greatest risk factor. |
| | Squamous cell carcinoma (most common type) represents 30–35% of bronchogenic carcinomas. Often starts out as a central hilar mass growing intraluminally in the bronchi. Easiest to detect cytologically by examining the sputum. Tends to metastasize first to the regional lymph nodes, then spreads widely to other organs. | Paraneoplastic hormone production. Hypercalcemia may result from parathyroid hormone–like hormone production. |
| | Adenocarcinoma represents 30–35% of bronchogenic carcinomas. Usually appears in the periphery of the lungs and, therefore, is more difficult to detect in the sputum. Bronchoalveolar cell carcinoma, a subtype of adenocarcinoma, accounts for about 2% and is a low-grade tumor. It tends to line the alveolar walls. | Adenocarcinoma. |
| | Small cell (oat cell) carcinoma represents 20–25% of bronchogenic carcinomas. Arises from neural crest cells (APUD), grows aggressively, and progresses rapidly. Tends to start centrally near the hilum. | Paraneoplastic production of antidiuretic hormone or adrenocorticotropic hormone. Cells have little cytoplasm and are organized into nests without squamous or adenocarcinoma characteristics. |
| | Large cell carcinoma accounts for 10–15% of bronchogenic carcinomas. This tumor behaves like adenocarcinoma and starts in the periphery. | May represent poorly differentiated squamous cell carcinoma or adenocarcinoma. |

*Continued*

## PRIMARY LUNG CANCERS (Continued)

| Type | Disease Description | Pathologic Process |
|---|---|---|
| Mesothelioma | Malignant or benign tumor arising in the pleura. Malignant form is strongly associated with prolonged asbestos exposure. There is no association between smoking and mesothelioma. | Pleural exudative effusion accounts for its preferred spread pattern along the pleura. Metastases are common to the pericardium, mediastinum, and the contralateral pleura. |
| Carcinoid Tumor | Also known as bronchial adenoma, this is a low-grade and malignant lesion (despite its name). Represents 1–5% of all primary lung cancers. It can produce serotonin (APUD tumor), but most tumors do not. It is centrally located. Cure rate is 90–95% with resection. Tumor rarely metastasizes. | Intrabronchial polyp consisting of uniformly sized round cells. |

# CHAPTER 6
# URINARY SYSTEM

**I. GLOMERULAR DISEASES**

Description of Glomerular Deposits

Nephrotic Syndromes

Nephritic–Nephrotic Syndromes

Nephritic Syndromes

Chronic Glomerulonephritis

**II. TUBULOINTERSTITIAL DISEASES**

Types of Tubulointerstitial Diseases

Urine Sediment Assisting Diagnosis

Vascular Kidney Disorders

Kidney Size Patterns in Disease States

Kidney Stones and Urinary Tract Obstruction

**III. OTHER RENAL DISORDERS**

Renal Cystic Diseases

Primary Renal Tumors

**IV. LOWER URINARY TRACT**

Lower Urinary Tract Diseases

Lower Urinary Tract Tumors

**ABBREVIATIONS**
**BUN** = blood urea nitrogen
**Ig** = immunoglobulin
**PMN** = polymorphonuclear leukocyte

**RBC** = red blood cell
**WBC** = white blood cell

## MOST COMMON Causes and Types

| Disorder | Common Cause |
|---|---|
| Nephrotic syndrome in children | Minimal-change disease |
| Nephrotic syndrome in adults | Membranous glomerulonephritis |
| Glomerulonephritis | IgA nephropathy |
| Acute renal failure | Ischemic acute tubular necrosis |
| Chronic renal failure | Diabetic nephropathy |

| Disorder | Common Type |
|---|---|
| Inherited kidney disease | Polycystic adult kidney disease |
| Childhood renal malignancy | Wilms tumor |
| Adult renal malignancy | Renal cell carcinoma |

| | |
|---|---|
| **Bilirubinuria** | Unconjugated bilirubin in the urine. Urine appears dark yellow, green, or brown. (See Chapter 10.) |
| **Glomerulonephritis** | Also known as glomerular nephritis, a noninfectious glomerular inflammation. Can cause nephrotic syndromes, nephritic syndromes, or both. Also divided into acute and chronic types. Both can cause renal failure; however, the chronic type is irreversible. Several patterns can be seen: diffuse global, diffuse segmental, focal global, or focal segmental. |
| | Diffuse and focal describe the number of glomeruli involved. Diffuse means all the glomeruli are affected; focal means some of the glomeruli are involved. Diffuse conditions cause hypoalbuminemia. |
| | Global and segmental describe the area of each glomerulus that is involved. Global means the entire glomerulus is affected; segmental means only part of the glomerulus is affected. |
| **Hematuria** | Blood in the urine. Urine appears red with gross hematuria and dark yellow to amber in microscopic hematuria. Blood in the urine is always abnormal. May be caused by glomerulonephritis; renal, ureter, or bladder carcinoma; renal stones; cystitis; vasculitis (polyarteritis nodosa or hemolytic-uremic syndrome); or bleeding disorders. |
| **Nephritic Syndrome** | Disorder that causes heavy hematuria, red cell casts, hypertension, and renal failure. |
| **Nephropathy** | Any disease that involves the kidney. |
| **Nephrotic Syndrome** | Includes 4 signs: proteinuria (albuminuria), hypoalbuminemia, hyperlipidemia, and generalized edema. Most often caused by glomerulonephritis. Pathology is due to increased basement-membrane permeability. All related disorders show mesangial proliferation in addition to the changes that are syndrome specific. |
| **Oliguria/Anuria** | Oliguria is decreased urine output (< 400 mL/d). The extreme condition is anuria (70–100 mL/d), caused by renal failure. |
| **Polyuria** | Excretion of more than 2000 mL (2 L) of urine per day. (See Chapter 8, Pancreatic Diseases and Diabetes Mellitus.) |
| **Proteinuria** | Protein in the urine. The urine looks normal, but protein in the urine is usually abnormal. Some patients are prone to postural or exercise-induced proteinuria, which is benign. Another cause is glomerulonephritis. Need indicator strips or laboratory analysis to detect protein. |
| **Pyuria** | Pus in the urine, composed of WBCs and cellular debris. Caused by pyelonephritis or cystitis. The urine may appear cloudy. |

*Continued*

## TERMS TO LEARN (Continued)

| | |
|---|---|
| **Renal Failure** | Decreased bilateral renal function. Causes are divided into prerenal, intrinsic, and postrenal failure. Also divided into acute and chronic. Acute failure is usually reversible unless the parenchyma has undergone necrosis. Chronic failure occurs when the number of glomeruli between both kidneys has decreased to 25% of normal. |
| | Prerenal type is caused by decreased glomerular filtration rate secondary to decreased perfusion of the kidney. Prolonged ischemia results in intrinsic kidney damage. |
| | Intrinsic (parenchymal) type includes tubular, interstitial, and glomerular damage. |
| | Postrenal type occurs when urine flow is obstructed. Prolonged obstruction results in intrinsic kidney damage. |
| **Renal Function Tests** | BUN is manufactured in the liver from amino acids and filtered in the kidneys. BUN increases when the glomerular filtration rate decreases. However, it is a nonspecific test because other causes can also increase it, including dehydration, high-protein diets, and gastrointestinal bleeding. |
| | Creatinine is produced at a steady rate from muscle creatine. Its clearance is a good estimate of the glomerular filtration rate. |
| | The BUN-creatinine ratio is a better predictor of renal function than creatinine alone. The ratio is increased in prerenal and postrenal failure but not in intrinsic failure (except for glomerulonephritis). |
| **Uremia** | Elevated BUN and other nitrogenous wastes. Acutely, patients present with nausea, vomiting, altered mental status, and death if uremia is not treated. A large portion of the kidneys' glomerular supply must be affected before patients become symptomatic. |
| **Urethritis** | Inflammation of the urethra, commonly due to infection. (See Chapter 7, Comparison of Sexually Transmitted Infections.) |
| **Urinary Tract Infection** | Encompasses upper-tract infections such as pyelonephritis and lower-tract infections such as cystitis and urethritis. |

# I. Glomerular Diseases

## DESCRIPTION OF GLOMERULAR DEPOSITS

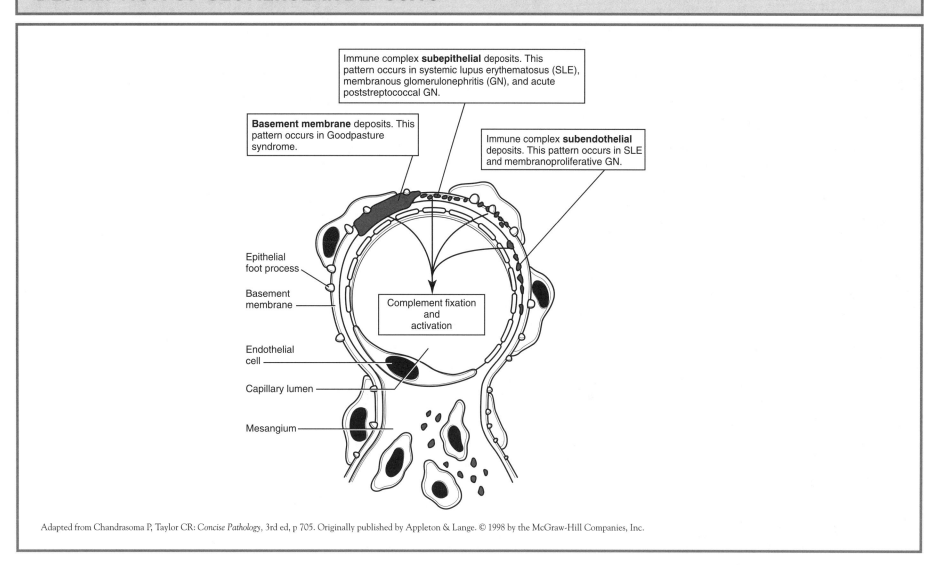

Immune complex **subepithelial** deposits. This pattern occurs in systemic lupus erythematosus (SLE), membranous glomerulonephritis (GN), and acute poststreptococcal GN.

**Basement membrane** deposits. This pattern occurs in Goodpasture syndrome.

Immune complex **subendothelial** deposits. This pattern occurs in SLE and membranoproliferative GN.

Epithelial foot process

Basement membrane

Endothelial cell

Capillary lumen

Mesangium

Complement fixation and activation

Adapted from Chandrasoma P, Taylor CR: *Concise Pathology*, 3rd ed, p 705. Originally published by Appleton & Lange. © 1998 by the McGraw-Hill Companies, Inc.

## NEPHROTIC SYNDROMES

| Condition | Description | Cause(s) | Pathologic Findings |
|---|---|---|---|
| **Minimal-Change Disease** | Also known as lipoid nephrosis. The most common cause of nephrotic syndrome in children, this is a glomerulonephritis that presents with massive proteinuria and fatty casts. No increased risk for chronic glomerulonephritis or renal failure. | Occurs after a respiratory viral infection. | Normal-appearing glomeruli with fused foot processes. No complement or immunoglobulin deposition. May remit with corticosteroids. |
| **Membranous Glomerulonephritis** | The most common cause of nephrotic syndrome in adults. Slowly progressive to chronic renal failure. | Most cases are idiopathic. Also secondary to tumors, systemic lupus erythematosus, drugs, hepatitis B, syphilis, malaria, or diabetes mellitus. | Initially appears as subepithelial deposits of antibody–complement complexes and foot-process fusion (on electron microscopy and light microscopy). In stage 2, basement-membrane spikes are evident on electron microscopy, again from deposition. In stage 3, basement membrane appears to be split and spikes form a "railroad track" (on electron and light microscopy). |
| **IgA Nephropathy** | Also known as Berger disease. Patients present from age 10 to their 30s with hematuria and proteinuria. Slowly progressive to renal failure. | Unknown. Associated with viral respiratory infections. | Focal mesangial proliferative glomerulonephritis. Mesangial immunoglobulin and complement deposits may be seen on electron microscopy. Sclerosis is seen in progressive disease. |
| **Diabetic Nephropathy** | The most common cause of chronic renal failure, seen after many years of uncontrolled diabetes mellitus. Diabetic retinopathy is often present as well. | Diabetes type 1 or type 2 (see Chapter 8). | Microangiopathy causes a focal diffuse glomerulosclerosis. Changes include glomerular capillary thickening with arteriolar sclerosis and focal hyaline nodules (Kimmelstiel-Wilson disease) in the glomerulus. No complement or immunoglobulin deposition. |
| **Renal Amyloidosis** | Progressive disease that results in chronic renal failure. | Primary or secondary amyloidosis. | Amyloid is deposited in the basement membrane, thickening it. Amyloid can be stained with Congo red and shows apple-green birefringence under polarized light. (See Chapter 1, Storage Diseases.) |
| **Henoch-Schönlein Purpura** | Rare progressive vasculitic disease in children. Affects the skin, joints, and gastrointestinal system. Presents with hematuria, nephrotic syndrome, and acute renal failure. | Follows childhood respiratory infection. | Focal and segmental distribution. Mesangial IgA deposits. |

## NEPHRITIC–NEPHROTIC SYNDROMES

| Condition | Description or Cause | Pathologic Findings |
| --- | --- | --- |
| Focal Segmental Glomerulosclerosis | Associated with heroin abuse or human immunodeficiency virus infection. | Loss of glomerular foot processes; focal segmental hyalinelike sclerosis; immunoglobulin and complement deposition. |
| Membranoproliferative Glomerulonephritis | Progressive disease. Type I can be associated with systemic lupus erythematosus or hepatitis B. | Thickened glomerular capillary walls and mesangial proliferation. Complement levels are decreased.<br><br>• In type I (65%), subendothelial deposits in basement membrane form a characteristic "tram track."<br><br>• In type II (35%), basement-membrane deposits and thickening are found. |
| Lupus Nephropathy | Chronic nephrotic syndrome with acute nephritic syndrome, eventually resulting in renal failure. | Basement-membrane and subendothelial deposits of immune complex and complement. Presents with no change, mesangial glomerulonephritis, focal proliferative glomerulonephritis (poor outcome), diffuse proliferative glomerulonephritis (poor outcome), or diffuse membranous glomerulonephritis. Serum complement is decreased. |

## NEPHRITIC SYNDROMES

| Condition | Description | Cause(s) or Association | Pathology |
| --- | --- | --- | --- |
| Acute Proliferative Poststreptococcal Glomerulonephritis | A self-limited disease commonly seen in children after "strep throat." Acute onset of fever and nephritic syndrome. Urine may be a characteristic "smoky urine" color. Elevated anti-streptolysin O. | Group A β-hemolytic streptococci | Diffuse global proliferative glomerulonephritis. Mesangial proliferation. Enlarged and bloodless glomeruli infiltrated with monocytes, eosinophils, lymphocytes, and PMNs. Epithelial proliferation may produce characteristic crescents in a few glomeruli. Subepithelial dense humps result from immune-complex deposition. |
| Rapidly Progressing Glomerulonephritis | Also known as crescentic glomerulonephritis. Rapidly progressing disease with renal failure within months of onset. | 50% from acute proliferative poststreptococcal glomerulonephritis; 10% from Goodpasture syndrome | Diffuse global proliferative glomerulonephritis. More than 70% of the glomeruli may have characteristic epithelial crescents that result in irreversible glomerular scarring. Electron microscopy may show glomerular basement-membrane rupture.<br><br>Crescent |
| Goodpasture Syndrome | Causes hematuria and hemoptysis, cough, or dyspnea secondary to lung involvement. Followed by a rapidly progressive glomerulonephritis. Renal failure occurs within 1 year of onset. | Antibody mediated | Focal proliferative glomerulonephritis that may evolve into rapidly progressing glomerulonephritis. Glomerular basement-membrane immunoglobulin and complement deposition. Linear pattern of immunofluorescence. |
| Alport Syndrome | Also known as hereditary nephritis. Presents with hematuria, blindness, and nerve deafness. More severe in males. | X-linked or autosomal dominant | Focal glomerulonephritis. Glomerular basement-membrane splitting with glomerulosclerosis. |

| | | | |
|---|---|---|---|
| Polyarteritis Nodosa | Vasculitis of the renal vessels. Presents with hematuria, proteinuria, and hypertension. Rapidly progressive renal failure may be seen. See Chapter 2, Types of Vasculitides (Vasculitis). | Hepatitis B and antineutrophil cytoplasmic autoantibodies | Renal infarction secondary to the vasculitis leads to renal atrophy and renal failure. Chronic lesions show fibrinoid necrosis of a circumferential section of the vessels. Associated with rapidly progressing glomerulonephritis. |
| Wegener Granulomatosis | Presents with pulmonary involvement and hematuria, proteinuria, and rapidly progressive renal failure. | Central antineutrophil cytoplasmic autoantibodies | Focal segmental proliferative glomerulonephritis. May cause epithelial crescents. Necrotizing granulomatous arterial vasculitis. May evolve into rapidly progressing glomerulonephritis. |

## CHRONIC GLOMERULONEPHRITIS

| Description | Cause(s) | Pathology |
|---|---|---|
| Presents with chronic renal failure, hypertension, microscopic hematuria, and proteinuria. Hypertension is due to a decrease in sodium (Na) excretion and fluid retention. | All progressive glomerular conditions may end here, including IgA nephropathy, renal amyloidosis, membranous glomerulonephritis, rapidly progressing glomerulonephritis, and Goodpasture syndrome. | Atrophied kidney(s) with a narrow cortex. Decreased nephrons with diffuse sclerosis and hyalinized nodules in the glomeruli. Tubular dilatation and interstitial fibrosis are also seen. |

## TYPES OF TUBULOINTERSTITIAL DISEASES

| Condition | Description | Cause(s) | Pathology |
|---|---|---|---|
| Acute Tubular Necrosis | Patients lose the ability to concentrate urine with loss of tubular function. Urine may contain RBCs and tubular epithelial cells. This is a reversible condition with 3 phases: oliguric phase—elevated BUN (2 weeks); diuretic phase—diuresis of dilute, isotonic urine; recovery phase—tubular function recovers and BUN and creatinine return to normal. Mortality rate is 25–50%. Causes are ischemic or nephrotoxic. | | |
| | Ischemic acute tubular necrosis | Ischemia is the most common cause of acute renal failure. Acute ischemia leads to parenchymal damage. Ischemia can occur with shock (the most common cause), severe hemorrhage, or congestive heart failure. | Patchy necrosis of proximal and distal convoluted tubules. In the ischemic type, the tubular epithelial cell brush border is no longer prominent (will not stain with periodic acid–Schiff). Tubules are filled with RBCs, myoglobin, hemoglobin, uric acid, or amyloid casts, depending on the cause. |
| | Nephrotoxic acute tubular necrosis (toxic nephrosis). Stop the offending agent. | • Extrinsic toxins include aminoglycosides, amphotericin B, radioactive contrast dye, cyclosporine, carbon tetrachloride, and mercury chloride. <br> • Intrinsic toxins include myoglobinuria, hemoglobinuria, hyperuricemia, and Bence Jones protein filtration secondary to multiple myeloma (amyloid nephrosis). | Same as above, except that in the nephrotoxic type, the brush border stains with periodic acid–Schiff. |

| Tubulointerstitial Nephritis | The acute form is also called allergic tubulointerstitial nephritis. Condition causes about 15% of acute renal failure and involves a sudden decrease in renal function after taking a new medication. Presents with fever, flank pain, maculopapular rash, and eosinophilia. Pyuria, proteinuria, and eosinophiluria may be present. Patient usually recovers on withdrawal of the offending drug. | | |
|---|---|---|---|
| | In the chronic form, polyuria and nocturia occur secondary to the decreased ability to concentrate urine. Urine may show mild proteinuria, few cells, and some granular casts. There may be salt wasting with significant volume depletion. | | |
| | Acute tubulointerstitial nephritis | Penicillin, ampicillin, and other beta-lactams; nonsteroidal anti-inflammatory drugs; rifampin; sulfa drugs; thiazides; furosemide; and cimetidine. | Interstitial infiltration with PMNs, plasma cells, and eosinophils with focal tubular necrosis. |
| | Chronic tubulointerstitial nephritis | Reflux nephropathy from prolonged urine flow obstruction (most common cause) (also see Kidney Stones and Urinary Tract Obstruction—Hydronephrosis below), chronic use of acetaminophen and nonsteroidal anti-inflammatory drugs, and lead or cadmium toxicity. | With reflux, urine components (Tamm-Horsfall proteins) escape into the interstitium and cause an inflammatory response. Chronic renal failure, small contracted kidneys, and renal papillary necrosis occur. Patients have increased risk for transitional cell carcinoma of the renal pelvis. |
| Renal Papillary Necrosis | See the respective causative diseases | Occurs because of ischemia, seen in chronic tubulointerstitial nephritis, diabetes mellitus, acetaminophen abuse, sickle cell disease, hydronephrosis, and acute pyelonephritis. | Necrosis and scarring of the renal calices and papillae. |

*Continued*

# TYPES OF TUBULOINTERSTITIAL DISEASES (Continued)

| Condition | Description | Cause(s) | Pathology |
|---|---|---|---|
| Pyelonephritis | Acute infection of the kidneys causes high fever, chills, flank pain, dysuria, frequency, and urgency. Urine has pyuria, bacteria, and WBC casts. | Infection with Escherichia coli (75%) from own fecal matter; also with Klebsiella, Proteus, and Enterococcus faecalis. Urinary stasis from bladder obstruction, shorter female urethra, pregnancy, diabetes mellitus, and urinary reflux all predispose. Women are affected more often than men. Associated with sexual activity. | Kidney is enlarged. Acute suppurative inflammation of the renal tubules leads to patchy liquefactive necrosis. Renal papillary necrosis may occur with severe disease. |
| | Chronic pyelonephritis accounts for 15–20% of chronic renal failure. Hypertension or chronic renal failure occurs if both kidneys are involved. Urine has pyuria and mild proteinuria. May or may not show bacteriuria. | Chronic vesicoureteral reflux (most common cause), chronic obstruction secondary to kidney stones, benign prostatic hyperplasia, tumors, or congenital anomalies. | Asymmetric kidney atrophy from scarring and fibrosis. Surviving tubules become distended with colloid casts resembling thyroid follicles. |
| Parenchymal Storage Diseases | Nephrocalcinosis is metastatic calcification of the renal interstitium. | See Chapter 1, Storage Diseases—Metastatic Calcification. | Calcium phosphate crystals are deposited in the interstitium and damage the tubules. |
| | Renal amyloidosis is a progressive disease that results in chronic renal failure. | See Nephrotic Syndromes—Renal Amyloidosis above. | Amyloid is deposited in the interstitium and obstructs the tubules. |
| | Urate nephropathy is slowly progressive; due to high serum uric acid levels. | See Chapter 12 for gout. | Urate crystals are deposited in the tubules and interstitium. |

## URINE SEDIMENT ASSISTING DIAGNOSIS

| Disease Category | Disorder | Urine Sediment |
|---|---|---|
| Glomerular Disease | Glomerulonephritis | RBC casts |
| Tubular or Interstitial Disease | Acute tubular necrosis | Tubular casts, RBCs |
| | Acute pyelonephritis | WBCs, WBC casts, and bacteria |
| | Tubulointerstitial nephritis | Tubular and WBC casts, eosinophils, and PMNs |
| Other | Chronic renal failure | Waxy and broad cell casts |

## VASCULAR KIDNEY DISORDERS

| Condition | Signs and Symptoms | Cause(s) | Pathologic Findings |
|---|---|---|---|
| Benign Nephrosclerosis | Usually asymptomatic. | Essential hypertension. (See Chapter 2, Hypertension.) | Bilateral kidney atrophy and cortex thinning. Hyaline arteriosclerosis of arterioles. Global sclerosis of the glomeruli, atrophy of the nephrons, and interstitial fibrosis are seen. Patients have increased risk of developing renal failure if they are volume depleted. |
| Malignant Nephrosclerosis | Proteinuria, hematuria, and rapidly progressive acute renal failure. Without treatment, most patients die. | Malignant hypertension. (See Chapter 2, Hypertension.) | Normal or enlarged kidneys show petechiae on the surface of the renal cortex; often called "flea-bitten kidneys." Fibrinoid necrosis of the arterioles with "onion skinning" of the vessel walls. |
| Renal Infarct | Acute onset of tenderness at the costovertebral angle followed by hematuria. If extensive, may cause renal failure. | Arterial embolism (most common cause) secondary to myocardial infarction, atrial fibrillation, infective endocarditis, or mitral stenosis. Renal artery thrombosis secondary to atherosclerosis. | Pale wedge-shaped infarct may be seen. Infarcted area shows coagulative necrosis and heals by scarring. Cholesterol clefts may be seen in renal artery or its branches after histologic fixation. |
| Renal Artery Stenosis | Hypertension or a renal infarct if the occlusion is complete. | Atheroembolic narrowing (often bilateral) in the elderly (most common cause). Fibromuscular dysplasia (unilateral) of the artery media in young females. | Diffuse ischemia of the affected kidney. If condition is bilateral, both kidneys undergo atrophy. If unilateral, the affected kidney atrophies and the other hypertrophies to compensate. Both types result in hypertension. (See Chapter 2, Hypertension.) |

## KIDNEY SIZE PATTERNS IN DISEASE STATES

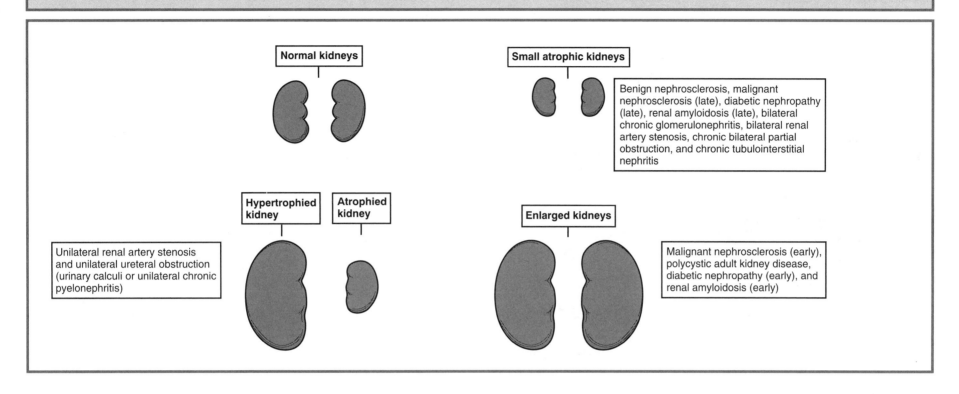

**Normal kidneys**

**Small atrophic kidneys**

Benign nephrosclerosis, malignant nephrosclerosis (late), diabetic nephropathy (late), renal amyloidosis (late), bilateral chronic glomerulonephritis, bilateral renal artery stenosis, chronic bilateral partial obstruction, and chronic tubulointerstitial nephritis

**Hypertrophied kidney**

**Atrophied kidney**

Unilateral renal artery stenosis and unilateral ureteral obstruction (urinary calculi or unilateral chronic pyelonephritis)

**Enlarged kidneys**

Malignant nephrosclerosis (early), polycystic adult kidney disease, diabetic nephropathy (early), and renal amyloidosis (early)

Kidney stones are also known as renal calculi, and their presence is known as urolithiasis. Acute ureteral obstruction occurs when one or more stones temporarily lodge in a ureter and obstruct urine flow. Patients present with acute renal colic (flank pain) and hematuria.

| Condition | Description | X-ray Appearance and Other Pathologic Findings |
|---|---|---|
| Calcium Stones (70%) | Stones are composed of calcium oxalate. May be caused by hypercalcemia from primary hyperparathyroidism, metastases to bone, multiple myeloma, vitamin D intoxication, and sarcoidosis. May also be caused by high oxalate excretion secondary to increased vitamin C intake, ingestion of ethylene glycol (antifreeze), or Crohn disease. Stone formation is not pH specific. | Radiopaque on X-ray |
| Triple Phosphate Stones (15%) | Stones are composed of magnesium ammonium phosphate. Stones are large and often fill the calices, forming a "staghorn" calculus. Caused by urea-splitting bacteria, such as *Proteus*, that create an alkaline urine. | Radiolucent on X-ray unless calcium is also present |
| Uric Acid Stones (10%) (variable shapes) | Stones are composed of sodium urate and are formed in acidic urine. May occur in patients with normal or elevated serum urate. Associated with gout. | Radiopaque on X-ray |
| Cystine Stones (rare) | Stones are composed of cystine. Seen in homocystinuria, a disease with a genetic defect in transporting cystine into the urine. Stone formation is not pH specific. | Radiopaque on X-ray |

| | | |
|---|---|---|
| **Urinary Tract Obstruction** | Obstruction may occur in the renal pelvis or calix, in the ureter, in the bladder, or in the urethra. Bilateral obstruction occurs if the urethra or the bladder is blocked. The other types involve unilateral obstruction.<br><br>• Acute ureteral obstruction is described at top of table.<br><br>• Chronic unilateral obstruction is often asymptomatic. See below.<br><br>• Chronic bilateral partial obstruction leads to progressive chronic renal failure. See below.<br><br>• Bilateral complete obstruction leads to acute renal failure. | |
| **Hydronephrosis** | Unilateral hydronephrosis (chronic unilateral obstruction) is caused by chronically lodged calculi, obstruction by necrotic debris, strictures, tumor compression, or congenital anomalies. Can lead to chronic tubulointerstitial nephritis. | Urine accumulates in the interstitium until increased pressure causes tubular dysfunction. Progressive cortical atrophy and irreversible loss of nephrons are seen over time. Renal pelvis dilates. No renal failure occurs because the other kidney can compensate. |
| | Bilateral hydronephrosis (chronic bilateral partial obstruction) is most commonly caused by benign prostatic hyperplasia in males and cystocele in females. Can also be caused by a neurogenic bladder (nonfunctional bladder) and pregnancy (relaxing effects of progesterone). | Same as above except that chronic renal failure occurs because both kidneys are involved. |

# III. Other Renal Disorders

## RENAL CYSTIC DISEASES

| Condition | Description | Cause | Pathology |
|---|---|---|---|
| Simple Cysts | Most common type of cyst; occurs in up to 50% of the population over 50 years old. Often found incidentally on ultrasound or autopsy. No clinical significance. | Unknown | Simple cyst lined by tubular epithelium. |
| Polycystic Adult Kidney Disease | Most common inherited kidney disorder. Causes 5–10% of cases of chronic renal failure. Asymptomatic for the first 40 years, but afterward, patients present with hematuria, polyuria, renal stones, and hypertension (cysts stretch the juxtaglomerular apparatus receptors). | Autosomal dominant | Bilateral cystic enlargement of the kidneys. The cysts are lined by proximal and distal tubular epithelium. 30% of patients also have liver, pancreatic, and splenic cysts, and 15% have berry aneurysms. Nephrons between the cysts are functional. Cysts continue to form. It takes years for renal failure to develop. |
| Infantile Polycystic Kidney Disease | Early manifestation of renal failure. Often results in death in infancy. | Autosomal recessive | Bilateral cystic enlargement of the kidneys. The entire renal parenchyma is composed of cysts. Condition is associated with liver cysts, and survivors may have liver fibrosis. |
| Medullary Sponge Kidney Disease | Patients present in their 40s to 60s, usually without symptoms. Renal function is normal but there is an increased incidence of urinary calculi. | Unknown | Can involve 1 or both kidneys. Examination shows small cystic dilatations of the medullary collecting ducts in the renal papillae. |
| Uremic Medullary Cystic Disease | Rare disorder in young adults that causes progressive chronic renal failure. Most common type is familial juvenile. | Autosomal recessive | Multiple cysts in the medulla, tubular atrophy, and interstitial fibrosis. |
| Dialysis Cystic Disease | Presents with hematuria from ruptured cysts. Often associated with dialysis in patients with end-stage renal failure. | Unknown | Associated with increased risk of renal adenocarcinoma. |

## PRIMARY RENAL TUMORS

| Condition | Description | Appearance of Tumor |
|---|---|---|
| **Benign Tumors** | | |
| Cortical Adenoma | Asymptomatic. Found incidentally on computed tomography scan or at autopsy. | Round, well-circumscribed, yellow mass. Composed of benign cells organized into a papillary or solid pattern. Oncocytoma (subtype of cortical adenoma) is composed of large uniform cells with small nuclei. |
| **Malignant Tumors**—responsible for 54,200 new cases per year in the United States and 11,900 deaths. It is the sixth most common type of cancer, but is not among the top 10 for mortality. | | |
| Renal Cell Carcinoma | The most common primary renal malignancy, accounting for 1–2% of adult cancers. Patients present in their 60s with painless hematuria. This is an aggressive tumor with early metastasis to lungs, bone, liver, and skin. (It metastasizes hematogenously rather than lymphatically.) Associated with smoking, male gender, von Hippel-Lindau disease (60%), and dialysis cystic disease (10%). | Solid or cystic yellow mass. Cut surfaces show hemorrhage, calcifications, and fibrotic areas. Infiltration is local, but invasion into renal vein causes early metastasis. Classically, tumor is composed of clear and polygonal cells. Tumor causes paraneoplastic syndrome and secretes parathyroid-like hormone, erythropoietin, or gonadotropins. |
| Wilms Tumor (Nephroblastoma) | Most common primary renal malignancy of childhood. Presents with a large abdominal mass. Most cases are hereditary (loss of the *WT-1* tumor suppressor gene). Metastases to the lung, liver, and brain are common. | Large soft tumor. Composed of either epithelial or mesenchymal cell types, when differentiated. Cells are organized into rosettes. |

# IV. Lower Urinary Tract

## LOWER URINARY TRACT DISEASES

| Disease | Description | Pathologic Findings |
|---|---|---|
| Acute Cystitis | Inflammation of the bladder, most commonly from infection with *E. coli*. (See Types of Tubulointerstitial Diseases—Pyelonephritis above for other pathogens and risk factors.) Patients present with the triad of urinary frequency, lower abdominal pain, and dysuria. May or may not have a low-grade fever. Urine has protein, RBCs, or PMNs but no casts. Cystitis is also caused by radiation and cyclophosphamide (hemorrhagic cystitis). | Bladder mucosal hyperemia with acute suppurative inflammation. If cystitis is caused by *Proteus*, may see triple phosphate stones. (See Kidney Stones and Urinary Tract Obstruction above.) |
| Urethritis | See Chapter 7, Comparison of Sexually Transmitted Infections. | |

# LOWER URINARY TRACT TUMORS

Tumors of the lower urinary tract are relatively rare. They cause 2300 new cases and 500 deaths per year due to cancer in the United States.

| Condition | Description | Cause(s) | Appearance of Tumor |
|---|---|---|---|
| Intestinal Metaplasia | Transitional epithelium changes into columnar. (See Chapter 1, Terms to Learn—Metaplasia.) | Chronic irritation | Development of nests of transitional epithelium called Brunn nests, with central cells becoming a columnar lining (cystitis cystica). There is an increased risk of carcinoma. |
| Transitional Cell Carcinoma | Most common bladder tumor. Patients present at age 40 years or older with painless hematuria. Tumor may obstruct the ureteral opening and cause bilateral hydronephrosis. | Cigarette smoking (the primary cause, with a 2- to 4-fold increase in risk), industrial aniline dye exposure, phenacetin use, and infection with *Schistosoma haematobium* (in Egypt) | Tumor occurs near the trigone or in a bladder-wall diverticulum. Flat and solid shape (most aggressive) or papillary tumor projecting into the lumen. Usually has more than 7 layers of transitional epithelium. |
| Squamous Cell Carcinoma | Can occur in the bladder or urethra. | Unknown | Composed of keratin pearls, if well differentiated. |

# CHAPTER 7
# MALE AND FEMALE REPRODUCTIVE SYSTEMS, THE BREAST, AND PREGNANCY

I. COMPARISON OF MALE AND FEMALE REPRODUCTIVE DISEASES

Comparison of Sexually Transmitted Infections

Comparison of External Genital Tumors

Comparison of Gonadal Tumors

II. UROLOGIC DISEASES

Testicular Diseases

Prostate Disorders

Prostate Disease Distribution

III. GYNECOLOGIC DISEASES

Uterine Conditions

Ovarian Cysts

Risk Factors, Incidence, and Mortality of Cancers in Women

Vaginal, Cervical, and Uterine Tumors

Cervical Carcinoma and Papanicolaou Smear Classification

Menstrual Cycle

Causes of Abnormal Uterine Bleeding

IV. DISEASES OF THE BREAST

Inflammatory Breast Conditions

Summary of Breast Lesions

Fibrocystic Disease

Common Features of Breast Cancer

Breast Tumors

V. GESTATIONAL DISORDERS

Diseases of Gestation

Gestational Tumors

**ABBREVIATIONS**

**CIN** = cervical intraepithelial neoplasia
**FSH** = follicle-stimulating hormone
**hCG** = human chorionic gonadotropin
**HIV** = human immunodeficiency virus

**HPV** = human papillomavirus
**LH** = luteinizing hormone
**PID** = pelvic inflammatory disease
**PMN** = polymorphonuclear leukocyte

## MOST COMMON Causes and Types

| Disorder | Common Cause |
|---|---|
| Testicular atrophy | Klinefelter syndrome |
| Orchitis | Mumps and syphilis |
| Epididymitis | Gonorrhea and tuberculosis |
| Vaginal or vulvar infection | Candidiasis |
| Sexually transmitted infection | *Chlamydia* |

| Disorder | Common Type |
|---|---|
| Testicular germ cell tumor | Seminoma |
| Prostate disorder | Benign prostatic hyperplasia |
| Vulvar and cervical tumors | Squamous cell carcinoma |
| Primary uterine benign tumor | Leiomyoma |
| Uterine malignancy | Adenocarcinoma |
| Primary ovarian malignancy | Serous cystadenocarcinoma |
| Benign ovarian tumor | Mature teratoma or serous cystadenoma |
| Breast disorder | Fibrocystic change of the breast |
| Fibrocystic change of the breast | Simple change |
| Primary malignancy of the breast | Invasive ductal carcinoma |
| Benign breast tumor | Fibroadenoma |

# I. Comparison of Male and Female Reproductive Diseases

## COMPARISON OF SEXUALLY TRANSMITTED INFECTIONS

| Disease | Male Disorder and Associated Findings | Female Disorder and Associated Findings |
| --- | --- | --- |
| Nongonococcal Urethritis/ Cervicitis | *Chlamydia trachomatis* is the most common sexually transmitted infection. Can be asymptomatic. Infected patients act as reservoirs for the infection. Can cause lymphogranuloma venereum, an infection of the lymph nodes with ulcerations in the rectal area. | |
| | Nonpurulent urethritis—Reiter syndrome (see Chapter 12 for arthritis). Can also be caused by *Mycoplasma genitalium* or *Ureaplasma urealyticum*. | Purulent cervicitis—May ascend and infect the fallopian tubes, causing salpingitis. |
| Gonorrhea | *Neisseria gonorrhoeae* is responsible. Condition is asymptomatic, with females affected more often than males. Can present with gonococcal pharyngitis, seen with oral sexual practices. | |
| | Acute purulent urethritis with dysuria and purulent urethral discharge. If not treated, may infect the prostate (prostatitis), seminal vesicles, and epididymis (epididymitis). Suppuration and fibrosis can cause sterility. | Purulent cervicitis. Can infect the urethra, Bartholin and Skene glands, and fallopian tubes (salpingitis). Complications include peritonitis, bacteremia, and infertility. |
| Vaginitis | Not applicable. | Caused by *Gardnerella vaginalis*, *Trichomonas*, or *Candida*. Presents with a malodorous vaginal discharge with or without itching. A wet smear of *Candida* shows pseudohyphae. *Candida* infection is more common with pregnancy, diabetes mellitus, chronic antibiotic use, oral contraceptive use, or immunocompromise. *Trichomonas* shows moving organisms on wet smear. |
| Herpes Genitalis | Most often caused by herpes simplex virus type 2. Ulcers heal spontaneously without scarring. May see recurrences with stress. | |
| | Small, red, painful papules on the penile shaft or glans that progress to vesicles and become ulcerated. | Small, red, painful papules on the vulva or cervix that progress to vesicles and become ulcerated. If there are active lesions at the time of delivery, the infant may become infected. (See Chapter 15, Congenital Infections.) |

*Continued*

## COMPARISON OF SEXUALLY TRANSMITTED INFECTIONS (Continued)

| Disease | Male Disorder and Associated Findings | Female Disorder and Associated Findings |
|---|---|---|
| Chancroid | Caused by *Haemophilus ducreyi*. Patients present with one to several soft, painful necrotic ulcers at the site of inoculation and regional painful lymphadenopathy. Most commonly occurs on the penile shaft. | Same except that the lesions occur on the vulva or labia. |
| Syphilis | Caused by *Treponema pallidum*. Primary syphilis presents with a painless ulcer (chancre) at the site of inoculation. Ulcer exudes bacteria-containing fluid and heals within a month. Secondary syphilis presents a few weeks to months later with fever, generalized lymphadenopa-thy, mucous membrane involvement, and a red maculopapular rash. A wartlike lesion (condyloma lata) may be found on the perineum. Ter-tiary syphilis (years after the initial infection) may cause neurosyphilis (see Chapter 13), gummas (painless granulomatous ulcers), or aortic disease (see Chapter 2, Aneurysms). | Primary syphilis presents at the penile glans or shaft. Primary syphilis presents on the vulva. Because *T. pallidum* can cross the placenta, the fetus is at risk for congenital syphilis. |
| Human Papillomavirus | Infects the surface epithelium of the skin of the penis. Forms a wartlike, benign papilloma lesion called condyloma acuminatum. (See Chapter 11, Skin Growths.) | Forms a wartlike papilloma on the vulva or asymptomatically infects the cervical mucosa. Predisposes to cervical carcinoma. |
| Other Infections | Other relevant infections include hepatitis B and HIV. | For hepatitis B, see Chapter 3; for HIV, see Chapter 10. Also see Chapter 15, Congenital Diseases, for infections that can be trans-mitted to infants during birth. |

## COMPARISON OF EXTERNAL GENITAL TUMORS

| Type of Tumor | Male (Penis or Scrotum) | Female (Vulva) | Pathologic Finding(s) |
|---|---|---|---|
| | There are 1400 new cases of penile tumors per year in the United States and 200 deaths. | There are 3300 new cases of vulvar tumors per year in the United States and 900 deaths. | |
| Squamous Carcinoma In Situ | Also called Bowen disease and erythroplasia of Queyrat. Causes a single red plaque on the scrotum or shaft with ulceration and crusting. | Causes a single red-brown plaque on the vulva. May present as leukoplakia. | Cells appear neoplastic with increased nuclear to cytoplasmic ratio and increased mitotic activity. Increased risk for invasive carcinoma over years. |
| Invasive Squamous Cell Carcinoma | Uncommon in the United States (< 1% of all cancers in males). Occurs on the glans or prepuce. | Most common neoplasm of the vulva (4% of all genital cancers). Occurs in women over 60 years old. Metastasizes early to the lymph nodes. It is unknown whether HPV is involved. | Early lesion may appear as leukoplakia, then a papule, then a painless ulcer. |
| | Verrucous carcinoma is a subtype that forms a wartlike lesion. Tends to remain localized. | Verrucous carcinoma is a polypoid wartlike growth that remains localized. | Squamous cell carcinoma. |
| Extramammary Paget Disease | No counterpart exists. | Rare lesion. Causes red, eczemalike crusted lesion resembling a map on the vulva of elderly women. | Anaplastic mucin-containing tumor cells in the epidermis; 30% of patients have an underlying invasive carcinoma. |

## COMPARISON OF GONADAL TUMORS

| Male (Testes) | | Female (Ovaries) | |
|---|---|---|---|
| Gonadal tumors cause 7400 new cases and 300 deaths per year in the United States. Germ cell tumors are the most common, and most are malignant (except for benign teratoma). They present as a painless growth or hydrocele on the testis and are easily detected and treated. | | Gonadal tumors cause 25,200 new cases and 14,500 deaths per year in the United States. They are the fifth most common cancer and cause of death in women. Epithelioid tumors (serous and mucinous) are the most common, and most are benign. Found incidentally on abdominal imaging or pelvic examination. Malignant tumors usually present after metastasis. | |
| **Name of Tumor** | **Description** | **Name of Tumor** | **Description** |
| **Germ Cell Tumors** | Represent > 95% of testicular tumors | **Germ Cell Tumors** | Represent 20% of all ovarian tumors |
| **Seminoma**—most common pure malignant germ cell tumor (30% of all testicular tumors) | Patients present at 30–50 years. Tumor is a partially circumscribed, firm, and solid mass composed of large polyhedral cells with a clear cytoplasm and a large central nucleus. | **Dysgerminoma** (5% of all ovarian tumors) | Patients present at 10–30 years. Tumor is a solid, firm, homogeneous mass. Identical to a seminoma. |
| **Embryonal Carcinoma** (20% of all testicular tumors) | Patients present at 15–30 years. Tumor is a solid, soft, and friable mass composed of undifferentiated malignant cells. | **Embryonal Carcinoma** (very rare) | Like the male counterpart. Focal necrosis gives a mottled appearance to the tumor. |
| **Teratoma** (10% of all testicular tumors) | Children most often get the mature, benign type. Includes derivatives of all three germ cell layers. Adults are more likely to get an immature, malignant type, which is less differentiated than the benign type. | **Teratoma**—most common germ cell ovarian tumor (15% of all ovarian tumors) | Both children and adults develop benign cystic teratoma (dermoid cyst). Consists of thick sebaceous material and hair. |
| **Yolk Sac Carcinoma** (rare) | Solid but soft and fleshy mass composed of cells with intracytoplasmic pink hyaline globules. Arranged into a lacy papular pattern. Produces $\alpha$-fetoprotein. | **Yolk Sac Carcinoma** (rare; < 1% of all ovarian tumors) | Patients are < 20 years old. Tumor is highly malignant, identical to the male version, and produces $\alpha$-fetoprotein. |
| **Testicular Choriocarcinoma** (rare) | Patients present at 10–30 years. Tumor is a solid hemorrhagic mass composed of cytotrophoblast and syncytiotrophoblast giant cells organized into villilike structures. Secretes hCG. | **Ovarian Choriocarcinoma** (very rare) | Small, aggressively growing nodule with syncytiotrophoblast and cytotrophoblast cells. Very malignant and aggressive. Produces hCG. |

| | | | |
|---|---|---|---|
| **Mixed Germ Cell Neoplasms** (35% of all testicular tumors) | Variable appearance. Contains cells originating from any of the above tumors. Tumors with a yolk sac component may secrete α-fetoprotein. Tumors with trophoblastic tissue may secrete hCG. | No counterpart exists. | |
| **Epithelial Tumors** | No counterpart exists. | **Epithelial Tumors** | Constitute 75% of all ovarian tumors. |
| No counterpart exists. | | **Serous Cystadenoma** (40% of all ovarian tumors) | Bilateral benign tumor (20%). Ranges from small cysts (germinal inclusion cysts or serous cystomas) to large multilocular cysts. Composed of a single layer of ciliated cuboidal or columnar cells. Psammoma bodies (concentric calcifications) are present. |
| No counterpart exists. | | **Serous Cystadenocarcinoma** (small subset of the above) | Bilateral malignant tumor with irregular solid and cystic areas arranged into papillary folds. Psammoma bodies are present. Capsular or stromal invasion is common, and tumor metastasizes early. May locally infiltrate the peritoneum or omentum. |
| No counterpart exists. | | **Mucinous Cystadenoma** (20% of all ovarian tumors) | Unilateral benign tumor (95%). Patients present at 15–50 years. Large cystic mass is filled with mucoid substance. Inner surface is lined with a single layer of nonciliated cuboidal or columnar cells. |
| No counterpart exists. | | **Mucinous Cystadenocarcinoma** (10% of all ovarian tumors) | Tumor appears as above but may have solid areas and invasion; 80% are bilateral. Has early infiltration of the peritoneum, causing a pseudomyxoma peritonei (organ adhesion). Metastasizes early and behaves like serous cystadenocarcinoma. |
| No counterpart exists. | | **Clear Cell Carcinoma** (5% of all ovarian tumors) | Composed of large clear cells arranged in a solid or papillary pattern. |

*Continued*

## COMPARISON OF GONADAL TUMORS (Continued)

| Male (Testes) | | Female (Ovaries) | |
|---|---|---|---|
| **Name of Tumor** | **Description** | **Name of Tumor** | **Description** |
| No counterpart exists. | | **Brenner Tumor** (2% of all ovarian tumors) | Most are benign. Solid mass contains small islands of epithelium that resemble transitional epithelium. |
| **Interstitial or Stromal Tumors** | Represent 3% of all testicular tumors. | **Interstitial or Stromal Tumors** | Represent 5% of all ovarian tumors. |
| **Sertoli Tumor** (2% of all testicular tumors) | Appears in children and young adults. Tumor is a well-circumscribed yellow mass composed of large sheets of cells. Contains rod-shaped intracellular crystalloids of Reinke. Most are benign. Androgen secretion causes precocious puberty. | **Sertoli-Leydig Tumor**—also known as androblastoma (rare) | Patients present at 10–30 years. Tumor is a solid white mass composed of large eosinophilic cells arranged in nests or tubules. Most are benign. Androgen secretion causes virilization (children) or masculinization (adults). |
| **Granulosa Cell Tumor** (rare) | May produce estrogens, causing gynecomastia. | **Granulosa–Theca Cell Tumor** (2% of all ovarian tumors) | Tumor is a solid, fleshy mass composed of granulosa and theca cells. Exner bodies are folliclelike structures filled with pink secretions. Estrogen secretion causes precocious puberty or endometrial hyperplasia (with postmenopausal bleeding in adults). Increased risk for uterine endometrial adenocarcinoma. |
| No counterpart exists. | | **Fibroma–Thecoma Tumor** (3% of all ovarian tumors) | Seen in postmenopausal women. Tumor is a hard, encapsulated white mass composed of fibroblasts and theca cells. Associated with Meigs syndrome as triad of ovarian fibroma, ascites, and hydrothorax. |
| **Metastatic Tumors** | Rare. | **Metastatic Tumors** | Common. |

# II. Urologic Diseases

| | |
|---|---|
| Balanitis | Inflammation of the penile glans and prepuce seen in children. Commonly associated with phimosis. Presents with redness and swelling of the glans. Prevented by circumcision. |
| Chylocele | Lymph fluid between the two layers of the tunica vaginalis. Can be due to lymphatic obstruction. |
| Epididymitis | Inflammation of the epididymis, caused most often by N. gonorrhoeae. Causes pain, swelling, and redness of the posterior part of the scrotum. |
| Epididymo-orchitis | Inflammation that presents like epididymitis and orchitis together. Acute cases are caused by Escherichia coli, N. gonorrhoeae, or C. trachomatis infections. Tuberculosis may cause infections in prevalent areas. Sterility occurs if both sides are affected. |
| Hematocele | Blood between the two layers of the tunica vaginalis of the testis, often secondary to trauma. Presents as scrotal enlargement. |
| Hydrocele | Fluid between the two layers of the tunica vaginalis. Presents as painless scrotal enlargement that is translucent with light transillumination. Associated with testicular tumors. |
| Orchitis | Inflammation of the testes, usually caused by mumps virus. Causes pain, redness, and swelling of the scrotum. |
| Phimosis | Tight, fibrotic foreskin. May increase the risk of infections and carcinoma. |
| Priapism | Painful, prolonged penile erection due to thrombosis in the corpus cavernosum. If not decompressed surgically, spongy tissue fibrosis of the corpus cavernosum will prevent further erections. |
| Prostatitis | Inflammation of the prostate, usually caused by an infection with E. coli. Can be acute or chronic. |
| Spermatocele | Cyst in the epididymal ducts containing sperm. Presents as a lump above the testis. |
| Varicocele | Distended veins in the spermatic cord. Usually asymptomatic, but can cause low sperm count. |

## TESTICULAR DISEASES

| Condition | Description | Cause | Pathology |
|---|---|---|---|
| Cryptorchism | Undescended testes (see Chapter 15) | | |
| Torsion of the Spermatic Cord | Sudden, severe scrotal pain and swelling | Trauma or incomplete testicular descent (cryptorchism) | Edematous, hemorrhagic testis undergoes venous infarction. Appears gangrenous, soft, and necrotic. |
| Testicular Atrophy | Asymptomatic | Klinefelter syndrome (most common cause), cryptorchism, mumps orchitis, hypopituitarism, or aging | Atrophy of the seminiferous tubules is seen, sparing the Sertoli and Leydig cells. Decreased number of seminiferous tubules and germ cells. |

## PROSTATE DISORDERS

| Condition | Description | Cause(s) | Pathologic Findings |
|---|---|---|---|
| Acute Prostatitis | Presents with painful urination or ejaculation. Prostate is tender on rectal palpation. | Infection with *E. coli* (most common), other coliform gram-negative bacteria, and gonococci | Acute suppurative inflammation of the prostate. |
| Chronic Prostatitis | Patient has vague complaints, possibly including low-back pain with dysuria. Irregular and firm prostate may mimic prostatic carcinoma. | Most causes are not bacterial, but cause is uncertain | Prostate is enlarged, firm, and infiltrated with plasma cells and macrophages, which are also present in prostatic secretions. |
| Benign Prostatic Hyperplasia | Most patients are asymptomatic. Often seen in patients > 50 years old. Compression of the urethra may cause urinary flow obstruction and incomplete bladder emptying. Patients have difficulty urinating and complain of decreased flow. Small increase in prostate-specific antigen is seen. | Unknown, but believed to be age-related cumulative androgen exposure, specifically to dihydrotestosterone | Gland is enlarged, firm, and rubbery, containing multiple nodules and cysts. Nodules are composed of hyperplastic glandular, fibrous, or muscular stroma. |
| Adenocarcinoma of the Prostate | Found at autopsy in 20–30% of men aged 50 and older and in 70% aged 90 years. Number 1 cancer in males and number 2 cause of cancer death. Hard, irregular nodule is found on rectal prostatic examination. Hematuria, altered urine flow, or frequency may be found. Metastases to bone cause an increase in alkaline phosphatase. | Unknown; possibly cumulative androgen exposure | Gritty, stone-hard tumor in the posterior part of the prostate. Composed of glands lined up back to back. Neoplastic cells produce high levels of serum prostate-specific antigen and acid phosphatase. |

## PROSTATE DISEASE DISTRIBUTION

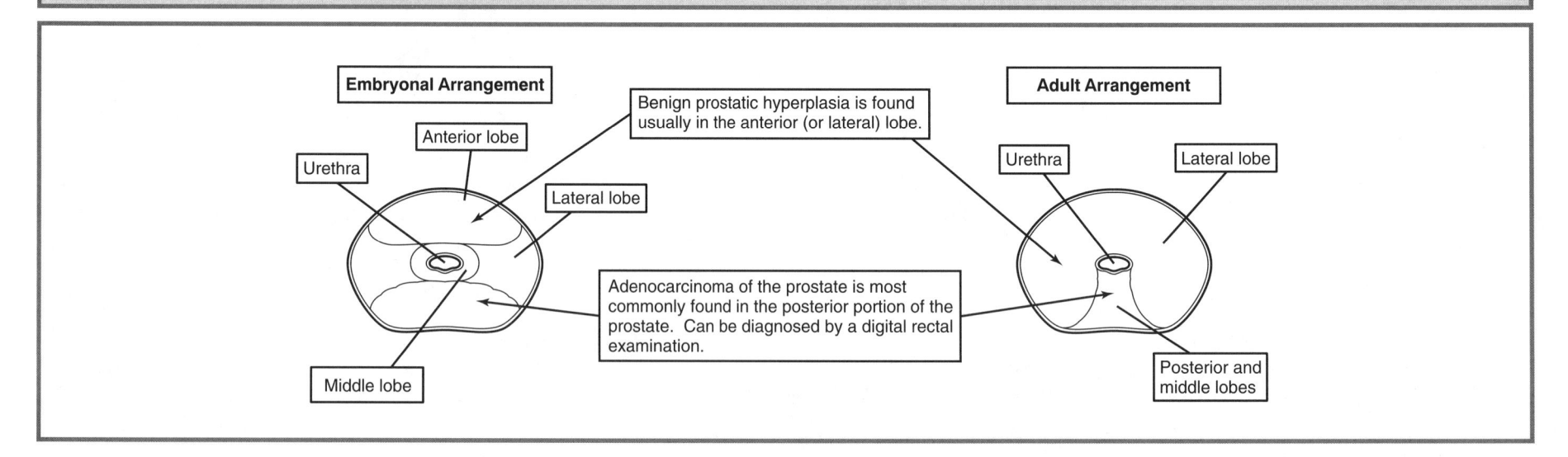

**Embryonal Arrangement**

Urethra

Anterior lobe

Lateral lobe

Middle lobe

Benign prostatic hyperplasia is found usually in the anterior (or lateral) lobe.

Adenocarcinoma of the prostate is most commonly found in the posterior portion of the prostate. Can be diagnosed by a digital rectal examination.

**Adult Arrangement**

Urethra

Lateral lobe

Posterior and middle lobes

# III. Gynecologic Diseases

## TERMS TO LEARN

| | |
|---|---|
| **Endometriosis Interna** | Also known as adenomyosis. Ectopic uterine endometrium found in the myometrium. At other sites, it is known as endometriosis externa (ovaries are the primary site). |
| **Endometritis** | Inflammation of the endometrium secondary to an infection. |
| **Gartner Duct Cyst** | Cyst of wolffian duct origin that characteristically appears on the anterolateral wall of the vagina. |
| **Krukenberg Tumor** | Bilateral metastasis from gastric carcinoma to the ovaries. Cells have ring-signet shape. |
| **Pelvic Inflammatory Disease** | Acute PID is also known as acute salpingitis. Caused by gonococci (60%), staphylococci, streptococci, or gram-negative bacilli. Causes fever and pelvic pain. Acute suppuration of the uterine tubes and abscess formation result. |
| | Chronic PID results after multiple attacks. Adhesions in the tubal lumen and fibrosis can cause chronic pelvic pain, infertility, or increased risk of ectopic pregnancy. |
| **Polyp** | Endocervical or endometrial polyps are benign lesions that may cause abnormal bleeding. |
| **Transformation Zone** | Boundary in the cervix between squamous and columnar epithelium; 95% of cervical cancers occur in this region. Transformation refers to the process of squamous epithelium (squamous metaplasia) replacing the cervical columnar epithelium. May obstruct openings of glandular cells (present only in the columnar epithelium), creating benign nabothian cysts. |
| **Vaginal Adenosis** | Presence of glandular epithelium instead of squamous in the vaginal walls. Associated with maternal diethylstilbestrol exposure during pregnancy and clear cell adenocarcinoma of the vagina. |

## UTERINE CONDITIONS

| Condition | Description | Cause(s) | Pathology |
|---|---|---|---|
| Endometritis | Acute endometritis can occur after elective abortions, uterine surgical procedures, pregnancy complications, or retention of placental fragments. Presents with fever and foul-smelling uterine discharge. | Streptococci or staphylococci. | Acute inflammation of the endometrium. |
| | Chronic endometritis is seen with an intrauterine device or retained placenta in the uterus. Presents with irregular uterine bleeding. Can also occur as an ascending infection. | Abnormally large stroma when compared with the endometrium. | Cessation of endometrial development. Stroma continues to grow, creating an unstable endometrium that is prone to bleeding. Plasma cells are found in the endometrium. |
| Endometriosis Externa | Asymptomatic or causes painful periods, menorrhagia (excessive bleeding), or infertility. Regresses during pregnancy or oral contraceptive use. After repeated episodes, fibrosis and peritoneal adhesions can increase the risk of ectopic pregnancy. | Hypothesis 1: regurgitation of blood and endometrial debris into the fallopian tubes. Hypothesis 2: metaplasia of epithelium into endometrial tissue. | Ectopic tissue on ovaries (most common) or fallopian tubes appears as chocolate cysts from cyclic bleeding. Composed of glandular tissue surrounded by stroma. |
| Endometriosis Interna | Also known as adenomyosis. May be seen in women aged 40 years and older. | Abnormal growth of the endometrium into the myometrium. | Endometrial islands of glands and stroma within the myometrium (stratum basalis extends into the myometrium). Responds cyclically to estrogen. |

## OVARIAN CYSTS

| Condition | Description | Cause(s) | Pathology |
|---|---|---|---|
| Follicular Cyst | Causes a pelvic mass and pelvic pain. May regress spontaneously, but may cause complications if persistent. Secondary anovulation is due to increased estrogen. Rupture causes severe abdominal pain. | Unruptured, unovulated ovarian follicle | Cysts are lined by granulosa cells. Fluid is rich in estrogen. |
| Theca-Lutein Cyst | Also known as a luteinized follicular cyst. Causes abdominal pain from ovarian torsion or cyst rupture. May produce estrogen. | Increased systemic hCG | Not a true corpus luteum. Resembles lutein cysts consisting of luteinized follicular cells. |
| Corpus Luteum Cyst | Transient cyst associated with the luteal phase of the menstrual cycle. Delayed menstruation occurs secondary to prolonged progesterone production. Persistent cyst may cause pelvic mass or pain and missed menses. | Abnormal degeneration of the corpus luteum | Cyst is derived from the corpus luteum and produces estrogen or androgens. |
| Polycystic Ovary Syndrome | Also known as Stein-Leventhal syndrome. Produces the triad of infertility, hirsutism, and obesity. Amenorrhea and anovulation occur from lack of the LH surge. Hirsutism is due to increased androgen secretion. Increased estrogens increase the risk of endometrial carcinoma. | Continuous excess of LH and FSH | Bilaterally enlarged ovaries contain multiple follicular cysts. Cysts form because of constant FSH and LH exposure. Thickened ovarian capsule (tunica albuginea) without a corpus luteum. |

## RISK FACTORS, INCIDENCE, AND MORTALITY OF CANCERS IN WOMEN[1]

| Cancer | Risk Factors | Incidence/year | Mortality/year |
|---|---|---|---|
| Breast Cancer | • Previous breast cancer (6×)<br>• Family history (mother or sister, 5×)<br>• Fibrocystic disease with epithelial atypia (ductal or lobular, 4–5×)<br>• Age > 40 years (2×)<br>• Nulliparity or late first pregnancy (> 35 years, 1.5×)<br>• Early menarche (< 12 years, 1.3×)<br>• Late menopause (> 50 years)<br>• *BRCA1* and *BRCA2* genes<br>• Endometrial cancer<br>• Ovarian cancer | 175,000 (highest of reproductive organ and breast cancers) | 43,300 (highest of reproductive organ and breast cancers) |
| Endometrial Cancer | • Obesity (3× if 21–50 lb overweight; 10× if > 50 lb overweight)<br>• Exogenous estrogens (4–8×)<br>• Diabetes (2.8×)<br>• Nulliparity (2–3×)<br>• Late menopause (> 50 years, 2.4×)<br>• Chronic hypertension<br>• Chronic anovulation, polycystic ovary syndrome, and granulosa–theca cell tumors<br>• Presence of breast, colon, or ovarian cancers | 37,400 (second highest) | 6400 (third highest) |

| Ovarian Cancer | • Family history (BRCA gene, p53 gene)<br>• Nulliparity or late first pregnancy (> 35 years) | 25,200 (third highest) | 14,500 (second highest) |
| Cervical Cancer | • HPV infection (early intercourse < 20 years, more than 2 sex partners, 20×)<br>• Multiparity or early age at pregnancy<br>• Low socioeconomic status<br>• Cigarette smoking<br>• Immunocompromise<br>• Diethylstilbestrol exposure | 12,800 (fourth highest) | 4800 (fourth highest) |

[1]Also see Chapter 1, Cancer Epidemiology.

## VAGINAL, CERVICAL, AND UTERINE TUMORS

| Condition | Description | Pathologic Findings |
| --- | --- | --- |
| **Vaginal Tumors**—account for 2300 estimated cases and 600 deaths per year in the United States | | |
| **Squamous Cell Carcinoma** | Most common vaginal tumor, occurring in women 55 years and older. Lesions are asymptomatic. | Polypoid, fungating, ulcerative mass composed of keratinized cells and keratin whorls. Tends to involve the posterior wall of the vagina. Local extension occurs early. |
| **Clear Cell Adenocarcinoma** | Rare vaginal tumor seen in daughters of mothers who took diethylstilbestrol while pregnant. Unlike squamous cell carcinoma, it occurs between 10 and 35 years of age. | Polypoid mass composed of clear cells. Commonly found on the anterior wall of the vagina. |
| **Botryoid Sarcoma** | Occurs in the first 5 years of life. Asymptomatic until metastasis, but may metastasize early. | Grapelike polypoid mass projecting into the lumen of the vagina. It is an anaplastic rhabdosarcoma. Highly malignant. |
| **Cervical Tumors**—account for 12,800 estimated cases and 4800 deaths per year in the United States | | |
| **Squamous Cell Carcinoma** | Nonspecific presentation. Patients may be asymptomatic but can present with postcoital bleeding or abnormal uterine bleeding. Associated with herpes simplex virus type 2 and HPV cervical infection. Local invasion is followed by lymphatic metastases. Papanicolaou smear is used to screen. (See Figure: Cervical Carcinoma and Papanicolaou Smear Classification.) <br><br> CIN I (mild)—dysplasia of 1/3 of the cervical epithelium <br><br> CIN II (moderate)—1/2 to 2/3 of the wall is dysplastic <br><br> CIN III (carcinoma in situ)—entire thickness is dysplastic <br><br> Invasive carcinoma—invasion into the basement membrane | Carcinoma usually occurs at the squamocolumnar junction (transformation zone) on preexisting dysplastic lesions. Mass appears as fungating, necrotic, and ulcerating. Usually composed of nonkeratinizing squamous cells (best prognosis). Keratinizing type is next most common. Some mild dysplastic lesions can resolve spontaneously. |

**Uterine Tumors**—account for 37,400 estimated cases and 6400 deaths per year in the United States

| | | |
|---|---|---|
| Leiomyoma | Most common benign tumor of the uterus, found in women aged 20–40, during the reproductive years. Also called uterine fibroids. Usually asymptomatic, but may present with excessive uterine bleeding and infertility. More common in black women. Abdominal pain occurs if the tumor undergoes necrosis. | Circumscribed, firm mass of uterine smooth muscle composed of spindle-shaped cells. Collagen may be present. Tumor grows during the reproductive years and pregnancy and shrinks postpartum and postmenopausally (it is estrogen sensitive). |
| Endometrial Carcinoma | Most common uterine malignancy. Most cases occur in postmenopausal women, aged 55–65 years. Presents with abnormal uterine bleeding and an enlarged uterus. | Unopposed estrogen causes endometrial hyperplasia (premalignant). Polypoid, fungating mass protrudes into the uterine cavity. Uterus is asymmetrically enlarged. Mass consists of glands lined by neoplastic cells. Degree of spread is the most important prognostic indicator. |
| Leiomyosarcoma | Rare cancer that causes postmenopausal bleeding or a uterine mass. | Fleshy mass with hemorrhage and necrosis composed of atypical-looking cells with mitotic figures. Occurs de novo. |
| Choriocarcinoma | See Gestational Tumors. | |

## CERVICAL CARCINOMA AND PAPANICOLAOU SMEAR CLASSIFICATION

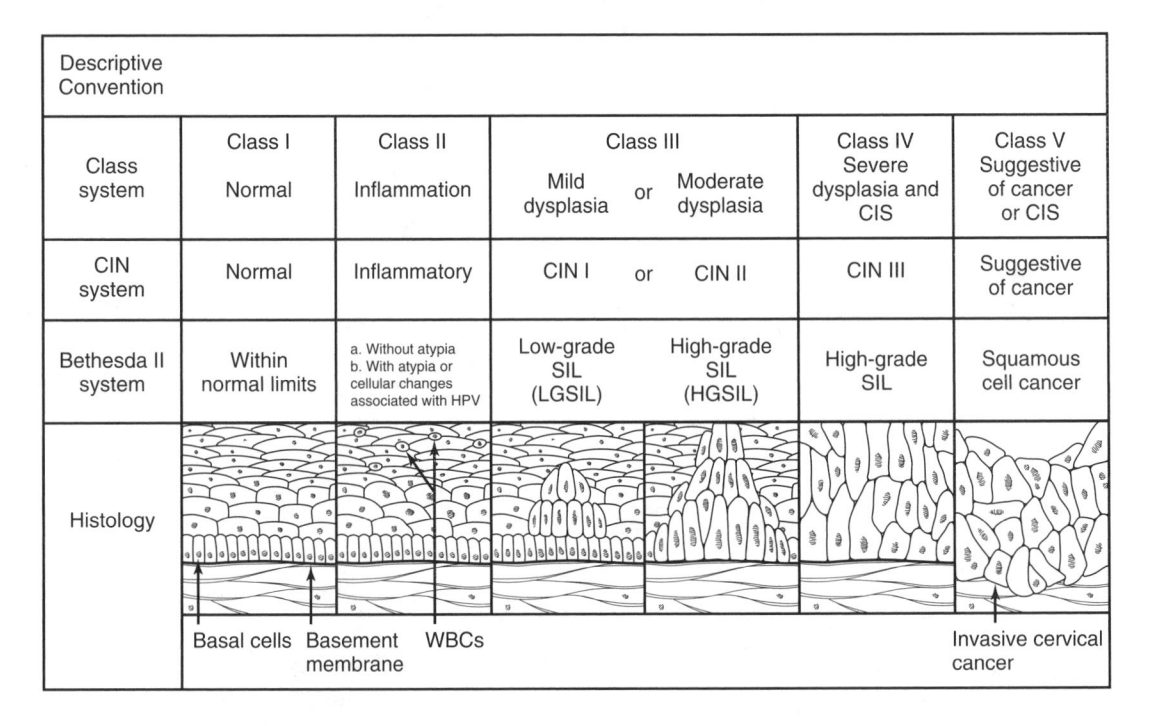

| Descriptive Convention | | | | | | |
|---|---|---|---|---|---|---|
| Class system | Class I<br>Normal | Class II<br>Inflammation | Class III<br>Mild dysplasia | or Moderate dysplasia | Class IV<br>Severe dysplasia and CIS | Class V<br>Suggestive of cancer or CIS |
| CIN system | Normal | Inflammatory | CIN I | or CIN II | CIN III | Suggestive of cancer |
| Bethesda II system | Within normal limits | a. Without atypia<br>b. With atypia or cellular changes associated with HPV | Low-grade SIL (LGSIL) | High-grade SIL (HGSIL) | High-grade SIL | Squamous cell cancer |
| Histology | | | | | | |

Basal cells  Basement membrane  WBCs  Invasive cervical cancer

CIN = cervical intraepithelial neoplasia; CIS = carcinoma in situ; HPV = human papillomavirus; SIL = squamous intraepithelial lesion; WBCs = white blood cells.

Adapted from Nieginski E (editor): *Obstetrics & Gynecology*, 3rd ed. Baltimore: Williams & Wilkins, 1998:518.

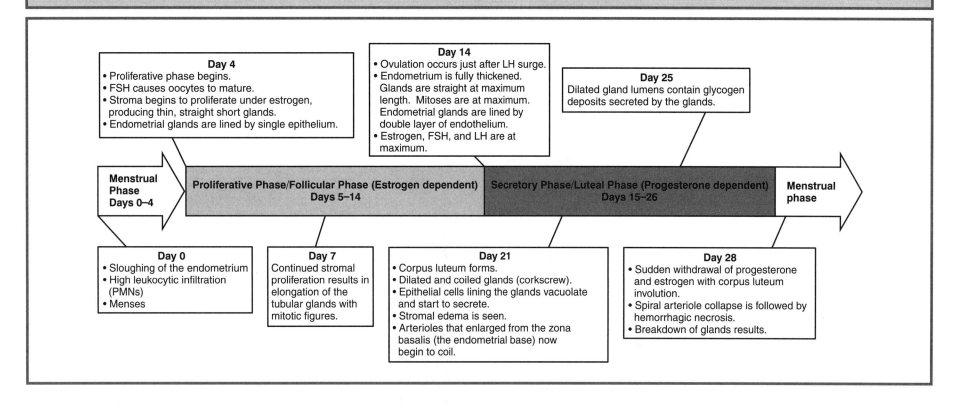

**Day 4**
- Proliferative phase begins.
- FSH causes oocytes to mature.
- Stroma begins to proliferate under estrogen, producing thin, straight short glands.
- Endometrial glands are lined by single epithelium.

**Day 14**
- Ovulation occurs just after LH surge.
- Endometrium is fully thickened. Glands are straight at maximum length. Mitoses are at maximum. Endometrial glands are lined by double layer of endothelium.
- Estrogen, FSH, and LH are at maximum.

**Day 25**
Dilated gland lumens contain glycogen deposits secreted by the glands.

**Menstrual Phase Days 0–4**

**Proliferative Phase/Follicular Phase (Estrogen dependent) Days 5–14**

**Secretory Phase/Luteal Phase (Progesterone dependent) Days 15–26**

**Menstrual phase**

**Day 0**
- Sloughing of the endometrium
- High leukocytic infiltration (PMNs)
- Menses

**Day 7**
Continued stromal proliferation results in elongation of the tubular glands with mitotic figures.

**Day 21**
- Corpus luteum forms.
- Dilated and coiled glands (corkscrew).
- Epithelial cells lining the glands vacuolate and start to secrete.
- Stromal edema is seen.
- Arterioles that enlarged from the zona basalis (the endometrial base) now begin to coil.

**Day 28**
- Sudden withdrawal of progesterone and estrogen with corpus luteum involution.
- Spiral arteriole collapse is followed by hemorrhagic necrosis.
- Breakdown of glands results.

## CAUSES OF ABNORMAL UTERINE BLEEDING

| Age Group | Disease or Condition | Pathogenesis |
|---|---|---|
| Prepuberty (< 12 years) | Precocious puberty | Early endometrial hyperplasia due to an increase in estrogens. |
| Puberty | Anovulatory cycle | Transient fluctuations in estrogen levels. Unopposed estrogen can cause nonuniform endometrial proliferation, which results in an unstable endometrium that is prone to bleeding. |
| Reproductive Age | Leiomyoma, endometriosis, pregnancy, PID, intrauterine device, diaphragm, anovulatory cycles, endometrial hyperplasia, or polyps (cervical or endometrial) | Erosion, infection, or irritation of the endometrium. |
| Perimenopause | Anovulatory cycle, endometrial carcinoma (> 35 years), and cervical carcinoma | Transient fluctuations in estrogen levels. Unopposed estrogen can cause nonuniform endometrial proliferation. Unstable endometrium is then prone to bleeding. Carcinoma causes erosion. |
| Postmenopause | Endometrial carcinoma, vaginal atrophy, and cervical carcinoma | Neoplastic erosion or ulceration. Atrophy leads to a fragile endometrium. |

# IV. Diseases of the Breast

## TERMS TO LEARN

| | |
|---|---|
| Congenital Inversion of Nipples | Benign condition that is clinically relevant because it can be confused with retraction of the nipple that can occur in breast malignancy. |
| Fibrocystic Change | Changes in breast tissue from constant cycling of estrogen. Most cases are benign, but some may cause an increased risk of breast carcinoma. |
| Gynecomastia | Abnormal increase of breast size in males, usually due to an increase in estrogen. |

## INFLAMMATORY BREAST CONDITIONS

| Condition | Description | Cause(s) | Pathologic Process |
|---|---|---|---|
| Acute Mastitis | Acute mastitis presents with painful inflammation. One area of a breast appears red, swollen, and tender. Occurs with breast-feeding. | Infection with *Staphylococcus aureus* | Unilateral acute inflammation with PMN infiltration. Bacteria can enter a fissure (break in the skin) near or at the nipple. |
| | Chronic mastitis is also known as plasma cell mastitis. Perimenopausal patients present with nipple retraction and a hard mass. | Lactiferous duct obstruction with impacted secretions | Obstruction leads to duct dilatation (mammary duct ectasia). Irregular fibrosis causes nipple retraction. |
| | Granulomatous mastitis is a chronic condition and presents similarly to above. | Rupture of small ductules causes granuloma formation | Granulomatous reaction to the secretions. |
| Fat Necrosis | Acute form presents with painful inflammation of the affected area of the breast. | Trauma or irradiation | Focal necrosis of fat with PMN infiltration. May cause a hemorrhagic focus with lipolysis. |
| | Chronic form presents with painless, hard, calcified scar tissue on the breast. | | Granulation tissue, collagen, fibrosis, and calcification produce a nodule clinically difficult to discern from carcinoma. May cause skin retraction over the mass. |

## SUMMARY OF BREAST LESIONS

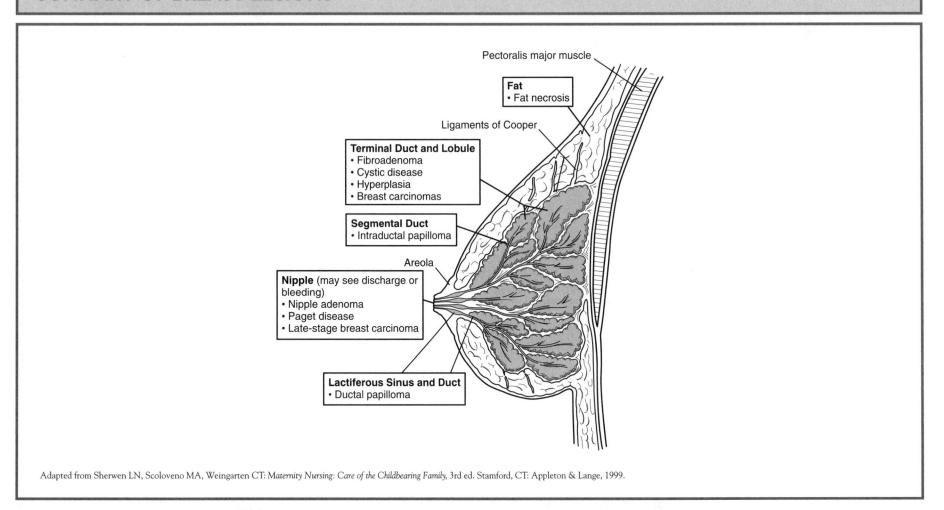

Pectoralis major muscle

**Fat**
• Fat necrosis

Ligaments of Cooper

**Terminal Duct and Lobule**
• Fibroadenoma
• Cystic disease
• Hyperplasia
• Breast carcinomas

**Segmental Duct**
• Intraductal papilloma

Areola

**Nipple** (may see discharge or bleeding)
• Nipple adenoma
• Paget disease
• Late-stage breast carcinoma

**Lactiferous Sinus and Duct**
• Ductal papilloma

Adapted from Sherwen LN, Scoloveno MA, Weingarten CT: *Maternity Nursing: Care of the Childbearing Family,* 3rd ed. Stamford, CT: Appleton & Lange, 1999.

## FIBROCYSTIC DISEASE

| Condition | Description | Pathologic Appearance |
|---|---|---|
| Simple Fibrocystic Change | Most common benign breast disease. May cause pain, nipple discharge, and irregular lumpy breast consistency. With the cystic component, blue-domed cysts may be seen. | Fibrosis is associated with duct dilatation (ductal ectasia) and formation of a masslike scar. Can mimic carcinoma. Also may cause cyst formation, which consists of apocrine epithelium. In apocrine metaplasia, ductal epithelium changes to large pink polyhedral cells with apocrine-type secretion. |
| Ductal or Lobar Hyperplasia | Presentation is the same as above. | Sclerosing adenosis consists of fibrosis and alteration of the stromal architecture. Lobule proliferation produces back-to-back glands. May be mistaken for invasive carcinoma. |
| Epithelial Hyperplasia With or Without Atypia | Risk of developing carcinoma depends on the level of atypia. | Increase in number of cell layers in the ducts. |
| | Atypical lobular hyperplasia, 4–5x increase in risk. | Proliferating atypical cells distend the lobules. Appearance falls short of lobular carcinoma in situ. |
| | Papillomatosis, 1–2x increase in risk. | Proliferating ductal cells appear with overlapping nuclei. |
| | Atypical ductal hyperplasia, 4–5x increase in risk; 8–10x if history of breast cancer. | Stratified atypical ductal cells often obstruct the lumen. |

# COMMON FEATURES OF BREAST CANCER

## Prognostic Indicators of Breast Cancer

5-year survival rate is 70%. Staging is the most important predictor of survival. Worst prognosis occurs with:

- Lymph node involvement (axillary node) and metastases

- Mass larger than 2 cm

- Presence of *NEU* gene

- Absence of estrogen and progesterone receptors

- Increased proliferation and aneuploidy

- High degree of angiogenesis

## Features Common to All Invasive Breast Cancers

- Painless breast mass (except in inflammatory carcinoma)

- Bloody nipple discharge

- Small and numerous microcalcifications

Most breast cancers are diagnosed and resected before late findings occur. When present, late findings include:

- Tumor fixed in place to the chest wall (adherence to fascia)

- Skin and nipple retraction secondary to fibrosis

- Lymphatic spread

## Breast Cancer Distribution Pattern

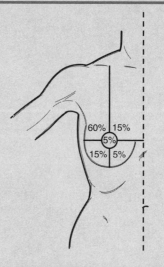

Adapted from Tierney LM, Jr., McPhee SJ, Papadakis MA (editors): *Current Medical Diagnosis & Treatment*, 36th ed, p 651. Originally published by Appleton & Lange. © 1997 by the McGraw-Hill Companies, Inc.

## BREAST TUMORS

| Condition | Description and Prevalence | Pathologic Findings |
|---|---|---|
| **Benign Tumors** | | |
| Fibroadenoma | Most common breast tumor in all ages, but more common at < 30 years. Presents as a free-moving and painless tumor. | Well-circumscribed, firm mass composed of glands that are compressed into clefts by proliferating fibrous stroma. Tumor size varies with pregnancy (estrogen sensitive). |
| Ductal Papilloma | Most common cause of bloody nipple discharge in women aged < 50 years. | Tumor originates in the lactiferous ducts, near the nipple. Papillary mass projects into the lumen of the duct. Composed of epithelial and myoepithelial cells. |
| **Malignant Tumors** | | |
| Responsible for 175,000 cases and 43,300 deaths per year in women in the United States. Most common cancer in women and the second most common cause of death due to cancer. Male breast cancers are rare, causing 1300 cases and 400 deaths per year. | | |
| **Phyllodes Tumor** | Low-grade malignant tumor that presents as a large mass. Skin ulceration may be seen. | Poorly circumscribed, fleshy tumor with cysts that resemble leaves. Composed of epithelial and myoepithelial cells. Locally infiltrating. |
| **Lobular Carcinoma In Situ** | Represents 2–3% of all breast cancers. No palpable mass is evident. Findings are incidental. | Tumor is often bilateral and multifocal. Composed of neoplastic lobular epithelial cells that do not infiltrate the basement membrane. Increases the risk of invasive lobular or ductal carcinoma by 10–12×. |
| **Ductal Carcinoma In Situ** | Represents 2–3% of all breast cancers. Also known as intraductal carcinoma. Nonpalpable except for the comedocarcinoma type. | Tumor may be bilateral. Composed of neoplastic ductal epithelium that does not infiltrate the basement membrane. Several types of growth patterns exist; the most striking is comedocarcinoma (high grade). Associated with invasive ductal carcinoma. Malignant cells can spread through the ducts. |

*Continued*

## BREAST TUMORS (Continued)

| Condition | Description and Prevalence | Pathologic Findings |
|---|---|---|
| Invasive Ductal Carcinoma | Most common breast malignancy (75%), occurring in women aged 50 years and over. Poorest prognosis of all the breast carcinomas. See Common Features of Breast Cancer above. | Tumor has hard and gritty consistency, with a characteristic grating sound when scraped. Yellow-white streaks surround ducts where elastic tissue is deposited. Massive fibrosis is present. Cells disseminate into the fibrous stroma. Lymphatic metastasis is common. |
| | Variant—Invasive medullary carcinoma represents 5% of all breast cancers. | Large, soft, well-circumscribed mass consisting of polygonal cells arranged into sheets with a lymphocytic infiltrate. Better prognosis than infiltrating ductal carcinoma. |
| | Variant—Invasive colloid or mucinous carcinoma represents 4% of all breast cancers. | Composed of large lakes of amorphous, pink-staining mucin that dissects through sheets of neoplastic cells. Better prognosis than infiltrating ductal carcinoma. |
| Invasive Lobular Carcinoma | Represents 10% of all breast cancers. See Common Features of Breast Cancer above. | Rubbery tumor with cells lining up single file, like beads on a string. Some tumors are bilateral. |
| Paget Disease (invasive) | Represents 1% of all breast cancers. Patients present with a scaly, red, and itchy nipple and areola. Nipple is fissured and ulcerated, with edema. | Tumor infiltrates the epidermis of the skin covering the breast. Composed of Paget cells, large and clear cells that stain positive for mucin. Signals an underlying ductal carcinoma in the affected breast. |
| Inflammatory Carcinoma | Represents 3% of all breast cancers. Presents with *peau d'orange* (orange-peel appearance of the skin overlying the breast). Breast is painful, red, and swollen without a mass. | Inflammation and blockage of the dermal lymphatics produce the characteristic *peau d'orange*. Very poor prognosis. |

# V. Gestational Disorders

## DISEASES OF GESTATION

| Condition | Definition and Symptoms | Predisposing Factors | Mechanism and Findings |
|---|---|---|---|
| Placenta Previa | Placenta attaches to the lower part of the uterus (abnormal) and may obstruct the internal cervical os. Presents late in the third trimester or at labor with premature placental separation and antepartum bleeding. Complications include fetal or maternal death. | Women with ≥ 4 cesarean sections, previous placenta previa, increasing parity (deliveries, abortions, ectopic pregnancies), and increasing age | Cervical effacement and stretching of the os separate the abnormally low placenta from the endometrium. The raw endometrial site hemorrhages. |
| Abruptio Placentae | Premature placental separation of a normally positioned placenta. Presents with antepartum bleeding (20% have concealed bleeding). Complications include disseminated intravascular coagulation, shock, and fetal or maternal death. | Cocaine use, trauma, or maternal hypertension | Separation of the placenta exposes a raw, hemorrhaging endometrial site. |
| Placenta Accreta | Failure of normal placental separation during the last part of labor, with continued hemorrhage after delivery (postpartum hemorrhage). Hysterectomy is frequently required to prevent maternal death. | Previous endometritis or cesarean section | Deeper than normal penetration of the placental villi into the endometrium prevents full uterine contraction necessary to stop the bleeding. |
| Toxemia of Pregnancy | Preeclampsia occurs in the third trimester of pregnancy. Presents with the triad of hypertension, proteinuria, and generalized edema. May also cause late jaundice. | Unknown | Placental degeneration with hyaline deposition and calcification is seen. Maternal side shows hemorrhagic necrosis. Placental infarcts follow. |
| | Eclampsia is a complication of preeclampsia in which convulsions and coma develop. | Unknown | Same as above. With eclampsia, renal cortical necrosis and liver periportal necrosis are seen. |

*Continued*

## DISEASES OF GESTATION (Continued)

| Condition | Definition and Symptoms | Predisposing Factors | Mechanism and Findings |
|---|---|---|---|
| Chorioamnionitis | Infection of the fetal membranes. Presents with fever before delivery. Fetal membranes can become infected after prolonged amnion rupture (> 24 hours) or prolonged labor. | Ascending infection with E. coli, β-hemolytic streptococci, or anaerobes | Thick membrane and cloudy amniotic fluid. Many PMNs are present. |
| Polyhydramnios | Increase in amniotic fluid. | Tracheoesophageal fistula, diabetes mellitus in the mother, duodenal atresia, fetal hydrops, or a neural tube defect (with leakage of cerebrospinal fluid) | Decreased fetal swallowing or gastrointestinal obstruction. |
| Oligohydramnios | Decrease in amniotic fluid. | Fetal renal agenesis, placental insufficiency, or maternal medications such as angiotensin-converting enzyme inhibitors | Renal dysgenesis or obstruction to urine flow. |
| Ectopic Pregnancy | Pregnancy outside of the uterus. Presents with a positive pregnancy test, vomiting, small uterus for gestational age, and a missed period 2–6 weeks after fertilization. Rupture of the uterine tube causes severe abdominal pain and massive intraperitoneal bleeding. | PID or endometriosis | Zygote implantation occurs outside of the uterus (usually in the fallopian tube). Tube cannot expand to accommodate fetal growth. |

## GESTATIONAL TUMORS

| Condition | Description | Pathology |
|-----------|-------------|-----------|
| Gestational Choriocarcinoma | Presents with a positive pregnancy test and abnormal uterine bleeding. Associated with a recent abortion, pregnancy, or hydatidiform mole. | Hemorrhagic mass without villi infiltrates into the uterine myometrium. Composed of malignant cytotrophoblast and syncytiotrophoblast cells. Highest hCG producer of all gestational tumors. Metastases to lungs, brain, liver, and bone marrow are common. With combined chemotherapy, 90% improve even with widespread metastases. |
| Hydatidiform Mole | Both moles present with signs of early pregnancy. Amenorrhea, vomiting, and a positive pregnancy test may be seen. Vaginal bleeding occurs by about the third month. Cystic swelling of placental villi without a fetus. May precede choriocarcinoma. | |
| | Partial mole occurs when two sperm fertilize an ovum. The karyotype is triploid (69,XXY). | Normal and abnormal placental villi are present. Abnormal villi are edematous and enlarged. Fetal parts may be present. hCG is mildly elevated. |
| | Complete mole occurs when one sperm fertilizes an ovum without chromosomes. Karyotype is 46,XX (from duplication of sperm DNA). Grapelike cysts are passed with bleeding after the third month. | Enlarged uterus fills with grapelike cystic structures. Cysts represent dilated chorionic villi. Mole is associated with high hCG levels and with bilateral theca-lutein ovarian cysts. |
| Invasive Mole | Hydatidiform mole that locally penetrates the uterine wall. Complications include villi embolism to the lungs and uterine rupture. | Villi may penetrate to the serosal surface of the uterus (entire thickness). Associated with hCG elevation. |

# CHAPTER 8
# ENDOCRINE SYSTEM

**I. PITUITARY DISORDERS**

Pituitary Hormones

Posterior Pituitary Hyperfunction

Pituitary Adenomas

Clinical Signs in Acromegaly

Hypopituitarism

**II. THYROID AND PARATHYROID DISORDERS**

Hypothyroidism and Hyperthyroidism (Thyrotoxicosis)

Clinical Signs in Hypothyroidism and Hyperthyroidism

Thyroiditis

Thyroid Goiters

Primary Thyroid Tumors

Parathyroid Gland Disorders

**III. ADRENAL DISORDERS**

Adrenal Structure

Adrenal Gland Disorders

Clinical Signs in Cushing Syndrome

Adrenal Tumors

Endocrine Disease Summary

**IV. PANCREATIC DISEASES AND DIABETES MELLITUS**

Diseases of the Endocrine Pancreas

Consequences of Chronic Uncontrolled Diabetes Mellitus

Pancreatic Islet Tumors

Multiple Endocrine Neoplasia Syndromes

**ABBREVIATIONS**

**ACTH** = adrenocorticotropic hormone
**ADH** = antidiuretic hormone
**FSH** = follicle-stimulating hormone
**GH** = growth hormone
**HLA** = human leukocyte antigen
**LH** = luteinizing hormone

**MEN** = multiple endocrine neoplasia
**MSH** = melanocyte-stimulating hormone
**PTH** = parathyroid hormone
$T_3$ = triiodothyronine
$T_4$ = thyroxine
**TSH** = thyroid-stimulating hormone

## MOST COMMON Causes and Types

| Disorder | Common Cause |
|---|---|
| Primary hypothyroidism | Primary idiopathic hypothyroidism |
| Primary hyperthyroidism | Graves disease |
| Thyroiditis | Hashimoto disease |
| Primary hyperparathyroidism | Parathyroid adenoma |
| Secondary hyperparathyroidism | Renal failure |
| Pituitary cachexia | Nonsecreting pituitary adenoma |
| Primary hypoparathyroidism | DiGeorge syndrome |
| Primary hypercorticoidism (Cushing syndrome) | Adrenal cortical adenoma |
| Secondary and overall hypercorticoidism (Cushing syndrome) | Corticotropic pituitary adenoma (Cushing disease) |
| Primary adrenal hypocorticoidism (Addison disease) | Autoimmune adrenalitis |
| Secondary adrenal hypocorticoidism | Exogenous corticosteroids |
| Primary hyperaldosteronism (Conn syndrome) | Functional adrenal adenoma |

| Disorder | Common Type |
|---|---|
| Pituitary tumor | Prolactinoma |
| Thyroid malignancy | Papillary carcinoma |
| Islet cell tumor | Insulinoma |

| Multiple Endocrine Neoplasia Syndromes | Group of hereditary syndromes that includes multiple tumors. See Multiple Endocrine Neoplasia Syndromes. |
|---|---|
| Thyroid Nodule | A small node in the thyroid, classified as either "hot" or "cold." Radionucleotide scanning measures radioactive iodine uptake by the thyroid. Hot nodules take up dye (active); cold nodules do not (inactive). (See Thyroid Goiters and Primary Thyroid Tumors.) Among solitary thyroid nodules, < 5% are malignant. Cold nodules are more likely to be malignant than hot nodules, but most cold nodules are still benign. Statistically, the breakdown for the cause of the nodules is as follows:<br><br>• 60% of nodules are benign colloid nodules.<br><br>• 30% of nodules are thyroid adenomas.<br><br>• 5% are Hashimoto thyroiditis or subacute thyroiditis. |
| Thyroiditis | Painful or painless inflammation of the thyroid gland. |
| Virilization | Excessive androgen production. In infant girls, produces ambiguous genitalia, clitoromegaly, and labioscrotal fusion. In adult women, produces defeminization with deeper voice, decreased breast size, frontal balding, muscularity, clitoromegaly, and hirsutism. Causes include familial polycystic ovary syndrome (see Chapter 7), adrenal enzyme defects (21-hydroxylase deficiency or, rarely, 11-hydroxylase deficiency), and ovarian tumors (Sertoli-Leydig or dysgerminomas). |

# I. Pituitary Disorders

## PITUITARY HORMONES

| Location in Pituitary | Hormone | Staining | Function |
|---|---|---|---|
| **Anterior Pituitary** | | | |
| Somatotrophs | GH | Acidophilic | GH causes somatomedin production (insulinlike growth factor) by the liver. Mediates growth in all tissues. GH antagonizes insulin. |
| Corticotrophs | ACTH and MSH | Basophilic | ACTH promotes adrenal cortisol and androgen secretion. Cortisol antagonizes insulin. MSH induces melanocyte proliferation and darker skin. |
| Thyrotrophs | TSH | Basophilic | TSH stimulates follicular thyroid cells to synthesize and secrete thyroid hormone. |
| Gonadotrophs | FSH and LH | Basophilic | FSH promotes growth of the ovarian follicles and estrogen secretion by the follicles. LH governs ovulation, maintenance of the corpus luteum, and progesterone secretion. In males, it causes testosterone production. |
| Lactotrophs | Prolactin | Acidophilic | Prolactin stimulates milk production and growth of breast ductal tissue. |
| **Posterior Pituitary** | | | |
| Hypothalamic Nuclei | Vasopressin (ADH) | None | ADH stimulates water retention by the renal collecting ducts. |
| Hypothalamic Nuclei | Oxytocin | None | Oxytocin stimulates milk ejection and smooth muscle contraction of the uterus and breast ducts. |

## POSTERIOR PITUITARY HYPERFUNCTION

| Condition | Description |
|---|---|
| Inappropriate ADH Secretion | Caused by cerebral trauma or tumors and small cell bronchogenic carcinoma of the lungs. High ADH levels cause water retention, diluting the plasma and lowering the plasma osmolarity. The dilution causes hyponatremia which, if severe, can cause seizures and death. |

## PITUITARY ADENOMAS

| Condition | Description | Pathology |
|---|---|---|
| **Primary Pituitary Tumors** are responsible for most of the hyperfunction of the anterior pituitary. Represent 10% of all primary intracranial tumors. | | |
| Prolactinoma | Represents 30% of pituitary tumors. The tumor secretes prolactin. In women, it causes secondary amenorrhea, infertility, and galactorrhea (inappropriate milk secretion). In men, it causes impotence, decreased libido, infertility, gynecomastia, and galactorrhea. | Microadenoma (< 1 cm). Tumor is a circumscribed, fleshy, necrotic mass with a thin fibrous capsule. Cellular composition resembles normal prolactin cells of the pituitary. |
| Somatotropic Adenoma | Represents 25% of pituitary tumors. The tumor secretes GH. In children, it causes bony epiphysial growth leading to gigantism. In adults, bone grows at articular cartilage and periosteum instead of at the epiphyses (acromegaly). Disproportionate enlargement of the bones distorts joints, coarsens facial features, and causes osteoarthritis. Also causes widespread organomegaly. (See figure below.) | Macroadenoma (> 1 cm) of somatotrophs. See above. |
| Corticotropic Adenoma | Represents 10% of pituitary tumors. The tumor secretes ACTH and MSH. High cortisol results in Cushing syndrome (see Adrenal Gland Disorders—Hypercorticoidism below). Hyperpigmentation occurs from MSH hypersecretion (Nelson syndrome). | Microadenoma of corticotrophs. See Prolactinoma above. |
| Nonfunctional Adenoma | Represents 30% of pituitary tumors and the most common cause of hypopituitarism. Causes visual disturbances by compressing the optic chiasm. All adenomas can compress the pituitary. | Chromophobic cells (not a specific cell type—any pituitary cell that lacks granules). Macroadenoma. See Somatotropic Adenoma above and Hypopituitarism below. |

## CLINICAL SIGNS IN ACROMEGALY

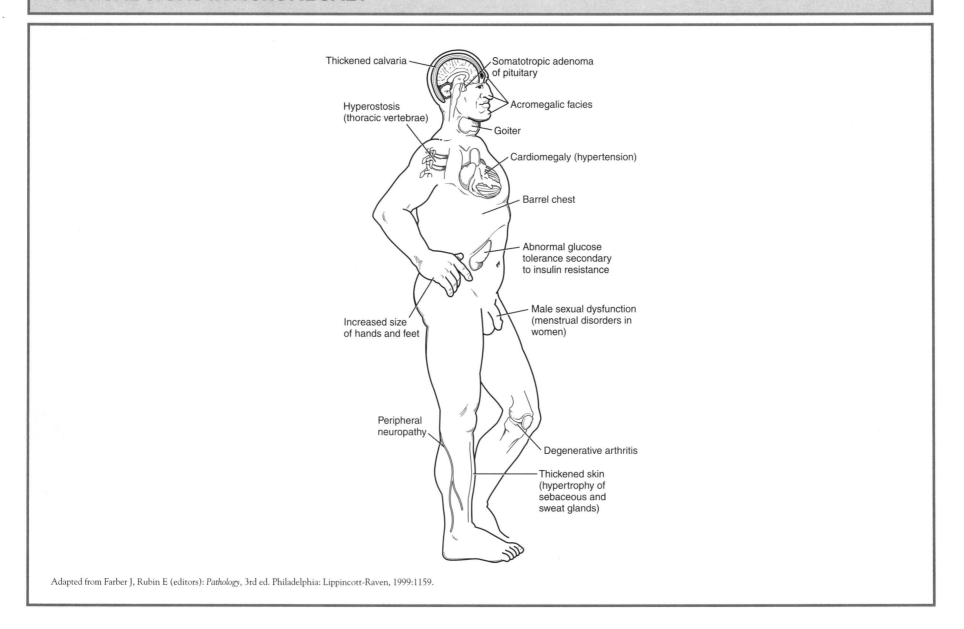

Adapted from Farber J, Rubin E (editors): *Pathology*, 3rd ed. Philadelphia: Lippincott-Raven, 1999:1159.

## HYPOPITUITARISM

| General Description | Pathologic Findings |
|---|---|
| Hypofunction of the pituitary is primarily due to ischemia (Sheehan syndrome or diabetes mellitus), tumors, or head trauma. The most common cause is nonfunctional, compressive pituitary tumors such as pituitary adenoma or craniopharyngioma. FSH and LH are the first to be lost; prolactin is last. Sheehan syndrome (postpartum necrosis) is due to pituitary hemorrhage and shock during childbirth. | Compressed normal pituitary tissue shows coagulative necrosis. Sheehan syndrome causes a hemorrhagic infarct that replaces normal pituitary with scar tissue. In diabetes, vascular ischemia causes necrosis. More than 90% of the pituitary must be destroyed before the condition is symptomatic. |

| Condition | Description |
|---|---|
| GH Deficiency | In children, causes pituitary dwarfism. Normal intelligence. |
| | In adults, causes increased insulin sensitivity, leading to hypoglycemia, and decreased muscle strength. |
| FSH and LH Deficiency | In preadolescents, causes delayed or absent secondary sexual maturation. |
| | In adult males, causes decreased libido, impotence, decreased muscle mass, and decreased facial hair. Causes amenorrhea in women. |
| TSH Deficiency | In infants, causes cretinism. Short, mentally retarded children. |
| | In older children and adults, results in myxedema. (See figure on hypothyroidism, p172.) |
| ACTH Deficiency | In children and adults, causes secondary adrenal failure (uncommon cause). Hypopigmentation occurs from MSH deficiency. Poor response to stress (e.g., infections, surgery, or trauma). Weakness, fatigue, weight loss, and hypotension result from cortisol deficiency. |
| ADH Deficiency | In both adults and children, causes diabetes insipidus with polyuria, dehydration, and polydipsia (excessive thirst). Causes include tumors, trauma, inflammation, or lysosomal storage diseases involving the hypothalamus or posterior pituitary. |

# II. Thyroid and Parathyroid Disorders

## HYPOTHYROIDISM AND HYPERTHYROIDISM (THYROTOXICOSIS)

| Condition | Laboratory Tests | Symptoms and Causes | Pathology |
|---|---|---|---|
| **Primary Hypothyroidism** | Low free $T_3$ and $T_4$; high TSH | In neonates, causes cretinism. Symptoms include lethargy, hypothermia, poor feeding, persistent neonatal jaundice, hypotonic muscles, large tongue, and growth and mental retardation. May be prevented if thyroid hormone is given early. In adults, causes myxedema. Symptoms include lethargy; cold intolerance; weight gain; constipation; hair loss; mental slowing; puffiness of the face, eyelids, and hands; normocytic anemia; effusions; increased serum cholesterol; and atherosclerosis. | |
| | | Primary idiopathic hypothyroidism is the most common cause in the United States. | |
| | | Hashimoto thyroiditis is the primary cause of goitrous hypothyroidism. This autoimmune condition is associated with HLA-DR5 and is common in women. Slow onset of thyroid enlargement. Graves disease may occur concurrently. Increased risk for papillary thyroid carcinoma or thyroid B-cell lymphoma. | Early findings include diffuse thyroid enlargement. With time, it atrophies with scarring, fibrosis, and dense focal lymphocytic infiltration (germinal centers). |
| | | Iodine deficiency is common in children (may cause cretinism). Normal compensatory enlargement. Also see Thyroid Goiters below. | Diffuse or nodular nontoxic goiter. |
| | | Can also be caused by thyroid agenesis, antithyroid drugs, irradiation, or surgical removal of the thyroid. | |
| **Secondary Hypothyroidism** | Low free $T_3$ and $T_4$; low TSH | Hypopituitarism (rare). Also see Hypopituitarism above. | Atrophy of the thyroid gland. |

| | | | |
|---|---|---|---|
| **Primary Hyperthyroidism** | High free T$_3$ and T$_4$; low TSH | Symptoms include nervousness, anxiety, tremors, and weight loss (with a good appetite). Complaints of sweating, palpitations, cardiac arrhythmias (atrial fibrillation), secondary amenorrhea, infertility, hair thinning, and dry skin. | |
| | | Graves disease is the primary cause. Symptoms as above plus exophthalmos (eye protrusion), periorbital inflammation, and pretibial myxedema. Autoimmune condition (thyroid receptor–stimulating antibodies) associated with HLA-DR3. More common in females (15–40 years). Associated with autoimmune diseases (pernicious anemia and Hashimoto disease). | Diffuse toxic goiter. "Too many" cells inside and around follicles. Colloid is scalloped from increased activity. Thyroid is very vascular. Lymphocyte infiltration and formation of germinal follicles. |
| | | Struma ovarii is an ovarian teratoma that consists of hyperfunctional thyroid tissue. | Ectopic thyroid tissue may be found in a mature teratoma. |
| | | Other causes include Plummer disease (multinodular toxic goiter), toxic thyroid adenoma, and subacute thyroiditis (note that TSH is normal). See the respective diseases. | |
| **Secondary Hyperthyroidism** | High free T$_3$ and T$_4$; high TSH | Pituitary thyrotropic adenoma (very rare). Diffuse goiter. | Diffuse thyroid enlargement. |

## CLINICAL SIGNS IN HYPOTHYROIDISM AND HYPERTHYROIDISM

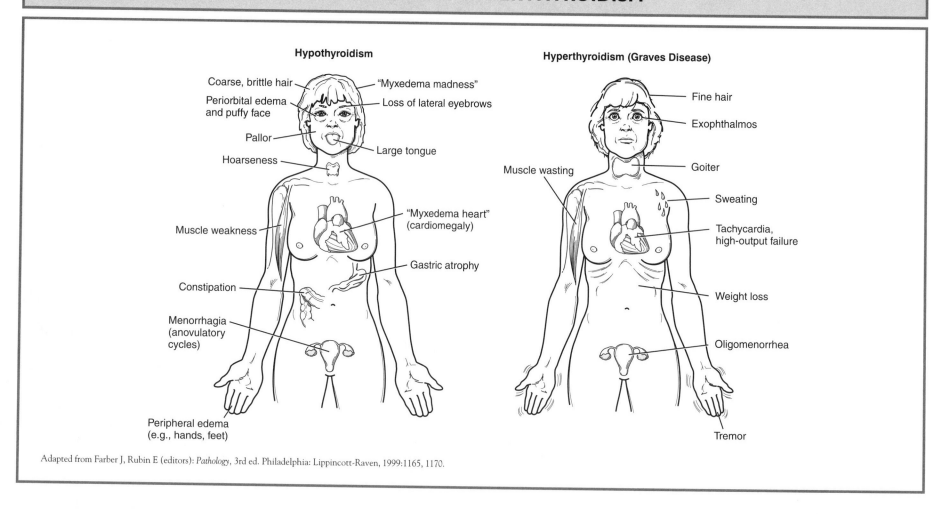

Adapted from Farber J, Rubin E (editors): *Pathology*, 3rd ed. Philadelphia: Lippincott-Raven, 1999:1165, 1170.

## THYROIDITIS

| Condition | Description | Cause(s) | Pathology |
|---|---|---|---|
| Hashimoto Thyroiditis | See Hypothyroidism and Hyperthyroidism—Primary Hypothyroidism. | | |
| Acute Infectious Thyroiditis | Painful thyroid goiter. | Infection with *Staphylococcus aureus*, streptococci, *Mycobacterium tuberculosis*, or *Salmonella* | Hematogenously spread infection causes acute inflammation. |
| Subacute Thyroiditis | Also called granulomatous thyroiditis (de Quervain thyroiditis). Soft, painful thyroid goiter, fever, and muscle aches. Self-limited to a few months without causing permanent thyroid dysfunction. | Follows an illness with Coxsackie or mumps virus | Diffuse thyroid enlargement with extensive fibrosis of thyroid follicles. Granulomatous inflammation around the colloid. |
| Subacute Lymphocytic Thyroiditis | Rare disorder in postpartum women. Painless goiter or hyperthyroidism. Self-limited, but may leave residual hypothyroidism after recovery. | Unknown | Lymphocytic infiltrate without germinal centers (compare with Hashimoto type). |
| Riedel Thyroiditis | Rare disorder. Painless, hard thyroid goiter. May compress the trachea or esophagus, causing stridor or dysphagia, respectively. Can be mistaken for thyroid adenocarcinoma. | Unknown | Hard fibrous tissue replaces the thyroid, leaving few residual functional follicles. Fibrosis may penetrate the thyroid capsule and cause adhesions. |

## THYROID GOITERS

| Condition | Description | Pathology |
|---|---|---|
| Goiter | Enlargement of the thyroid from hyperthyroidism or hypothyroidism. In hypothyroidism, goiter compensates for the decrease in thyroid hormone production. In hyperthyroidism, goiter forms because of thyroid hyperactivity. | |
| Nontoxic Goiters | With diffuse goiters, patients remain euthyroid. Presents as a painless diffuse enlargement without nodules. Multinodular goiter occurs after years of fibrosis of a diffuse goiter. | Small follicles lined with columnar cells become flattened and cuboidal. Different areas undergo different stages. May see calcification, fibrosis, and hemorrhage on a chronic basis. |
| | Physiologic goiter forms because of increased demand at puberty or during pregnancy. Endemic goiter occurs in certain geographic areas because of iodine-deficient diets or iodine-antagonizing foods (e.g., cabbage). | |
| Toxic Goiters | Hyperthyroidism (increased serum $T_3$ and $T_4$) results from a "hot" nodule. Nodular goiter has autonomous production of thyroid hormone. Hot nodules may rarely form in nontoxic multinodular goiters. Small risk for thyroid carcinoma. | Similar to above. |

## PRIMARY THYROID TUMORS

| Condition | Description and Prevalence | Pathology |
|---|---|---|
| **Benign Tumor** | | |
| **Follicular Adenoma** | Represents 30% of solitary thyroid nodules. More common in women. Is a firm, painless thyroid nodule. | Firm, gray-red, fully encapsulated nodule that compresses normal thyroid tissue. Composed of various sizes of follicles. Variants include embryonal adenoma (well-developed, small follicles and amyloid stroma) and Hürthle cell adenoma (Hürthle cells are large, pink, granular cells). Most adenomas are nonfunctional (do not produce hormone). |
| **Malignant Tumors** | Responsible for 18,100 cases and 1200 deaths per year in the United States. It is the 10th most common cancer in women. | |
| **Papillary Adenocarcinoma** | Most common type of thyroid carcinoma. More common in young women (15–35 years). Painless and "cold" thyroid nodule. Metastasizes especially to the cervical nodes. In 10%, there is a history of early childhood thyroid irradiation. 90% survive 5 years. | Mass is usually infiltrating or partially circumscribed. Arranged into a papillary pattern (fingerlike projections). Nuclei have a ground-glass appearance with "orphan Annie" eyes (artifact of tissue fixation). Psammoma bodies are found (round, laminated, and calcified bodies). Slow-growing, locally infiltrating tumor, preferring lymphatic metastasis. |
| **Follicular Adenocarcinoma** | Second most common type of thyroid carcinoma. More common in middle-aged women. Painless and "cold" thyroid nodule. Metastasizes especially to the bone or lungs. 65% survive 5 years. | Encapsulated tumor; resembles follicular adenoma. Uniformly sized follicles. Rarely, follicles are lined by clear cell or Hürthle cell variants. Slow-growing tumor with early hematogenous metastasis (an exception for carcinoma, which usually metastasizes via the lymphatics). |
| **Anaplastic Carcinoma** | Third most common type of thyroid carcinoma. Patients are usually over 50 years. Very aggressive and highly metastatic. Usually fatal within a year. | Massive, hard, and gritty infiltrating tumor without a capsule. Composed of spindle cells and giant cells. |
| **Medullary Carcinoma** | Infrequent cause of thyroid carcinoma. Painless and "cold" thyroid nodule. 50% survive 5 years. | Derived from parafollicular (C type) neuroendocrine cells. Hard, gray, infiltrative mass. Arranged into sheets or cords. Produces calcitonin and has an amyloid stroma. 10% of tumors occur as part of MEN IIa or IIb (III). Tumor is slow-growing but metastasizes. |

## PARATHYROID GLAND DISORDERS

| Condition | Laboratory Tests | Description | Pathology |
|-----------|------------------|-------------|-----------|
| Hypoparathyroidism | Low serum calcium; high serum phosphate; low PTH | Uncommon. Severely low calcium causes muscle tetany and numbness of the hands, feet, and lips. Metastatic calcification occurs (see Chapter 1). Caused by congenital DiGeorge syndrome, accidental excision or injury during thyroid surgery, or hypomagnesemia (low magnesium prevents PTH release). | No parathyroid glands = no PTH. Tetany is due to increased neuromuscular excitability. Serum phosphate accumulates from decreased renal excretion (no PTH). |
| Primary Hyperparathyroidism | High serum calcium; low serum phosphate; high PTH | Hypercalcemia can cause urinary calculi (stones) from hypercalciuria. Metastatic calcification and bone resorption cause osteoporosis. See Chapter 12, Metabolic Bone Diseases. | Parathyroid gland does not shut down when it senses high serum calcium. Chief cell receptor is malfunctional. |
| | | Parathyroid adenoma is the most common cause of hyperparathyroidism. In parathyroid adenoma, a solitary nodule affects one gland; the other three glands appear normal. Adenoma secretes PTH autonomously. | Small, well-encapsulated mass composed of chief and oxyphyl cells arranged in sheets or glandular structures. Little fat is present in adenoma. Adenoma compresses normal tissue against the capsule. |
| | | In diffuse hyperplasia of all four glands, glands secrete PTH autonomously. | Proliferation of all cell types crowding out the fat. Composition of the cells is identical to that of adenoma. |
| | | Parathyroid carcinoma is a rare condition involving one gland. Secretes PTH autonomously. | Infiltrating mass with fibrosis. Locally infiltrates or metastasizes. |
| | | Ectopic PTH production can be caused by squamous cell carcinoma of the lung. | See Chapter 5, Primary Lung Cancers. |

| Secondary Hyperparathyroidism | Normal to high serum calcium; high PTH | Normal response to normalize low serum calcium. Low serum phosphate and high alkaline phosphatase are present from bone resorption. | All four glands undergo hyperplasia. Chief cell is the major cell type. |
|---|---|---|---|
| | | Chronic renal failure is the most common cause. Vitamin D is not activated and calcium is not adequately absorbed in the intestine. Decreased serum calcium leads to a compensatory increase in PTH. Serum phosphate is elevated. | Leads to osteomalacia and osteitis fibrosa cystica, both metabolic bone diseases. See Chapter 12. |
| Hypercalcemia without Hyperparathyroidism | High serum calcium; low PTH | Hypercalcemia not caused by high PTH can be due to metastatic bone disease, sarcoidosis, vitamin D toxicity, and multiple myeloma. | PTH is suppressed by high serum calcium. Reaction is normal; hypercalcemia is not. |

**Primary Parathyroid Hyperplasia** affects all four glands equally.

- Each gland has fat cells.
- Gland has no capsule of its own.

Posterior aspect of the thyroid gland

Parathyroid glands

**Parathyroid Adenomas** affect only one or two glands.

Solitary nodule, involving only one gland

- Has its own capsule
- Small proportion of or no fat cells

# III. Adrenal Disorders

## ADRENAL STRUCTURE

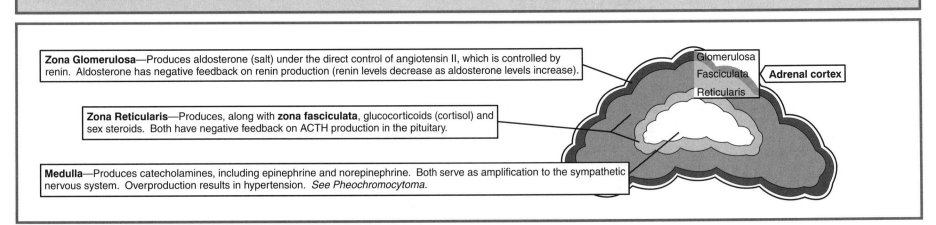

**Zona Glomerulosa**—Produces aldosterone (salt) under the direct control of angiotensin II, which is controlled by renin. Aldosterone has negative feedback on renin production (renin levels decrease as aldosterone levels increase).

**Zona Reticularis**—Produces, along with **zona fasciculata**, glucocorticoids (cortisol) and sex steroids. Both have negative feedback on ACTH production in the pituitary.

**Medulla**—Produces catecholamines, including epinephrine and norepinephrine. Both serve as amplification to the sympathetic nervous system. Overproduction results in hypertension. *See Pheochromocytoma.*

Glomerulosa
Fasciculata
Reticularis
**Adrenal cortex**

# ADRENAL GLAND DISORDERS

| Condition | Laboratory Tests | Description and Common Causes | Pathology |
|---|---|---|---|
| **Primary Hypocorticoidism (Addison Disease)** | Low cortisol; low aldosterone; high or low ACTH and MSH | Also known as adrenal insufficiency (addisonian crisis). Symptoms include fatigue, weakness, and weight loss. Complications may occur with stress (e.g., infection, surgery, or trauma). Also causes circulatory collapse and hypotension, hyponatremia, and hyperkalemia. MSH increases skin pigmentation. | |
| | | Autoimmune adrenalitis is the most common cause of primary hypocorticoidism (60–70%). Autoimmune disease causes chronic adrenal insufficiency. Associated with Hashimoto thyroiditis, Graves disease, and pernicious anemia. | Atrophy of the adrenal cortex. Cortex is narrow, fibrotic, and infiltrated with lymphocytes. |
| | | Second most common cause is rapid withdrawal from chronic exogenous steroid use. | Corticosteroids (prednisone) suppress pituitary ACTH secretion. Adrenal atrophy results. With abrupt discontinuation, adrenals lack the time to resume producing cortisol. Prednisone regimens must be tapered slowly. |
| | | Waterhouse-Friderichsen syndrome causes adrenal infarct from meningococcal sepsis and disseminated intravascular coagulation. Presents with fever, petechial rash, shock, and death. | Hemorrhagic infarct in the adrenal cortex. |
| | | Infections (tuberculosis and histoplasmosis), infiltrative diseases (sarcoidosis, amyloidosis, hemochromatosis), and metastases destroy the adrenals, causing chronic adrenal insufficiency. | See respective diseases. |
| **Secondary Hypocorticoidism** | Low cortisol, low ACTH | Caused by hypopituitarism. See Hypopituitarism above. | Atrophic adrenal cortex secondary to decreased ACTH stimulation. |

*Continued*

## ADRENAL GLAND DISORDERS (Continued)

| Condition | Laboratory Tests | Description and Common Causes | Pathology |
|---|---|---|---|
| Primary Hypercorticoidism (Cushing Syndrome) | High cortisol; low ACTH | Presents with redistribution of body fat resulting in a "buffalo hump," thin extremities, and hypertension. May cause diabetes mellitus from cortisol's antagonistic effect on insulin. Muscle wasting, easy bruising, and poor wound healing are due to protein catabolism. Cortisol is immunosuppressive. Androgenic effects cause hirsutism, infertility, and amenorrhea.[1] | |
| | | Adrenal cortical adenoma is the most common cause of primary hypercorticoidism (second most common endogenous[1] cause of primary hypercorticoidism). Occurs in one adrenal gland and produces cortisol. | Well-circumscribed, yellow nodule that may contain hemorrhage and fibrosis. Composed of uniform large, lipid-filled cells. Other adrenal gland is atrophied. |
| | | Adrenal adenocarcinoma is the second most common cause (fourth most common endogenous[1] cause). Produces cortisol. | Poorly circumscribed mass that may infiltrate the kidney. Composed of large pleomorphic cells. Abundant mitotic activity. |
| Secondary Hypercorticoidism (Cushing Syndrome) | High cortisol; low or high ACTH | Adrenal cortical adenoma is the most common endogenous[1] cause of secondary hypercorticoidism. Also may result from corticosteroid use in the treatment of disorders (most common exogenous[1] cause of secondary hypercorticoidism). | Bilateral adrenal cortical atrophy is due to exogenous[1] corticosteroid suppression of pituitary ACTH. |
| | | Corticotropic pituitary adenoma is the second most common cause (most common endogenous[1] cause). Produces ACTH. | Bilateral adrenal hyperplasia of the zona fasciculata and reticularis is due to ACTH stimulation. |
| | | Ectopic ACTH production is the third most common cause (third most common endogenous[1] cause). It is produced by small cell bronchogenic carcinoma of the lung. | Bilateral adrenal cortical hyperplasia. |

[1]Endogenous = internally produced. Exogenous = originating outside the body.

| | | | |
|---|---|---|---|
| **Primary Hyperaldosteronism** | High aldosterone | Also known as Conn syndrome. Rare disorder results in salt and water retention, potassium excretion, and hypertension. | Aldosterone-secreting adrenal adenoma. Appears identical to the cortisol-secreting adenoma. |
| **Secondary Hyperaldosteronism** | High aldosterone | The most common cause of high aldosterone levels. Results in salt and water retention, potassium excretion, and generalized edema. Normal compensatory response. | |
| | | Also may be due to renal ischemia from malignant hypertension or renal artery stenosis. | Causes high renin release (kidney acts as if there is not enough perfusion) and increases aldosterone production. |
| | | Reduced circulating plasma volume is seen in congestive heart failure and nephrotic syndrome. | Results in high renin release. |

## CLINICAL SIGNS IN CUSHING SYNDROME

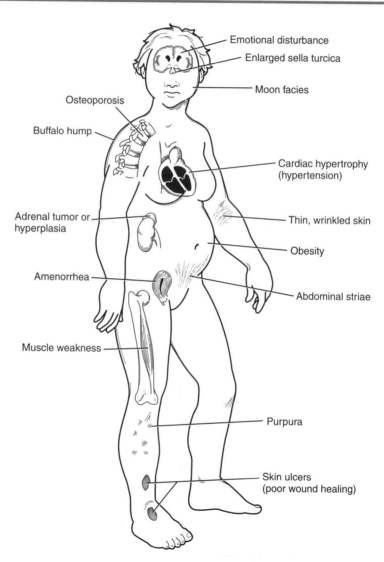

Adapted from Farber J, Rubin E (editors): *Pathology*, 3rd ed. Philadelphia: Lippincott-Raven, 1999:1193.

## ADRENAL TUMORS

| Condition | Description | Pathology |
|---|---|---|
| **Cortical Tumors** | | |
| Adrenal Cortex Adenoma | Functional adenomas secrete cortisol, aldosterone, or, rarely, androgens. May be part of MEN I, IIa, and IIb (III) syndromes. | See Adrenal Gland Disorders—Hypercorticoidism and Hyperaldosteronism above. |
| | Nonfunctional adenomas produce no symptoms. May be part of MEN I, IIa, and IIb (III) syndromes. | |
| **Medullary Tumors** | | |
| Pheochromocytoma | The most common adrenal medullary tumor (however, an uncommon adrenal tumor). Symptoms include intermittent hypertension with palpitations, tachycardia, anxiety, and excessive sweating (from norepinephrine and epinephrine). Complications include death from heart failure. | Tumor is unilateral (alone) or bilateral (part of MEN IIa, IIb, or other inherited conditions). Mostly benign and well circumscribed. Composed of large chromaffin cells in a rich vascular stroma. Produces epinephrine and norepinephrine. In the adrenal, 10% of tumors are malignant; outside the adrenal, 40% are malignant (10% occur outside the adrenal). Metastasis determines whether it is benign or malignant. |
| Neuroblastoma | Occurs in children under 5 years as an enlarging abdominal mass. Metastases are common to bone, liver, and bone marrow. | Large, soft, infiltrating mass composed of small neoplastic cells arranged into rosettes (cells in a circle). May become a more differentiated ganglioneuroma. |

## ENDOCRINE DISEASE SUMMARY

| Disorder | Cause of Primary Condition | Cause of Secondary Condition |
|---|---|---|
| Hyperparathyroidism | Parathyroid adenoma (most common) or parathyroid hyperplasia | Chronic renal failure (most common) |
| Hypoparathyroidism | Accidental excision or DiGeorge syndrome | None |
| Hyperthyroidism | Graves disease | TSH-secreting pituitary adenoma (rare) |
| Hypothyroidism | Hashimoto thyroiditis or idiopathic | Hypopituitarism affecting the TSH cells |
| Cushing Syndrome (Adrenal Hypercorticoidism) | Adrenal cortical adenoma (most common) | • Exogenous (most common): therapeutically administered corticosteroids<br>• Endogenous (most common): ACTH-secreting pituitary adenoma (Cushing disease) |
| Adrenal Hypocorticoidism | Addison disease | Hypopituitarism affecting the ACTH cells (note that this is partial hypocorticoidism because aldosterone secretion is not under ACTH control) |

# IV. Pancreatic Diseases and Diabetes Mellitus

## DISEASES OF THE ENDOCRINE PANCREAS

| Condition | Causation and Symptoms | Pathologic Process |
|---|---|---|
| **Primary Diabetes Mellitus** | Most common type of diabetes (95%). Unknown cause, but hereditary. | |
| | Diabetes mellitus type 1—presents in adolescence with hyperglycemia, polyuria, polydipsia, muscle wasting, and weight loss. Associated with HLA-DR4 or -DR3, pernicious anemia, Graves disease, and Addison disease. Complications include:<br><br>• Diabetic ketoacidosis—extreme hyperglycemia, ketone bodies, and altered mental status<br><br>• Hypoglycemic coma—overdose of insulin | Antibody-mediated destruction of the pancreatic β cells (decreased number of islets). Because of decreased insulin, the body prepares for starvation. Results in gluconeogenesis and glycogenolysis (hyperglycemia = osmotic polyuria), lipolysis (free fatty acids = ketones and ketoacidosis), and proteolysis (muscle wasting). |
| | Diabetes mellitus type 2 (most common)—associated with a strong family history. Patients present similarly but are obese and older than 40 years. Patients do not get diabetic ketoacidosis. Complications include:<br><br>• Hyperosmolar nonketonic coma—in elderly patients with uncontrolled diabetes. Hyperglycemia is responsible for severe fluid depletion. | Two mechanisms include impaired rapid insulin release after meals and increased insulin resistance by muscle and fat cells. Obesity and pregnancy predispose to insulin resistance. |
| **Secondary Diabetes Mellitus** | Causes 5% of cases of diabetes mellitus | |
| | Insulin antagonists—increased levels of cortisol (Cushing syndrome), exogenous corticosteroids, and increased GH (acromegaly). | |
| | Pancreatitis—islet cell destruction. | |
| | Gestational diabetes—increased insulin resistance during the third trimester or soon after birth. | |
| | Idiopathic hemochromatosis—"bronze diabetes"—excess iron deposits (hemosiderin) within pancreatic islets destroy the cells. | |
| | Other causes include carcinoma of the pancreas, glucagonoma, and pheochromocytoma (catecholamine mediated). | |

## CONSEQUENCES OF CHRONIC UNCONTROLLED DIABETES MELLITUS[1]

| Organ Affected | Pathologic Process |
|---|---|
| Kidney | Nodular glomerulosclerosis with hyaline arteriolar thickening, leading to progressive diabetic nephropathy, chronic nephrotic syndrome, and chronic renal failure |
| Cardiovascular System | Hypertension and atherosclerosis are hastened. Predisposes to myocardial infarction and peripheral arterial insufficiency. |
| Eyes | Cataracts (the lens absorbs sorbitol) and diabetic retinopathy secondary to hypertension and hyperglycemia |
| Nervous System | Peripheral and autonomic neuropathy. See Chapter 13, Peripheral Neuropathies. |
| Skin | Xanthomas (due to hyperlipidemia) and increased risk of infections such as furuncles, abscesses, and fungal infections (because of poor macrophage function). Also poor healing of wounds. |

[1]Diabetes control refers to controlling the hyperglycemia over the long term. Keeping serum glucose levels close to normal slows down or prevents many of the above complications. Glucose levels can be monitored by checking immediate serum levels or by measuring HgbA1c or glycosylated hemoglobin levels. This level correlates well with the average glucose level over 3 months, the life span of red blood cells. In type 2 diabetes, hyperinsulinemia is responsible for the complications as well as glucose.

## PANCREATIC ISLET TUMORS

| Tumor Type | Description | Pathology |
|---|---|---|
| Insulinoma (β-Cell Tumor) | Most common islet cell adenoma. Presents with Whipple's triad—transient hypoglycemia, central nervous system dysfunction, and reversal of central nervous system symptoms with glucose administration. | Tumor is composed of β cells and secretes insulin. C peptide should be elevated because of increased insulin production. |
| Gastrinoma | Second most common islet cell tumor. Presents with Zollinger-Ellison syndrome—gastric acid hypersecretion with recurrent peptic ulcer disease. | Tumor contains G cells and secretes gastrin; 70% are malignant. |
| Glucagonoma (α-Cell Tumor) | Rare tumor of glucagon-secreting cells. Presents with mild diabetes mellitus secondary to glucagon's antagonizing effects on insulin. Produces necrotic migratory erythema (skin lesions). | Most tumors are malignant. |
| Vipoma | Rare tumor that causes watery diarrhea, hypokalemia, and achlorhydria. | Tumor secretes vasoactive intestinal polypeptide. |

## MULTIPLE ENDOCRINE NEOPLASIA SYNDROMES

| Tumor Type | MEN I (Wermer Syndrome) | MEN IIa (Sipple Syndrome) | MEN IIb (or III) |
|---|---|---|---|
| Parathyroid neoplasm | ✓ | ✓ | |
| Pancreatic islet cell neoplasm | ✓ | | |
| Pituitary neoplasm | ✓ | | |
| Medullary thyroid carcinoma | | ✓ | ✓ |
| Adrenal pheochromocytoma | | ✓ | ✓ |
| Neuromas, ganglioneuromas of oral cavity | | | ✓ |

☞ PPP. All start with P.

# CHAPTER 9
# GASTROINTESTINAL TRACT AND THE ORAL CAVITY

**I. DISEASES OF THE ORAL CAVITY**

Oral Cavity Lesions

Oral Cavity Tumors or Growths

Salivary Gland Diseases

Salivary Gland Tumors

**II. ESOPHAGEAL DISORDERS**

Esophageal Diseases

Inflammatory Esophageal Changes and Tumors

**III. STOMACH DISORDERS**

Stomach Diseases and Tumors

**IV. INTESTINAL DISORDERS**

Small Intestine Diseases and Tumors

Peptic Ulcer Comparison

Colon Inflammatory Diseases

Bowel Obstruction

Inflammatory Bowel Disease Comparison

Inflammatory Bowel Disease Characteristics

Intestinal Polyps

Intestinal Tumors

**V. DIARRHEA, MALABSORPTION, AND INTESTINAL INFECTIONS**

Mechanisms of Diarrhea

Malabsorption Syndromes

Infectious Diarrhea

Bacterial Diarrheas

Other Intestinal Infections

**VI. MISCELLANEOUS DISORDERS**

The Appendix

The Peritoneum

**ABBREVIATIONS**

**CMV** = cytomegalovirus

**HIV** = human immunodeficiency virus

**HSV** = herpes simplex virus

**NSAID** = nonsteroidal anti-inflammatory drug

**PMN** = polymorphonuclear leukocyte

## MOST COMMON Causes and Types

| Disorder | Common Cause |
|---|---|
| Oral leukoplakia | Chewing tobacco |
| Oral lesions | Aphthous ulcers |
| Congenital anomaly of the small intestine | Meckel diverticulum |

| Disorder | Common Type |
|---|---|
| Benign oral epithelial tumor | Papilloma |
| Oral cancer | Squamous cell carcinoma |
| Salivary gland tumor | Pleomorphic adenoma (mostly parotid) |
| Appendix tumor | Carcinoid tumor |

## TERMS TO LEARN

| | |
|---|---|
| Dysphagia | Difficulty swallowing |
| Glossitis | Beefy, red, inflamed tongue due to deficiency of vitamin $B_{12}$, riboflavin ($B_2$), niacin, pyridoxine ($B_6$), or iron |
| Malabsorption Syndromes | Intestinal malabsorption of iron; folate; magnesium; calcium; vitamins A, D, E, and K; as well as proteins, carbohydrates, and fats. Caused by intestinal mucosal damage, lack of bile salts, or lack of pancreatic enzymes. If distal ileum is involved, vitamin $B_{12}$ is malabsorbed. Excess fat causes fatty, yellow stools that float. |
| Mucosal Erosion | Destruction of the superficial part of the mucosa. Gastritis and esophagitis are examples. |
| Mucosal Ulceration | Full-thickness destruction of the mucosa, submucosa, or the surrounding muscle. Peptic ulcers are examples. |

# I. Diseases of the Oral Cavity

## ORAL CAVITY LESIONS

| Disease | Description | Cause(s) | Pathology |
|---|---|---|---|
| Aphthous Stomatitis | Also known as canker sores, the most common oral lesion in the United States (up to 40% of the population). Self-limited, painful, shallow ulcers on the oral mucosa. | Unknown. May be associated with inflammatory bowel disease. | Acute inflammation. Early lesions contain mononuclear inflammatory cells. |
| Herpes Stomatitis | Up to 20% of the population is affected.<br><br>• Primary lesions: gingivostomatitis with multiple red, edematous, ulcerative lesions on the oral mucosa, tongue, and gingiva (self-limited).<br><br>• Recurrence (reactivation): herpes labialis (cold sore or fever blister) is a shallow ulcer or blister on the lips. Precipitated by respiratory infections, allergies, sunlight, or cold weather. | HSV type 1 | Lesions contain giant cells and inclusions. |
| Oral Thrush | Common in neonates and immunocompromised patients. Superficial curdy, white-gray membrane covers red and inflamed, ulcerated oral mucosa. | *Candida albicans* | Lesions contain *Candida*. Organism may be seen with staining. |
| Acute Necrotizing Ulcerative Gingivitis | Also known as Vincent angina (trench mouth). Severe ulcerative gingivitis that causes pain and bleeding in the gums. Affects immunocompromised and malnourished patients. | *Fusobacterium* and *Bacteroides* | Inflammation and necrosis of the gingival mucosa. |

## ORAL CAVITY TUMORS OR GROWTHS

| Disease | Description | Predisposing Factors | Pathology |
|---|---|---|---|
| Mucocele | Painful cystic mass; not a true neoplasm | Salivary duct or gland rupture | Mucus cyst lined by granulation tissue near a salivary gland, producing a localized inflammatory reaction. A ranula is a large mucocele on the floor of the mouth. |
| Pyogenic Granuloma | Also called pregnancy tumor, although it is not a true tumor. A small, bright red nodule with overlying mucosal ulceration found on the gingiva. Resolves spontaneously. | Unknown | Reactive inflammatory proliferation of granulation tissue. |
| Benign Tumors | Squamous papilloma, fibroma, lipoma, neurofibroma, or hemangioma may all involve the oral cavity. | Unknown | Findings are tumor specific. See Chapter 12, Soft Tissue Tumors; and Chapter 11, Viral Skin Infections—Verrucae Vulgaris, for papilloma. |
| **Malignant Tumors** | | | |
| Leukoplakia | A painless, white, oral mucosal plaque that cannot be removed by scraping. Self-limited leukoplakia is associated with chronic irritation. Persistent leukoplakia can be precancerous. | Smoking, tobacco chewing, alcohol use, human papillomavirus infection, and Epstein-Barr virus | Findings range from hyperkeratosis to lesions bordering on carcinoma in situ. If erythroplakia (red eroded plaque) is seen, it has dysplasia to squamous cell carcinoma. |
| | Hairy leukoplakia is a similarly appearing oral lesion in patients with AIDS. | HIV infection | Areas of white hyperkeratotic thickening on the mucosa. Increased risk of squamous cell carcinoma. |
| Squamous Cell Carcinoma | The most common primary oral malignancy, responsible for 29,800 cases and 8100 deaths per year in the United States, and the seventh most common cause of cancer in males. Involves the tongue (30%), lower lip (17%), and the floor of the mouth (17%). Begins as leukoplakia or as an indurated plaque that ulcerates. | Tobacco chewing (most common cause), alcohol use, and cigarette and pipe smoking | Squamous cell carcinoma; lymphatic spread with lymph node involvement. |

## SALIVARY GLAND DISEASES

| Disease | Description | Predisposing Factors | Pathology |
|---|---|---|---|
| Sialolithiasis | Painful, unilateral glandular enlargement from mucus stone impaction in a salivary duct. | Thickened secretions (cystic fibrosis) | Predisposes to sialadenitis (from inflammation or metastatic infiltration) |
| Parotiditis | Parotid gland infection and inflammation, causing painful gland enlargement. Caused by mumps virus (most common cause), *Staphylococcus aureus*, and *Streptococcus viridans*. | None | Inflammation |
| Sjögren Syndrome | Autoimmune disease of the lacrimal and salivary glands associated with malignant lymphomas of the salivary glands. | Autoimmune mechanism | Lymphocytic and plasma cell infiltrates of the salivary glands with destruction and fibrosis |

## SALIVARY GLAND TUMORS

| Tumor | Description | Pathology |
|---|---|---|
| **Benign Tumors** | | |
| Pleomorphic Adenoma | Most common primary salivary gland tumor (45% of all salivary gland tumors). High recurrence rate. (Represents 60% of parotid gland tumors.) | Mixed tumor (epithelial and mesenchymal). Circumscribed, partially encapsulated, firm yellow-white tumor. Composed of cords and nests of epithelial cells in a hyalinelike mucoid stroma. Glands may be distended with colloidlike substance. |
| Warthin Tumor | Second most common primary salivary gland tumor (11%). Mostly found in the parotid gland, forming a parotid mass. May be bilateral. More common in males. | Cysts lined by double layer of pink epithelial cells, surrounded by dense masses of lymphocytes. |
| **Malignant Tumors** | | |
| Adenocarcinoma (not otherwise specified) | Slow-growing salivary gland mass. | Adenocarcinoma with or without mucus-secreting glands. |
| Mucoepidermoid Carcinoma | Most common primary malignant salivary gland tumor. | Solid areas lined by squamous cells and cystic areas lined by mucous cells (if well differentiated). |
| Adenoid Cystic Carcinoma | Slow-growing but highly infiltrative; tends to invade along nerves. | Small, round epithelial cells line the cystic spaces. |

# II. Esophageal Disorders

## ESOPHAGEAL DISEASES

| Disease | Description | Mechanism or Cause | Pathologic Findings |
|---------|-------------|--------------------|--------------------|
| Esophageal Diverticulum | A diverticulum is an out-pocketing. In the esophagus, it causes dysphagia. Zenker diverticulum occurs in the upper esophagus. | • False herniation (pulsion): herniation of mucosa through weak muscular layer<br>• True herniation (traction): herniation of entire esophageal-wall thickness | True herniation is caused by inflammation or fibrosis of the diverticulum. |
| Achalasia | Dysphagia of solids and liquids; can be caused by Chagas disease (trypanosomiasis) | Peristalsis is absent from loss of ganglion cells in the esophageal wall. Tonic contraction of lower esophageal sphincter occurs. | Increased risk of squamous cell carcinoma. |
| Esophageal Varices | Painless hematemesis (vomiting of blood) | Dilation of submucosal esophageal veins secondary to portal hypertension. | Portosystemic-venous anastomoses. See Chapter 10, Portal Hypertension. |
| Mallory-Weiss Syndrome | Common in alcohol users and pregnant women; may cause severe hematemesis. | Rupture of the esophagus from severe retching or vomiting. | Esophageal mucosal tear causes hemorrhage. |
| Plummer-Vinson Syndrome | Triad of iron-deficiency anemia, glossitis, and esophageal dysphagia. More common in women, but generally rare in the United States. | Iron-deficiency anemia. Dysphagia and glossitis resolve when the anemia is corrected. | Degeneration of the pharyngeal mucosa from iron deficiency. Increased risk of squamous cell carcinoma of the esophagus, oropharynx, and posterior tongue. |

## INFLAMMATORY ESOPHAGEAL CHANGES AND TUMORS

| Syndrome | Description | Cause and Association | Pathology |
|---|---|---|---|
| Reflux Esophagitis | Also known as gastroesophageal reflux ("heartburn"). Causes persistent coughing, hoarseness, and substernal burning pain, which are worse on lying supine. | Associated with hiatal hernia, incompetent lower esophageal sphincter, pregnancy, or scleroderma | Red and superficially eroded esophageal mucosa. Mucosal hyperplasia, elongation of the lamina propria papillae, and infiltration with eosinophils and some PMNs. With chronic reflux, the mucosa may become ulcerated or fibrotic or form Barrett's esophagus (intestinal metaplasia), which has an increased risk of esophageal adenocarcinoma. |
| Candida Esophagitis | White adherent patches on the esophagus causing dysphagia. Opportunistic infection in immunocompromised patients. | C. albicans | White patches with shallow ulcerations underneath contain fungi. |
| Viral Esophagitis | Opportunistic infection in immunocompromised patients. Causes dysphagia. | HSV type 1 and CMV | In HSV, multinucleated giant cells with inclusions are present. In CMV, can see large intranuclear or cytoplasmic inclusions in enlarged cells. |
| Esophageal Squamous Cell Carcinoma | Responsible for 12,500 cases and 12,200 deaths per year in the United States (seventh cause of cancer mortality in men). Patients present in their 50s with severe dysphagia, weight loss, and anorexia. Cancer is often unresectable at time of presentation. Risk of cancer increases with strictures, Plummer-Vinson syndrome, and achalasia. | Chronic alcoholism (20×) and smoking (10×) | Usually affects the middle third of the esophagus. Early plaque thickening in the mucosa may become polypoid, protruding into the lumen; may grow laterally, invading the mucosa; or may ulcerate. Lymphatic spread occurs early. |

# III. Stomach Disorders

## STOMACH DISEASES AND TUMORS

| Disease | Description | Cause(s) | Pathology |
|---|---|---|---|
| **Acute Erosive Gastropathy** | Common in the United States. Often asymptomatic but may be associated with dyspepsia (indigestion). Can cause epigastric pain and hematemesis. | NSAIDs (most common cause), corticosteroids, smoking, heavy alcoholism, bile reflux, chemotherapy, Curling ulcers from burn injury, and Cushing ulcers from intracranial lesions | Process is traditionally called acute gastritis, although it is noninflammatory. Multiple small erosions and ulcers are seen on the gastric mucosa, with variable necrosis of the superficial glands. Epithelium regenerates during healing. |
| **Chronic Gastritis** | Also known as atrophic gastritis. It is not an erosive process. Fundal (type A) is an autoimmune process that causes pernicious anemia. It can also be associated with chronic thyroiditis and Addison disease. Increased risk of gastric adenocarcinoma. | Autoantibody to parietal cells | Mucosal inflammation and hyperplasia with or without dysplasia and atrophy of the glands; intestinal metaplasia. Lymphocytic and plasma cell mucosal infiltrate surrounds parietal cells, destroying them. See Chapter 4 for megaloblastic anemia and pernicious anemia. |
| | Antral (type B) is the most common. Can be asymptomatic or causes mild pain and abdominal discomfort. Associated with chronic ulcers, gastric adenocarcinoma, and malignant gastric lymphoma. | *Helicobacter pylori* | PMN infiltration of the mucous glands, followed by deeper infiltration, destruction, and atrophy. Intestinal metaplasia and reactive lymphoid hyperplasia. |
| **Gastric Ulcers** | Gastric ulcers are less common than duodenal ulcers. Both are called peptic ulcers. Ulcer commonly affects the antral and prepyloric regions, with recurrent burning or gnawing epigastric pain that is worse with eating. | *H. pylori* (most common cause), aspirin, NSAIDs, steroids, caffeine, and cigarette smoking | Normal to low acid production, except in Zollinger-Ellison syndrome (see Chapter 8). Mechanism involves decreased mucosal resistance to acid or *H. pylori* stomach infection. Solitary, large, round ulcers having margins flush with the mucosa. Folds radiate from the ulcer. Ulcer is composed of superficial necrosis covering granulation tissue. Chronic ulcers develop fibrosis. |

*Continued*

## STOMACH DISEASES AND TUMORS (Continued)

| Disease | Description | Cause(s) | Pathology |
|---|---|---|---|
| Gastric Adenocarcinoma | The most common primary gastric malignancy and the 10th cause of cancer death. Antral and prepyloric regions are most commonly affected. Patients are asymptomatic early on. Late cancer presents as weight loss and early satiety. Early lymphocytic metastasis occurs to the lymph nodes and liver. | > 50 years, males, blood group A, pernicious anemia, chronic type B gastritis, and exposure to nitrites (food preservatives) in smoked fish and pickled vegetables | Muscle-invading gastric ulcer can be polypoid, ulcerative, flat, or diffusely infiltrating (most common type). Virchow node: metastases to the supraclavicular nodes. Krukenberg tumor metastasizes to both ovaries. If ulcer is flat, it has everted edges not flush with the mucosa (compare with Gastric Ulcer above). Has signet ring cells (nucleus displaced to one side by mucin). |
| Gastric Lymphoma | Two kinds exist: low grade, associated with lymphoid tissue in the mucosa, and high-grade immunoblastic B-cell lymphoma. Nonspecific symptoms. Increased incidence in patients with AIDS. | H. pylori | Polypoid, ulcerating, or infiltrating. Lymphoma cells stain negative for mucin. |

# IV. Intestinal Disorders

## SMALL INTESTINE DISEASES AND TUMORS

| Disease | Description | Cause(s) | Pathology |
|---|---|---|---|
| Duodenal Ulcers | The most common type of peptic ulcer. (Also see Stomach Diseases and Tumors—Gastric Ulcers above.) Similar to gastric ulcers, except that food relieves rather than worsens the pain (probably neutralizes the acid). | *H. pylori* (most common cause), aspirin, NSAIDs, steroids, caffeine, cigarette smoking, blood type O, family history, and Zollinger-Ellison syndrome | Mechanism is similar to that of gastric ulcers except that hypersecretion of gastric acid is more common in duodenal ulcers. Appearance resembles gastric ulcers. |
| Intestinal Infarction | Most common cause is thrombosis in the superior mesenteric artery from atherosclerosis. Second most common cause is non-occlusive mesenteric ischemia from decreased cardiac output.<br><br>• Acute infarction: fever, sudden abdominal pain, vomiting, and abdominal distention; then shock and peritonitis. Without surgery, mortality rate is 100%.<br><br>• Chronic infarction: patients present in their 60s with abdominal angina (ischemic abdominal pain 10–30 minutes following a meal). Weight loss occurs from fear of eating. | Atherosclerosis (most common cause), emboli from infective endocarditis, mural emboli, and cardiac events (e.g., myocardial infarction, congestive heart failure, and arrhythmias) | Affected bowel undergoes hemorrhagic necrosis of the entire wall, which appears black. Luminal infection leads to wet gangrene. |

## PEPTIC ULCER COMPARISON

| Type and Gender Prevalence | % of Ulcers | Predisposes to Cancer? | Decrease in Mucosal Barrier | Most Common Cause | Pain | Other Characteristics |
|---|---|---|---|---|---|---|
| Gastric (male = female) | 25% | No | Yes | H. pylori | ↑ with eating | No family history. |
| Duodenal (female = male) | 75% | No | No | H. pylori | ↓ with eating | Family history; blood type O. Ulcer commonly perforates. |

## COLON INFLAMMATORY DISEASES

| Disease | Description | Predisposing Factors | Pathology |
|---|---|---|---|
| Colonic Diverticula | Patients present in their 60s with diverticulum usually in the sigmoid colon. It is not a true herniation (only the mucosa herniates). Diverticulosis is a diverticulum without inflammation and without symptoms. Complications include obstruction or perforation. | Low-fiber diet | Recurrent high intraluminal pressures occur during defecation from chronic constipation. |
| | Diverticulitis is an inflammation of the diverticulum that may become infected. Causes fever and abdominal pain (left lower quadrant). Complications include perforation with peritonitis and bright red rectal bleeding. | | Inflammation of the diverticulum. |
| Ischemic Colitis | Occurs from atherosclerotic narrowing of the inferior mesenteric artery at the splenic flexure or rectosigmoid area ("watershed areas"). Patients present at age > 60 years with acute onset of abdominal pain, fever, and bloody diarrhea. | Atherosclerotic narrowing | Patchy mucosal necrosis followed by ulceration. Healing occurs by fibrosis and epithelial regeneration. |
| Hemorrhoids | Dilated internal or external venous plexuses in the anal canal. External hemorrhoids are usually painful after undergoing thrombosis. Internal hemorrhoids are painless but can bleed extensively. | Low-fiber diet, chronic constipation, pregnancy, and portal hypertension | Dilated hemorrhoidal veins can undergo thrombosis, bleed, or strangulate. |

## BOWEL OBSTRUCTION

| Type | Description | Pathology |
|------|-------------|-----------|
| **Hernias** | Many types of hernias exist: hiatal hernias, umbilical hernias, incisional hernias, and inguinal hernias (the most common type). All can cause bowel ischemia or strangulation. | |
| | In umbilical hernias, peritoneum, omentum, or bowel protrudes through a weak fascial wall. Incisional hernias are identical except that weakness in the fascia is created by prior abdominal surgery. | Bowel strangulation can occur if venous drainage or arterial supply is occluded. Infarction is followed by infection and wet gangrene. |
| | In inguinal hernias, direct hernias protrude through the posterior wall of the inguinal canal. Indirect hernias enter the internal ring of the inguinal canal. | |
| | Femoral hernias protrude below the inguinal ligament, into the femoral canal. | |
| **Volvulus** | Twisting of bowel loop around the mesentery. Usually occurs in the sigmoid colon, but also in the cecal colon. Causes abdominal pain. | |
| **Intussusception** | One segment of bowel telescopes into another at the ileocecal junction (the most common cause). In neonates, small-bowel polyps can cause it. In adults, a tumor or polyp can cause it. Palpable mass may be felt. Abdominal pain, vomiting, and rectal bleeding may occur. | Intussuscepted part becomes ischemic and necrotic. |

## INFLAMMATORY BOWEL DISEASE COMPARISON

Certain characteristics are common to both types of inflammatory bowel disease: fever, enteropathic arthritis, chronic bloody diarrhea, iritis or uveitis, aphthous ulcers, and weight loss.

| Disease and Gender Prevalence | Part of Bowel Affected | Type of Lesion | Wall Thickening | Strictures or Obstructions | Transmural Inflammation | Risk for Colon Adenocarcinoma | Fistulas | Pseudopolyps |
|---|---|---|---|---|---|---|---|---|
| Crohn Disease (male = female) | Gastrointestinal tract (most commonly in the distal ileum) | Skip | "Lead pipe" appearance | Yes | Yes | 6× | Yes | No |
| Ulcerative Colitis (female > male) | Colon | Continuous | None to marginal | Rare | Slight | 25× | Rare | Yes |

## INFLAMMATORY BOWEL DISEASE CHARACTERISTICS

| Disease | Description | Associations | Pathology |
|---|---|---|---|
| Crohn Disease | Involves the terminal ileum (most common site) and colon. Acute condition causes fever, diarrhea, and abdominal pain (if right-sided, it may mimic appendicitis). In the chronic phase, patients are asymptomatic or have weight loss. | Unknown cause. Runs in families and occurs in young adults. Common in Jews. Affects whites more often than blacks. | Acute condition causes patchy lesions of edematous, red, and ulcerated intestinal mucosa (skip lesions). Chronic condition causes intestinal wall thickening, fibrosis, and narrowing of the lumen. Also may see fissures, cobblestoning, and ulcers separated by fibrosis. Noncaseous granulomas and crypt destruction can be seen. |
| Ulcerative Colitis | Involves the colon and the rectum. Patients have fever, abdominal pain, and bloody diarrhea with mucus. A complication specific to ulcerative colitis is toxic megacolon (dilated colon). | Unknown cause. Affects whites more often than blacks. More common in Jews. | Acute condition causes diffuse erythema, inflammation, and mucosal ulcerations. Crypt abscesses are seen. In the chronic condition (during remission), ulcers reepithelialize, forming small polyps (pseudopolyps). Remainder of the mucosa appears atrophic. Crypt atrophy and distorted architecture may be seen. |

## INTESTINAL POLYPS

| Disease | Description | Pathology |
|---|---|---|
| Non-neoplastic Polyps | Hyperplastic polyp is the most common type of benign polyp. Asymptomatic and incidental. | Small sessile polyps attached to the mucosa without a stalk, composed of hyperplastic colonic epithelial cells. No increased risk for carcinoma. |
| | Inflammatory polyps are pseudopolyps. Seen in ulcerative colitis. | Pseudopolyps consist of regenerating mucosa, inflammation, and often granulation tissue. |
| | Other polyps include lymphoid polyps and hamartomatous polyps, including Peutz-Jeghers syndrome. | Hamartomatous polyps are composed of intestinal epithelium, glandular tissue, and smooth muscle cells. No neoplastic cells or increased risk for gastrointestinal carcinoma. Lymphoid polyps are composed of hyperplastic lymphoid tissue. |
| Adenomatous Polyps | Tubular adenoma is the most common type of colon adenoma (90%). Usually asymptomatic, although some patients may have occult bleeding. Premalignant lesion, with risk calculated by size (> 4 cm), architecture, and severity of dysplasia. | 50% are a small single polyp; 50% are multiple. Polyps are pedunculated on a thin stalk (stalk is not neoplastic; compare with Polypoid Adenocarcinoma below). May be sessile. Composed of neoplastic glands containing hyperchromatic cells with or without mucin. Epithelial dysplasia precedes malignancy. |
| | Villous adenoma is uncommon (< 10% of colon adenomas). Most patients are asymptomatic, although some may have occult bleeding. Increased risk of malignancy (if polyp is sessile and > 4 cm). | Polyp is usually sessile. Soft, large mass with a large number of villi is attached to the muscularis mucosa without a stalk. Composed of colonic neoplastic epithelium. ☞ Think of villous adenoma as the biggest villain (most malignant). |

| Disease | Description | Cause(s) and Association | Pathology |
|---------|-------------|--------------------------|-----------|
| Multiple Polyposis Syndromes | Familial adenomatous polyposis is the most common type. May cause many adenomatous polyps (> 100), appearing in teens to young adulthood (usually by the late 30s). Main symptom is rectal bleeding. Risk for malignancy is 100% (usually in the sigmoid colon). | Autosomal dominant | See Intestinal Polyps—Adenomatous Polyps above. |
| | Peutz-Jeghers syndrome is the second most common type. Pigmented macules on the oral mucosa, lips, hands, and genitalia, and benign hamartomatous polyps in the small intestine. Increased risk of carcinoma of the stomach, breast, and ovaries. | Autosomal dominant | See Intestinal Polyps—Non-neoplastic Polyps above for hamartomatous polyps. |
| | Gardner syndrome causes many adenomatous polyps in the small and large intestine. Associated with osteomas and fibromas in extraintestinal tissues. Risk for malignancy is 100% (usually in the sigmoid colon). Nearly all patients have cancer by their late 30s. | Autosomal dominant | See Intestinal Polyps—Adenomatous Polyps above. Also see Chapter 12 for osteoma and fibroma. |
| | Turcot syndrome causes many adenomatous polyps in the colon, with a similar 100% risk of malignancy. Associated with astrocytoma (glioblastoma multiforme). | Autosomal recessive | See Intestinal Polyps—Adenomatous Polyps above. Also see Chapter 13 for astrocytoma. |
| Colorectal Adenocarcinoma | Most common intestinal malignancy (95% of all intestinal malignancies). Responsible for 129,400 cases and 56,600 deaths per year in the United States; second most common cause of cancer mortality. Presents in the 50s to 70s, and asymptomatic in the early stage. Carcinoembryonic antigen is elevated (nonspecific sign). Tumor on the right side (cecal) presents with fatigue, iron-deficiency anemia, weight loss, and anemia. Tumor on the left side (colorectal) presents with changes in bowel habits and occult bleeding. | Adenomatous polyps, inherited multiple polyposis syndromes, chronic ulcerative colitis, family history, female > male, > 50 years, low-fiber diet, and high-fat diet | Right-sided lesions are usually polypoid and fungating. Left-sided lesions present as napkin-ring lesions (annular encircling mass). Most lesions start in adenomatous polyps. |
| Small Intestine Adenocarcinoma[1] | Most common primary small intestine malignancy, responsible for 4800 cases and 1200 deaths per year in the United States. Duodenum is the most common site. | Crohn disease (4× increase in risk) | Adenocarcinoma. |

*Continued*

## INTESTINAL TUMORS (Continued)

| Disease | Description | Cause(s) and Association | Pathology |
| --- | --- | --- | --- |
| Carcinoid Tumor[1] | Benign or malignant, depending on origin, size, and depth of invasion. Appendix is the most common site (99% benign). Mostly malignant in the ileum, colon, and stomach. With gastrointestinal carcinoid tumors, carcinoid syndrome occurs only with metastasis to the liver. Carcinoid syndrome causes flushing, watery diarrhea, cramps, bronchospasm, and valvular fibrosis on the right side of the heart. | Unknown | Firm, yellow, ulcerating masses that infiltrate the mucosa. See Chapter 2, Noninfective Endocarditis—Carcinoid Syndrome. |
| Lymphoma[1] | See Stomach Diseases and Tumors—Gastric Lymphoma above. | AIDS, heavy-chain disease (see Chapter 4), and celiac disease | See Stomach Diseases and Tumors—Gastric Lymphoma above. |

[1]Small intestine malignancies represent < 1% of all gastrointestinal malignancies.

# V. Diarrhea, Malabsorption, and Intestinal Infections

## MECHANISMS OF DIARRHEA

| Type | Symptoms and Pathogenesis | Cause(s) and Mechanism |
|------|---------------------------|------------------------|
| Secretory | Constant isotonic high-volume diarrhea. Caused by irritation of the small intestine. | Intrinsic intestinal secretions stimulated by *Vibrio cholerae*, serotonin from carcinoid tumor, and several viruses. Also see Infectious Diarrhea below. |
| Osmotic | High-volume diarrhea that occurs only during meals. Pathogenesis involves the colon. | Hypertonic luminal contents, such as undigested fats, magnesium, mannitol, sorbitol and other complex sugars, and cathartics, draw water into the colon. |
| Exudative | Constant purulent, bloody diarrhea due to invasive colon infections. | Infection with invasive bacteria, including *Shigella*, *Salmonella*, *Escherichia coli* O157:H7, *Yersinia*, and *Campylobacter*. See Bacterial Diarrheas below. |
| Motility | Constant diarrhea caused by increased intestinal motility. | Post-gastrectomy, carcinoid syndrome (serotonin), irritable bowel syndrome, spastic colon. |
| Malabsorptive | Stools are loose, fat laden, greasy, bulky, and pale gray-yellow (steatorrhea). Occurs only during meals. | |
| | Lack of bile salts in the small intestine. | Cholestasis. See Chapter 10, Obstructive Jaundice. Deconjugation of bile acids (bacterial overgrowth). Failure to reabsorb bile acids in the terminal ileum (Crohn disease). |
| | Lack of pancreatic enzymes, lipase, amylase, and trypsin in the small intestine. Similar to osmotic diarrhea. | Chronic pancreatitis. |
| | Mucosal abnormalities, including atrophy of intestinal villi. | See Malabsorption Syndromes below. |

## MALABSORPTION SYNDROMES

| Disease | Description | Cause(s) | Pathology |
|---|---|---|---|
| Celiac Disease | Also known as nontropical sprue (gluten-induced enteropathy). Causes severe malabsorption with weight loss, weakness, and diarrhea with pale, foul-smelling stools. May occur in children as growth retardation or failure to thrive. Associated with intestinal T-cell lymphoma and dermatitis herpetiformis. | Eating gluten contained in wheat products | Atrophy of small intestinal villi and increased number of lymphocytes in the lamina propria. See Chapter 14, Nutritional and Diet-Related Disorders. |
| Tropical Sprue | Similar to celiac disease. Malabsorption of vitamin $B_{12}$ and folate. Megaloblastic anemia occurs. | Chronic bacterial infection of the intestines | Atrophy of small intestinal villi. |
| Whipple Disease | Rare disease seen in adult men. Similar to celiac disease. Causes fever, polyarthritis, or ascites. | Possible infectious etiology | On electron microscopy, villi are distended with macrophages containing rod-shaped bacilli. On light microscopy, granules stain with periodic acid–Schiff. Other organs also have bacterial inclusions. |

## INFECTIOUS DIARRHEA

| Disease | Description | Cause(s) | Pathology |
|---------|-------------|----------|-----------|
| Traveler's Diarrhea | Mild illness that presents in travelers with cramps and watery diarrhea. Also occurs in neonatal units. | Toxinogenic *E. coli* (most common cause), viruses, parasites, and other bacteria | Depends on the etiologic agent. |
| Nosocomial Diarrhea | Occurs in hospital-bound patients receiving chronic antibiotic treatment. Causes fever, purulent bloody diarrhea, and cramps. Also called pseudomembranous enterocolitis. Rapidly progressive and fatal if not treated with antibiotics. | *Clostridium difficile* | Exotoxin-mediated superficial necrosis of colonic mucosa. Mucosa is covered by exudative yellow plaques. |
| Diarrhea and AIDS | Severe chronic watery diarrhea. | Cryptosporidium, microsporidium, and *Isospora* | Cryptosporidium attaches to surface mucosal cells and is visualized with acid-fast stain. Microsporidium infects mucosal cells of the small intestine. |
| | Severe chronic diarrhea that may be fatal. Intestinal perforations may be seen. | CMV | CMV infects the mucosa and vascular endothelium of the entire intestinal tract. Infected cells have intranuclear and cytoplasmic inclusions. |
| | Severe chronic diarrhea. | *Mycobacterium avium-intracellulare* | Organism accumulates in intestinal macrophages and in lymph nodes. No inflammation occurs. |
| Non–HIV-Related Chronic Diarrhea | Occurs after ingestion of food containing *Amoeba* cysts. Causes fever and bloody, mucus-containing diarrhea. May infest the liver (see Chapter 10, Other Infections of the Liver). | *Entamoeba histolytica* | Trophozoites invade the colonic mucosa and submucosa. Enzymatic necrosis leads to multiple ulcers with overlying necrotic debris. Amoeba may contain swallowed red blood cells. |
| | Occurs after ingestion of food containing *Giardia* cysts. Patients present with cramping, abdominal pain, watery diarrhea, and malabsorption. | *Giardia lamblia* | *Giardia* attaches itself to the duodenal mucosa by a sucker. Causes partial villus atrophy. |
| | Chronic bloody diarrhea | Inflammatory bowel disease | See Inflammatory Bowel Disease—Crohn Disease and Ulcerative Colitis above. |
| Viral Diarrhea | Presents as gastroenteritis ("stomach flu") with fever, diarrhea, vomiting, and abdominal pain. Symptoms last approximately 3–4 days. | *Rotavirus, Calicivirus*, and enteric adenoviruses | Infection and inflammation of small intestine epithelial cells. Plasma cells and lymphocytes infiltrate the villi and cause blunting. |

## BACTERIAL DIARRHEAS

| Type | Description | Cause(s) | Foods Involved and Pathologic Process |
|---|---|---|---|
| Preformed Exotoxin (Food Poisoning) | Affects the small intestine. Self-limited illness that occurs 1–6 hours after eating, with nausea, vomiting, abdominal cramps, and diarrhea. Toxin is found in food. | S. aureus | Multiplies in unrefrigerated food, releasing its toxin. Food smells and looks normal. Common in dairy products and pies. |
| | | Bacillus cereus | Occurs in reheated fried rice. Spores germinate and produce the toxin. |
| | | Clostridium perfringens | Occurs in poorly cooked or reheated food. Food is foul smelling. |
| | | Clostridium botulinum | Occurs in sausage or home-canned foods. See Chapters 12 and 15 for botulism. |
| Noninvasive Enterotoxin (Toxinogenic Gastroenteritis) | Affects the small intestine. After 1–2 days of incubation, produces abdominal cramps and watery diarrhea with or without a fever. Toxin is manufactured within the intestines. | V. cholerae | Found in shellfish. Cholera toxin is produced within the small intestine, where it irreversibly increases cyclic adenosine monophosphate, causing a secretory, profuse, watery diarrhea. No mucosal damage occurs. May be fatal from fluid and electrolyte imbalance. |
| Invasive Enterocolitis | Affects the colon after 3–5 days of incubation. Causes fever, abdominal cramps, tenesmus (sensation of having to defecate), small and frequent bowel movements, and diarrhea containing blood, mucus, and white blood cells. | Salmonella species | Found in unpasteurized milk and contaminated water. The only bacteria that invade the small intestine. Acute inflammation, mucosal hyperemia, and focal mucosal ulceration may be seen. |
| | | Shigella species | Found in shellfish and contaminated water. Invades the colon, producing acute inflammation and shallow ulcers. |
| | | Campylobacter | Infects the colonic mucosa of children. Is associated with hemolytic-uremic syndrome. See Chapter 4, Hemolytic Anemias. |
| | | Yersinia enterocolitica | Infects the colon. Invades the lymph nodes, producing mesenteric adenitis with high fever. May mimic appendicitis. |
| | | E. coli O157:H7 | Occurs in unpasteurized dairy products. Can cause fatal necrotizing enterocolitis in neonates. It is associated with hemolytic-uremic syndrome. In adults, causes extensive necrosis of the colonic mucosa. |

# OTHER INTESTINAL INFECTIONS

| Disease | Cause | Description | Pathology |
|---------|-------|-------------|-----------|
| **Typhoid Fever** | *Salmonella typhi* | Intestinal stage causes fever, headache, and muscle aches. Bacteremic stage causes rose-colored macular rash, bradycardia, splenomegaly, and neutropenia. Bacteremic stage is fatal if not treated. | *S. typhi* enters the intestinal tract and multiplies in lymphoid tissue. Also enters the blood, causing widespread symptoms (bacteremia). Reenters the intestines and causes necrosis from direct invasion and enterotoxin. |
| **Tapeworms** | *Diphyllobothrium latum* | Results from eating raw fish that contain larvae. Patients may be asymptomatic or have vague abdominal complaints and megaloblastic anemia (vitamin $B_{12}$ deficiency). | Organism attaches to the small intestine and consumes vitamin $B_{12}$. |
| **Whipworm** | *Trichuris* | Results from ingesting eggs found in contaminated soil. Usually asymptomatic, but can mimic chronic appendicitis. May also cause bloody diarrhea. | Organism attaches to the colon. |
| **Hookworm** | *Necator americanus* | Soil-living larvae burrow through the skin, creating itchy entry sites. Causes asthma (with lung entry), iron-deficiency anemia, and growth retardation. | Organism attaches to the small intestine and consumes red blood cells. |
| **Trichinosis** | *Trichinella spiralis* | Results from eating pork infected with larvae. Early symptoms are nausea, vomiting, and diarrhea. Late symptoms are fever, myalgias, myocarditis, and encephalitis. | Organism attaches to the small intestine. Larvae cannot mature into adults because humans are accidental hosts. |

# VI. Miscellaneous Disorders

## THE APPENDIX

| Disease | Description | Cause(s) | Pathology |
| --- | --- | --- | --- |
| Acute Appendicitis | Acute onset of mild fever, anorexia, nausea, and periumbilical abdominal pain that localizes to the right lower quadrant. Appendix must be resected. | Obstruction of appendiceal lumen by a fecal mass (fecalith). Infection with *E. coli*, *Streptococcus faecalis*, or anaerobes. | • Early appendicitis—acute inflammation of the full wall thickness with a few PMNs. Serosa looks dull and red.<br><br>• Suppurative appendicitis—many PMNs, purulent serosal exudate, perforation, necrosis, and luminal abscess formation.<br><br>• Gangrenous appendicitis—further necrosis and rupture. |

## THE PERITONEUM

| Disease | Description | Cause(s) | Pathology |
| --- | --- | --- | --- |
| Sterile Peritonitis | Severe abdominal pain, with voluntary and involuntary guarding of the abdominal muscles. Rebound tenderness from peritoneal irritation. | Chemical irritation from bile, pancreatic juices, surgical debris, blood, or ascites | Acute inflammation. |
| Peritoneal Infection | Fever in addition to the symptoms above. | Appendicitis, ruptured peptic ulcer, cholecystitis, or diverticulitis | Dull gray membrane with exudate. May cause a persistent abscess. |
| Peritoneal Tumors | Primary cancers of the peritoneum are rare (i.e., mesothelioma). The most common peritoneal neoplasm is secondary to diffuse peritoneal seeding by metastatic tumors. | | |

# CHAPTER 10
# HEPATOBILIARY SYSTEM AND THE EXOCRINE PANCREAS

I. LIVER ARCHITECTURE AND PATTERNS OF NECROSIS

II. JAUNDICE
   Mechanisms of Jaundice
   Categories of Jaundice
   Obstructive Jaundice

III. HEPATITIS, LIVER FAILURE, PORTAL HYPERTENSION, AND TUMORS
   Acute Viral Hepatitis
   Acute Hepatitis B Serology
   Recovery From Hepatitis B
   Alcoholic Hepatitis
   Other Infections of the Liver
   Chronic Hepatitis

Progression of Chronic Hepatitis
Fatty Liver
Acute Liver Failure
Liver Cirrhosis
Portal Hypertension
Hepatic Tumors

IV. GALLBLADDER DISORDERS
   Obstructive Diseases of the Gallbladder
   Other Gallbladder Diseases
   Biliary Tree and Gallbladder Cancers

V. PANCREATIC DISORDERS
   Diseases of the Exocrine Pancreas

## ABBREVIATIONS

**ALP** = alkaline phosphatase
**ALT (SGPT)** = alanine aminotransferase (serum glutamic-pyruvic transaminase)
**AST (SGOT)** = aspartate aminotransferase (serum glutamic oxaloacetic transaminase)
**GGTP** = gamma-glutamyl transpeptidase
**HBcAb** = antibody to hepatitis B core antigen
**HBeAb** = antibody to hepatitis B early antigen
**HBeAg** = hepatitis B early antigen

**HBsAb** = antibody to hepatitis B surface antigen
**HBsAg** = hepatitis B surface antigen
**HBV** = hepatitis B virus
**HCV** = hepatitis C virus
**HDV** = hepatitis D virus
**HELLP** = hemolysis, elevated liver enzymes, low platelets
**HLA** = human leukocyte antigen
**Ig** = immunoglobulin
**IV** = intravenous

## MOST COMMON Causes and Types

| Disorder | Common Cause |
|---|---|
| Liver disease | Alcoholism |
| Micronodular cirrhosis | Alcoholism |
| Macronodular cirrhosis | Hepatitis B and C |
| Chronic hepatitis | Hepatitis C |

| Disorder | Common Type |
|---|---|
| Benign liver tumor | Hemangioma |
| Primary liver malignancy | Hepatocellular carcinoma |
| Gallbladder tumor | Adenocarcinoma |
| Cholelithiasis (gallbladder stones) | Mixed cholesterol stones |
| Liver malignancy | Metastasis from breast, ovaries, and lungs |

| | |
|---|---|
| **Alcoholic Liver Disease** | Most common liver disease in the United States, consisting of hepatic steatosis, alcoholic hepatitis, and alcoholic cirrhosis. Each can exist independently or together. |
| **Aminotransferases** | Markers of hepatocellular damage.<br>• ALT (SGPT)—specific liver enzyme. ☞ Remember L in ALT stands for LIVER.<br>• AST (SGOT)—nonspecific liver enzyme<br>In alcoholic hepatitis, AST > ALT. In viral hepatitis, both increase, with AST marginally higher than ALT. |
| **Cholestasis Markers** | In the liver, ALP and GGTP are elevated with obstruction of the intrahepatic canaliculi, main hepatic ducts, common hepatic duct, or common bile duct. |
| **Hepatitis** | Inflammation of the liver from viral infection, toxins, alcohol abuse, or autoimmune processes. Acute hepatitis is often self-limited, but may become chronic (depending on the cause). Chronic hepatitis increases the risks of liver cirrhosis and failure and hepatocellular carcinoma. ☞ To remember the transmission of viral hepatitis, use "ABCDE": A and E are the Ends (mouth and anus, where water and food pass); BCD stands for BlooD acquired). |
| **Hepatomegaly** | Enlargement of the liver from heart failure (see Chapter 2), infiltration by malignancies, or hepatitis. |
| **Jaundice** | Yellowing of the skin and sclera (icterus). |
| **Liver Cirrhosis** | Irreversible liver damage that presents with portal hypertension, hematemesis from esophageal varices (caused by portal hypertension), and ascites. Increased risk for hepatocellular carcinoma. Fibrotic bands and nodules cause an enlarged liver. Persistent cycling of hepatocyte regeneration and destruction causes diffuse parenchymal disorganization, forming a small atrophic liver. |
| **Liver Failure** | Occurs after > 80% of the liver parenchyma is destroyed. Acute liver failure is caused by acute massive hepatocyte necrosis, as seen with fulminant hepatitis, toxins, drugs, and acute fatty liver change. Chronic liver failure is related to liver cirrhosis. |
| **Liver Function Tests** | Albumin and clotting factors (except factor VIII) are manufactured by the liver. Can decrease with chronic liver failure or cirrhosis. |
| **Pruritus** | Itchy skin. One cause is bile acids. For other causes, see Chapter 11. |
| **Steatosis** | Fatty change in the liver. See Chapter 1, Steatosis (Fatty Change). |

# I. Liver Architecture and Patterns of Necrosis

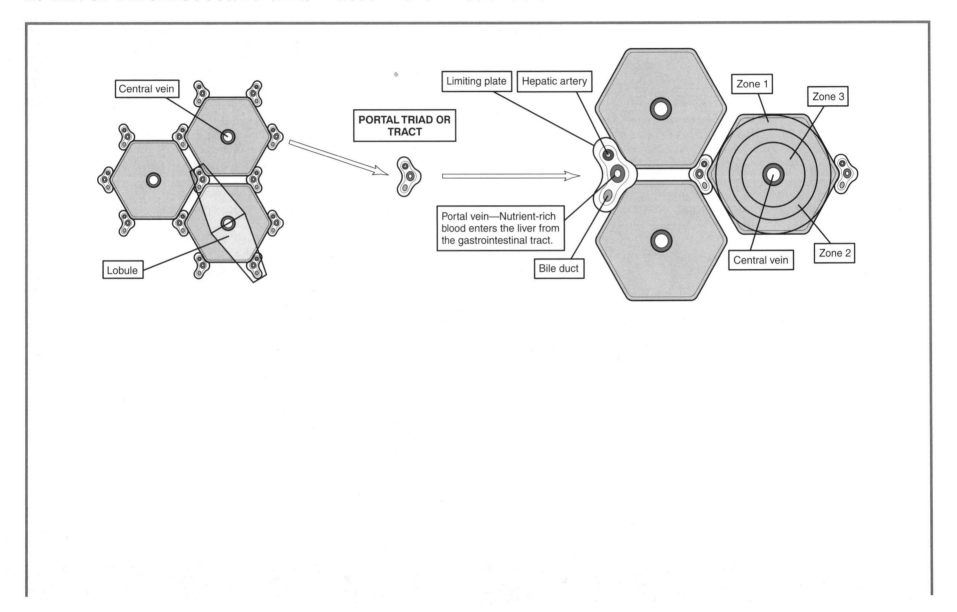

| Zone | Description and Location of Necrosis | Representative Diseases |
|---|---|---|
| 1 | Closest to the portal triads. Damage in this zone is known as peripheral zonal necrosis. | Phosphorus toxicity and eclampsia |
| 2 | Uncommonly damaged. Damage in this zone is called midzonal necrosis. | Yellow fever |
| 3 | Farthest from the portal vein and hepatic artery and closest to the central vein. Damage in this zone is known as centrilobular necrosis. | Viral hepatitis; toxicity from acetaminophen, tetracycline, carbon tetrachloride, and chloroform; alcoholic fatty liver damage; and hypoxic damage from cardiac failure or cardiogenic shock |

**Types of Liver Necrosis**

- Focal—random necrosis of single or multiple cells
- Submassive necrosis (bridging necrosis)—crosses lobular boundaries and the limiting plate includes portal to portal triad, portal to central vein, or central vein to central vein
- Massive necrosis—affects large areas of the liver, usually all three zones

# II. Jaundice

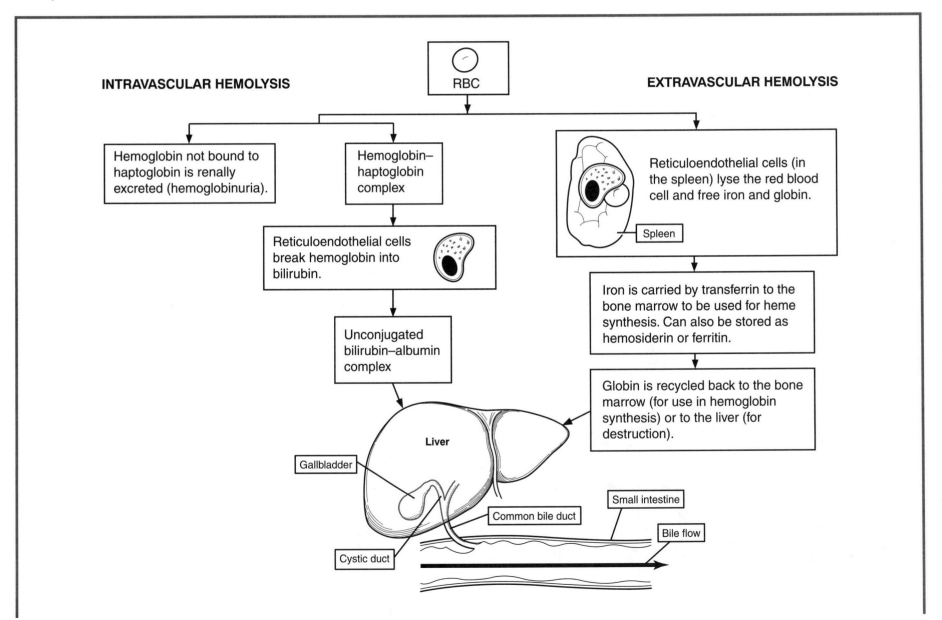

## MECHANISMS OF JAUNDICE

| Type of Bilirubin | Description | Pathology |
|---|---|---|
| Unconjugated Bilirubin | Hemoglobin is broken down into bilirubin, conjugated with glucuronic acid, secreted into bile, and stored in the gallbladder. | Excessive unconjugated bilirubin (hyperbilirubinemia) accumulates in the blood. It is stored in skin and organs but cannot be excreted in the urine (only the conjugated form is excreted). |
| Conjugated Bilirubin | Hepatic bile duct conducts bile from the liver to join with the cystic duct, forming the common bile duct. Conjugated bilirubin is both resorbed and excreted. In the colon, resident bacteria convert it to urobilinogen. | Conjugated bilirubin accumulates in the blood. It is then stored in skin (jaundice) and organs. It is excreted in urine (bilirubinuria). |

| Unconjugated Hyperbilirubinemia | Conjugated Hyperbilirubinemia |
|---|---|
| (1) Overproduction of unconjugated bilirubin as seen in intravascular hemolytic disease, transfusions, and ineffective hematopoiesis | (1) Reduced excretion of conjugated bilirubin as seen in hepatocellular damage (conjugated bilirubin escapes into the circulation from the bile ducts) |
| (2) Impaired conjugation of bilirubin by the liver as seen in Crigler-Najjar syndrome or in diffuse hepatocellular damage (poor conjugation by damaged hepatocytes) | (2) Bile flow obstruction |
| (3) Reduced liver uptake of unconjugated bilirubin as in Gilbert syndrome | |

## CATEGORIES OF JAUNDICE

| Category | ALT | AST | ALP / GGTP | Conjugated Bilirubin | Unconjugated Bilirubin | Urobilinogen in the Urine | Description | Representative Diseases |
|---|---|---|---|---|---|---|---|---|
| **Hemolytic or Iron Overload** | Normal | Normal | Normal | Normal | ↑ | ↑ | See Chapter 4. | Hemolytic anemias, thalassemia major, and multiple transfusions |
| **Hepatocellular** | ↑ | ↑ | ↑ or Normal | ↑ | ↑ | ↑ or Normal | Aminotransferases increase except in congenital conjugation disorders (see Chapter 15), in which only unconjugated bilirubin accumulates. | Acute hepatitis, cirrhosis, drug toxicity (tetracycline, salicylates), and Reye syndrome |
| **Obstructive** | Normal or ↑ | Normal or ↑ | ↑ | ↑ | Normal | ↓(complete obstruction) | See Obstructive Jaundice below. | |

# OBSTRUCTIVE JAUNDICE

| Disease | Description | Cause(s) | Pathology |
|---|---|---|---|
| **Primary Biliary Cirrhosis** | Late onset of intrahepatic obstructive jaundice, pruritus, and hypercholesterolemia. | Autoimmune mechanism | Antimitochondrial antibody is elevated, causing granulomatous reaction, inflammation, and destruction of bile canaliculi with fibrosis. |
| **Secondary Biliary Cirrhosis** | More common than primary biliary cirrhosis. Occurs with prolonged bile duct obstruction, causing early intrahepatic obstructive jaundice. Reversible until fibrosis leads to liver cirrhosis. | Obstruction from gallstones and compressive tumors (especially pancreatic head cancer) | Bile stasis in "bile lakes" (necrotic foci with acute and chronic inflammatory cells and pigment). |
| **Primary Sclerosing Cholangitis** | Rare, chronic, progressive intrahepatic and extrahepatic cholestatic disease that is associated with chronic ulcerative colitis. | Autoimmune mechanism | Inflammatory obliterative fibrosis and bile duct narrowing; bile duct onion-skin appearance. |
| **Choledochal Cyst** | Focal dilatation of the common bile duct (extrahepatic) causing jaundice, abdominal pain, and a mass. Predisposes to gallstone formation, pancreatitis, extrahepatic biliary duct adenocarcinoma, and biliary obstructions. | Unknown | Common bile duct wall is thick and fibrotic. |
| **Cholestasis of Pregnancy** | Occurs in the third trimester of pregnancy with severe pruritus and intrahepatic obstructive jaundice. Aminotransferases are mildly elevated. May cause fetal death. Jaundice reverses at the end of pregnancy. | Estrogenic hormones; altered hepatocyte bile secretion and bile metabolism | Mild intrahepatic obstruction without necrosis. |
| **Other Causes** | Other extrahepatic obstructions can be found in acute cholecystitis, ascending cholangitis, and in compressive cancers such as pancreatic carcinoma. | | |

# III. Hepatitis, Liver Failure, Portal Hypertension, and Tumors

## ACUTE VIRAL HEPATITIS

| Type of Hepatitis | Causative Virus and Description of Disease | Mode of Transmission |
| --- | --- | --- |
| | Anicteric hepatitis (the most common presentation) causes a flulike illness without jaundice. Other symptoms may include acute onset of fever, vomiting, jaundice, and tender hepatomegaly. All viral hepatitis involves diffuse hepatocyte swelling, focal hepatocyte necrosis (Councilman bodies—coagulated pink cytoplasm and nuclear pyknosis), inflammatory infiltrate, and regenerating hepatocytes. Submassive or massive necrosis may occur (see Figure: Liver Architecture and Patterns of Necrosis above). Infrequently may become fulminant hepatitis, with acute liver failure and a high mortality rate. If patient recovers, liver completely regenerates itself. | |
| Hepatitis A | Picornavirus—RNA. Mild, self-limited illness that is most infectious before the onset of jaundice. No chronic state exists. | Fecal-oral route. Virus is found in contaminated water, milk, or shellfish. |
| Hepatitis B | Hepadnavirus—DNA. Asymptomatic to severe. Disease may progress to a chronic state, but most patients recover. There is a risk for hepatocellular carcinoma and cirrhosis if disease progresses to the chronic state. | Infants congenitally infected are often chronic carriers. May be passed by blood (transfusions or IV drug use), by sexual intercourse, or tattoos. |
| Hepatitis C | Flavivirus—RNA. Presentation is similar to above, but 50% of cases become chronic (most common cause of chronic hepatitis). Greater risk for hepatocellular carcinoma and liver cirrhosis (20%). | Blood transfusions, IV drug use, or renal dialysis. |
| Hepatitis D | Hepatitis delta virus—RNA. Occurs with hepatitis B (needs HBV viral envelope to replicate). Increases the severity of both the acute and chronic states. | Blood transfusions and IV drug use. |
| Hepatitis E | Calicivirus—RNA. Uncommon, mild, self-limited illness. See Hepatitis A above. | See Hepatitis A above. |

## ACUTE HEPATITIS B SEROLOGY

Acute infection is suggested by rising HBsAg or HBcAb (IgM).

Resolution of the acute phase is suggested by a falling HBsAg titer and rising HBcAb titer. (Also see Figure: Recovery From Hepatitis B.)

Recovery is suggested by rising HBsAb.

Chronic infection is suggested by persistence of HBsAg.

| Serology | Description | Serology | Description |
|---|---|---|---|
| HBsAg | First serology to be detected. | HBsAb (Anti-HBs) | Indicates recovery and immunity. |
| HBcAb (Anti-HBc) | IgM marks acute infection or window period. IgG is present with resolution and recovery. | Window Period | Period in which HBcAb is elevated but HBsAg (already declined) and HBsAb (not yet formed) are undetectable. |
| HBeAg | Indicates infectious state. Absence does not mean non-infectivity. | HBeAb | Indicates resolving hepatitis and reduced infectivity. |

## RECOVERY FROM HEPATITIS B

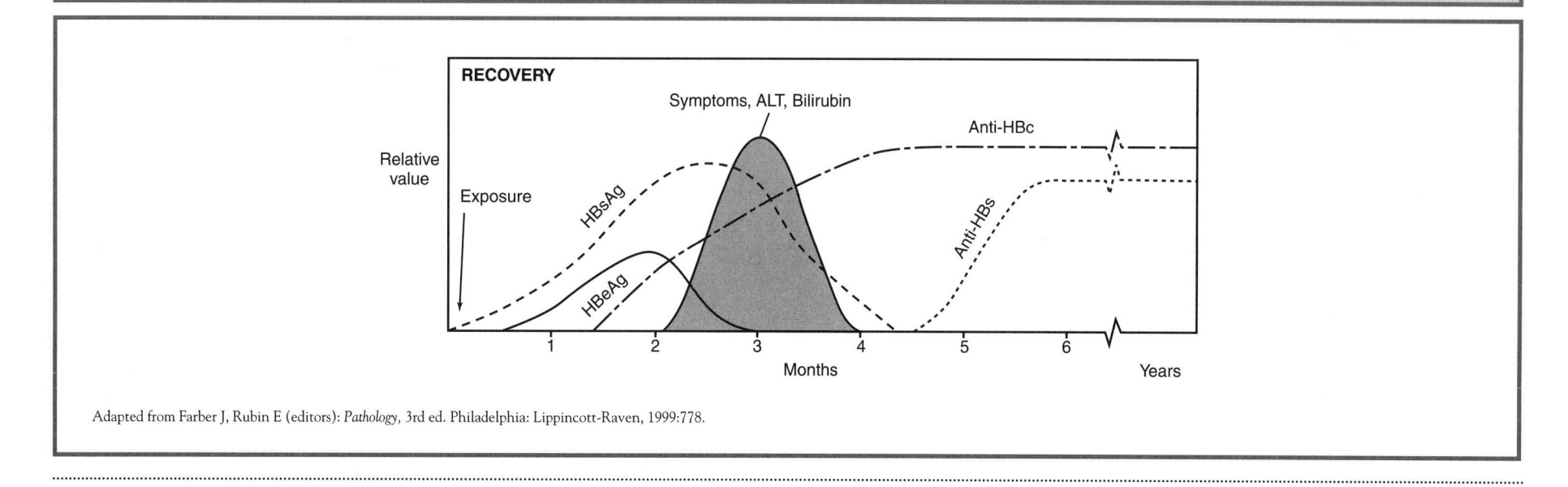

Adapted from Farber J, Rubin E (editors): *Pathology*, 3rd ed. Philadelphia: Lippincott-Raven, 1999:778.

## ALCOHOLIC HEPATITIS

| Disease | Description | Pathology |
|---|---|---|
| **Alcoholic Hepatitis** | Acute onset of fever, jaundice, tender hepatomegaly, and ascites after a bout of heavy drinking. Symptoms resolve with the cessation of drinking, but the liver damage is cumulative. Characteristically, AST > ALT. Also see Liver Cirrhosis below for alcoholic cirrhosis. | Focal hepatocyte necrosis with infiltration by polymorphonuclear leukocytes, sclerosis around the central venules, and intracytoplasmic waxy hyaline Mallory bodies |

## OTHER INFECTIONS OF THE LIVER

| Disease | Causation and Description | Pathology |
|---|---|---|
| **Other Viral Hepatitis** | Herpes simplex virus type 1 or 2, cytomegalovirus, and Epstein-Barr virus may cause hepatitis in immunocompromised patients and in infants (congenital). | See Chapter 15, Congenital Infections. |
| **Yellow Fever** | Caused by a bacterium, *Leptospira*, and transmitted by rats, dogs, pigs, and cattle. Patients may present with jaundice. | Infected hepatocytes appear as Councilman bodies (see Acute Viral Hepatitis above). |
| ***Echinococcus granulosus*** | Accidental ingestion of tapeworm causes hydatid cysts in the liver. Cysts become calcified. | Large cysts with walls that contain a germinal layer from which the larvae grow. |
| **Schistosomiasis** | Infection with *Schistosoma*. Adult worms live and produce eggs in the intestinal portal venous plexus. | Granulomas form around eggs, producing scarring and possible portal hypertension. |
| **Hepatic Amebiasis** | Complication of primary *Entamoeba histolytica* intestinal infection. They reach the liver via the portal vein, causing amebic hepatitis. | Amebic microabscesses and focal hepatocyte necrosis may be seen. Abscesses are filled with liquefied liver and ameboid trophozoites. |

## CHRONIC HEPATITIS

| Disease | Description | Cause(s) | Pathology |
|---|---|---|---|
| **Chronic Viral Hepatitis** | Patients may be asymptomatic or experience fatigue, anorexia, intermittent jaundice, and elevated ALT and AST. Death may occur from liver cirrhosis, chronic liver failure, portal hypertension, or hepatocellular carcinoma. (See Figure: Progression of Chronic Hepatitis below.) | | |
| | Healthy carrier state is asymptomatic. | HCV (most common cause), HBV, and HDV (only with concurrent HBV infection) | No inflammatory changes. HBsAg is positive. |
| | Minimal chronic hepatitis (previously called chronic persistent hepatitis) produces minimal symptoms. | | Inflammation is limited to the portal triad with an intact limiting plate. No active hepatocyte necrosis. |
| | Progressive disease (previously called chronic active hepatitis) is the active infectious disease. | | Inflammation progresses past the limiting plate with hepatocyte necrosis. Hepatocytes at the lobule periphery undergo piecemeal necrosis (most common finding). May show bridging necrosis (see Figure: Liver Architecture and Patterns of Necrosis above). May lead to post-necrotic cirrhosis of the liver. |
| **Autoimmune Hepatitis** | Progressive disease similar clinically to chronic active hepatitis. Lupoid hepatitis (autoimmune chronic active hepatitis) is associated with rheumatoid arthritis, Hashimoto thyroiditis, Sjögren disease, and ulcerative colitis. | Autoimmune mechanism | Antimitochondrial antibody, anti–smooth muscle antibody, or antinuclear antibody. Necrosis is similar to that in chronic active hepatitis. |
| **Other Causes of Chronic Hepatitis** | Hepatitis plus disease-specific symptoms. | Wilson disease, use of isoniazid, and $\alpha_1$-antitrypsin deficiency | Pathology is similar to that of viral hepatitis. |

## PROGRESSION OF CHRONIC HEPATITIS

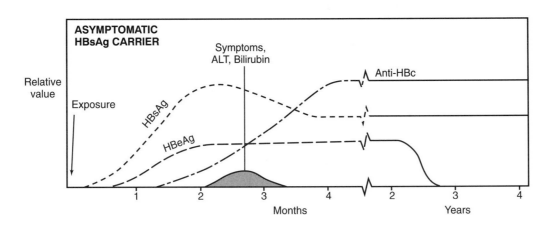

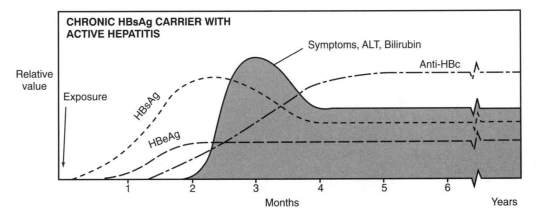

Adapted from Farber J, Rubin E (editors): *Pathology*, 3rd ed. Philadelphia: Lippincott-Raven, 1999:778.

## FATTY LIVER

| Disease | Description | Pathology |
|---|---|---|
| **Alcoholic Hepatic Steatosis** | Most patients are asymptomatic. May or may not cause mild elevation of serum bilirubin and alkaline phosphatase. | Hepatic steatosis (microvesicular, then macrovesicular changes). Enlarged fatty liver. Steatosis results from increased hepatocyte accumulation of lipids. Alcohol disrupts mitochondrial function and allows free-radical damage. |
| **Other Causes of Fatty Liver** | Can also be caused by Reye syndrome, acute fatty liver of pregnancy, tetracycline overdose, and Wilson disease. Also see Chapter 1, Figure: Steatosis. | |

## ACUTE LIVER FAILURE

| Condition | Description | Pathology |
|---|---|---|
| **Reye Syndrome** | Occurs mainly in children, with acute liver failure and encephalopathy. Associated with aspirin use during viral infections (chickenpox or influenza). | Microvesicular fatty change of the liver, heart, and kidneys. |
| **Liver Failure of Pregnancy** | Occurs in the third trimester of pregnancy. Risk of fetal and maternal mortality with severe preeclampsia and eclampsia unless pregnancy is terminated. | Eclampsia can cause renal cortical necrosis and liver periportal necrosis. In HELLP syndrome, hepatocyte necrosis and fibrin deposition occur. Also see Chapter 7, Diseases of Gestation. |
| | Preeclampsia—hypertension, proteinuria, and peripheral edema. Eclampsia—convulsions and coma in addition to preeclamptic signs. HELLP syndrome (hemolysis, elevated liver enzymes, and low platelets) presents with nausea, vomiting, and abdominal pain, and indicates liver disease seen with severe preeclampsia or eclampsia. | |
| | Acute fatty liver of pregnancy can cause nausea, vomiting, jaundice, abdominal pain, disseminated intravascular coagulation, hyperbilirubinemia, and even coma or death. High association with preeclampsia. | Microvesicular fatty liver change. |
| **Tetracycline Toxicity** | Unpredictable hypersensitivity reaction that can result in acute liver failure. | Microvesicular fatty liver change. |

# LIVER CIRRHOSIS

| Type | Description | Cause(s) | Pathology |
|------|-------------|----------|-----------|
| **Micronodular Cirrhosis** | Alcoholic cirrhosis—most common type of liver cirrhosis (30–60% of all cirrhosis). Condition progresses with continued drinking. Damage is irreversible. | Chronic alcohol abuse. | Micronodular pattern (nodules < 3 mm). Fibrous bands span the liver parenchyma. Regenerating nodules appear (abnormal masses of hepatocytes completely surrounded by fibrosis). |
| | Biliary cirrhosis—slowly progressing disease of the bile ducts. Prolonged cholestasis causes late liver failure. Also see Obstructive Jaundice—Biliary Cirrhosis above. | Primary: caused by portal fibrosis. Secondary: caused by large bile duct obstruction. | Regenerating nodules are present once liver cirrhosis develops. |
| | Hemochromatosis—excessive accumulation of iron (5% of all cirrhosis). Can cause liver cirrhosis, secondary diabetes mellitus, cardiomyopathy, skin color change (bronze), arthritis, hypopituitarism, or Addison disease. Highest risk for hepatocellular carcinoma. | Primary: inherited increase in iron absorption. Associated with HLA-A3. Secondary: iron overload, as with multiple transfusions, alcoholic cirrhosis, and chronic hemolytic anemias. | Hemosiderin deposits in hepatocytes and Kupffer cells. Prussian blue stains positive for iron. |
| | Galactosemia—rapidly progressive liver failure, mental retardation, and cataracts in children. Prevented with a milk-free diet. See Chapter 14, Diet-Related Disorders. | Inherited metabolic disorder. | Cholestasis and fatty change are seen in addition to liver cirrhosis. |
| | $\alpha_1$-Antitrypsin deficiency (rare cause of cirrhosis)—abnormal antitrypsin molecules accumulate in the liver. Also causes lung emphysema (see Chapter 5). | Pathogenesis is unknown. Occurs in homozygous PiZZ individuals. | Abnormal antitrypsin molecules appear as eosinophilic globules in hepatocyte cytoplasm. Stain red with periodic acid–Schiff and are diastase resistant. |
| **Macronodular Cirrhosis** | Results from chronic viral hepatitis (10–30% of all cirrhosis). Progression is rapid. | HCV (most common cause) or HBV with or without HDV. | Patchwork of variably sized nodules separated by broad septal scars. Impossible to tell the etiology of the cirrhosis by pathology alone. |
| | Autoimmune chronic active hepatitis (10% of all cirrhosis). | Autoimmune mechanism. | |
| | Wilson disease—acute hepatitis or Parkinson-like extrapyramidal symptoms. Kayser-Fleischer ring is found (copper deposition around the cornea). | Autosomal recessive disorder with poor bile excretion of copper. | Copper deposition in hepatocytes causes fatty liver change and hepatocyte necrosis. Chronic deposition causes cirrhosis. |

## PORTAL HYPERTENSION

Resistance to portal blood flow is due to 1 of 3 mechanisms:
- Posthepatic a functional obstruction in the inferior vena cava can occur if the right ventricle can no longer accept returning blood from the liver as in right ventricle failure or constrictive pericarditis. Thrombosis of the hepatic veins or inferior vena cava also causes an obstruction, called Budd-Chiari syndrome. Obstruction can also result from hepatocellular carcinoma.

- Intrahepatic (most common cause) obstruction in the vascular sinusoids, creates arteriovenous fistulas. Can also be caused by liver cirrhosis.

- Prehepatic obstruction of the portal vein by thrombosis, cancer, or inflammation. Can also occur with biliary cirrhosis.

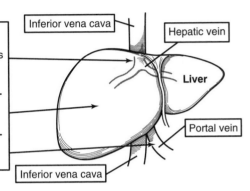

**Consequences:**

- Portosystemic—venous blood flow bypasses the portal circulation—engorged and dilated systemic veins form around the esophagus (esophageal varices), rectum (hemorrhoids), and umbilicus (caput medusae). Entry of "nondetoxified" portal blood into the systemic circulation may cause hepatic encephalopathy.

- Ascites—from increased hydrostatic pressure across the peritoneal membrane. If portal hypertension is due to cirrhosis, then hypoalbuminemia may contribute to the edema. See Chapter 1 for edema.

- Congestive splenomegaly—drainage from the splenic vein into the portal system is obstructed. Results in a large, blood-filled spleen.

## HEPATIC TUMORS

| Disease | Description | Causes | Pathology |
|---|---|---|---|
| **Benign Tumors** | | | |
| **Hemangioma** | Most common benign primary liver tumor. Asymptomatic; found incidentally on abdominal X-rays, during surgery, or at autopsy. | Unknown | Cavernous hemangioma. See Chapter 2, Primary Vascular Tumors or Tumorlike Conditions—Hemangioma. |
| **Adenoma** | Rare solitary or multiple tumor. Asymptomatic unless a mass or abdominal pain is felt. May rupture and bleed. If caused by steroid use, tumor may regress once steroids are withdrawn. | Male anabolic steroid use; female oral contraceptive use | Benign hepatocytes arranged into thick cords. No bile ducts or portal tracts within these cords. |
| **Malignant Tumors** | Along with biliary tree cancers, malignant hepatic tumors are responsible for 14,500 cases and 13,600 deaths per year in the United States. They are the seventh most common cause of cancer mortality in men and the ninth most common cause overall. | | |
| **Hepatocellular Carcinoma** | Also known as hepatoma. The most common primary liver malignancy. Causes weight loss, abdominal pain, hepatomegaly, and increasing ascites. Up to 90% of patients have elevated serum $\alpha$-fetoprotein. The tumor can secrete erythropoietin. Metastasizes early via the lymphatics; prognosis is poor. | Common in Asia and Africa. Liver cirrhosis due to alcoholic cirrhosis (most common cause in the United States), HBV (most common cause worldwide), hemochromatosis, HCV, or aflatoxin B. | Yellow-green tumor. If well differentiated, bile pigment and sinusoids are seen. If poorly differentiated, anaplastic cells with mitotic figures are seen. |
| **Cholangiocarcinoma** | An intrahepatic bile duct tumor that rarely occurs in the United States or Europe. Presents as a liver mass. Slow progression to metastasis. | Liver fluke: *Clonorchis sinensis* | Pale gray tumor. Adenocarcinoma with mucin production. |
| **Hemangiosarcoma** | Rare vascular tumor. Appears as a rapidly growing liver mass. | Polyvinyl chloride and thorium exposure | Solid, large, hemorrhagic mass. Tumor consists of vascular spaces lined by malignant endothelium. |
| **Metastatic Tumors** | Most common cause of liver malignancy. Metastases are most commonly seen from breast, gastrointestinal tract, lung cancer, and malignant melanoma. | | |

# IV. Gallbladder Disorders

## OBSTRUCTIVE DISEASES OF THE GALLBLADDER

| Disease | Symptoms | Associated Conditions | Mechanism | Pathology |
|---|---|---|---|---|
| **Cholelithiasis (Gallstones)** | Asymptomatic. | Diabetes and liver cirrhosis | Cholesterol: cholesterol concentration is greater than the bile salts necessary to dissolve it. Pigment: precipitation of unconjugated bilirubin calcium salts. | Two kinds of stones: cholesterol (most common) and pigment. |
| **Biliary Colic** | Nausea, vomiting, and epigastric abdominal pain 1–2 hours after eating. Pain remits once the stone has become disimpacted. | Female gender, age > 40 years, obesity, and previous pregnancies | Temporary obstruction of the cystic or common bile duct. Gallbladder contracts and stone becomes impacted. | No permanent changes. |
| **Acute Cholecystitis** | Fever, nausea, vomiting, right upper-quadrant pain, and a palpable gallbladder. May cause mild jaundice. | Previous bouts of biliary colic | Stone impaction. Concentrated bile is very inflammatory. Bile may become infected with coliform bacteria (i.e., *Escherichia coli*). | Inflamed, congested gallbladder with wall thickening and edema. May see mucosal ulcerations. Distended cystic duct. |
| **Ascending Cholangitis** | Charcot triad: fever, intermittent right upper-quadrant pain, and jaundice. May cause pancreatitis from gallstone impaction in the pancreatic duct. | Previous bouts of biliary colic; gallstone impaction (common bile duct = choledocholithiasis) | Bile duct obstruction allows bile stasis and proliferation of coliform bacteria. | Infection of intrahepatic biliary ducts. |

## OTHER GALLBLADDER DISEASES

| Disease | Description | Pathology |
|---|---|---|
| **Chronic Cholecystitis** | Vague abdominal pain or intermittent indigestion, with occasional bouts of biliary colic. Intolerance of fatty foods. Most common complication is acute cholecystitis. | Extensive fibrosis and thickening of the gallbladder wall, possibly with wall calcifications. If extensive, may see a calcified "porcelain gallbladder," which predisposes to gallbladder carcinoma. Rokitansky-Aschoff sinuses are outpocketings of mucosa. Condition may be associated with cholesterolosis. |
| **Cholesterolosis** | Also called a strawberry gallbladder. Not inflammatory and, by itself, it has no clinical importance. | Yellow cholesterol pockets are seen on the mucosal surface of the gallbladder and resemble the seeds of a strawberry. Foamy macrophages are seen in the mucosa. |

## BILIARY TREE AND GALLBLADDER CANCERS

See Hepatic Tumors above for statistics.

| Disease | Description | Associated Conditions | Pathology |
|---|---|---|---|
| **Adenocarcinoma of the Gallbladder** | Most common tumor of the gallbladder. Asymptomatic unless disease is advanced. Patients may present with weight loss or a palpable gallbladder. If tumor penetrates the gallbladder wall, the prognosis is very poor. | Gallstones (80%) and chronic cholecystitis | Polypoid or infiltrating mass of the gallbladder wall. Adenocarcinoma. |
| **Adenocarcinoma of the Extrahepatic Biliary Ducts** | Occurs at the ampulla of Vater (most common), common bile duct, or near the liver (Klatskin tumor). Causes early progressive obstructive jaundice and a palpable, enlarged gallbladder (from obstruction of the common bile duct). | Choledochal cysts, ulcerative colitis, or chronic fluke or *Giardia* infection | Slow-growing, well-differentiated adenocarcinoma. |

# V. Pancreatic Disorders

## DISEASES OF THE EXOCRINE PANCREAS

| Disease | Description | Predisposing Factors | Pathology |
|---|---|---|---|
| **Acute Pancreatitis** | Causes severe pain in the upper abdomen radiating toward the back, vomiting, mild jaundice, and shock. Serum amylase and lipase (specific) are elevated. | Associated with alcoholism and gallstones (70–80%), hypercalcemia (10%), hyperlipidemia, thiazides, and steroids | Pancreatic enzymes are released into the parenchyma and surrounding tissues. Massive inflammation causes hemorrhage and thrombosis. Coagulative necrosis leads to liquefied parenchyma, fat, and omentum digestion. Peritoneal effusion contains high amylase levels. |
| **Chronic Relapsing Pancreatitis** | Causes constant or intermittent severe abdominal pain, vomiting, attacks of acute pancreatitis, pancreatic insufficiency, malabsorption, and weight loss. May cause diabetes mellitus in 30% of patients. | Chronic alcoholism (40%), gallstones (20%), acute pancreatitis | Progressive parenchymal fibrosis causes atrophy. In end-stage disease, acini cannot be distinguished from extensive fibrosis. Ducts are dilated. Islets may or may not be involved. |
| **Pancreatic Adenocarcinoma** | Responsible for 28,600 cases and 28,600 deaths per year in the United States; the fifth most common cause of cancer mortality. Patients present in their 50s with common bile duct obstruction or chronic pancreatitis (if it is a pancreatic head tumor). Body and tail tumors present late. Paraneoplastic Trousseau sign may be seen (superficial migratory leg vein thrombophlebitis). | Diabetes in women (6×), smoking (5×), K-ras oncogene | Tumors usually occur in the head of the pancreas (70%). Hard infiltrative mass obstructs the pancreatic duct. Poorly differentiated adenocarcinoma with fibrosis. Metastasizes early and prognosis is poor. |

# CHAPTER 11
# THE SKIN

I. RASHES

Immune-Mediated Rashes

Rashes of Uncertain
Pathogenesis

Pigmented Lesions

Sunlight-Caused Lesions

II. SKIN INFECTIONS

Bacterial Skin Infections

Viral Skin Infections

Superficial Fungal Skin
Infections

Arthropod-Caused Skin
Infections

Desquamation Syndromes

III. SKIN GROWTHS

Skin Cysts

Benign Skin Tumors

Premalignant and Malignant
Skin Tumors

**ABBREVIATIONS**

**HSV** = herpes simplex virus

**Ig** = immunoglobulin

**PMN** = polymorphonuclear leukocytes

## MOST COMMON Causes and Types

| Disorder | Common Cause |
|----------|--------------|
| Malignant skin tumor | Basal cell carcinoma |
| Skin infection | Bacterial pathogens (*Staphylococcus* and *Streptococcus*) |

| Disorder | Common Type |
|----------|-------------|
| Malignant melanoma | Superficial spreading |

## TERMS TO LEARN

| | |
|--|--|
| Acantholysis | Epidermal cell separation resulting in a vesicle or bullae. |
| Acanthosis | Thickening of the stratum Malpighi (basal, squamous, and granular layers). |
| Bulla (Blister) | Elevated, thin-walled, fluid-filled lesion of > 5 mm. Seen in eczematous dermatitis. |
| Crust | Dried exudate after seeping from a bulla, vesicle, or pustule. |
| Cyst | Nodule filled with semisolid material. |
| Eczema | Also known as eczematous dermatitis, or simply dermatitis. Superficial skin inflammation. |
| Erosion | Shallow wound created by partial or complete epidermal loss. No dermal loss. |
| Erythema | Skin redness from dilated capillaries in the dermis. Blanches when compressed. Seen in cellulitis. |
| Excoriation | Linear deep scratch. |
| Hyperkeratosis | Thickened stratum corneum. |

| | |
|---|---|
| Lichenification | Thickened skin with accentuation of skin markings, as seen in atopic dermatitis. |
| Macule | Small, circumscribed, colored flat lesion. |
| Melanoma | Malignant pigmented skin lesion, with two types of growth patterns:<br><br>• Radial growth—growth is confined within the epidermis and dermal papillae. Metastasis is rare. The longer this phase lasts, the better the prognosis.<br><br>• Vertical growth—grows into the deep dermis. Prognosis is based on the thickness of invasion. See Premalignant and Malignant Skin Tumors below for melanoma. |
| Nevus | Congenital or acquired skin tumor. See Chapter 15, Rashes and Skin Lesions—Birthmarks. |
| Nodule | Elevated, indurated firm lesion of > 5 mm. |
| Papule | Elevated solid lesion of ≤ 5 mm. Seen with insect bites. |
| Parakeratosis | Keratinocytes retain their nuclei in the stratum corneum. |
| Patch | Circumscribed, colored flat lesion of > 5 mm with surface changes such as scaling. |
| Plaque | Elevated, flattened lesion of > 5 mm. |
| Pruritus | Itchy skin. |
| Purpura | Black-purple skin lesion from bleeding in the dermis. Does not blanch when compressed. Seen with vasculitis. |
| Pustule | Elevated, pus-filled lesion, commonly seen in acne. |
| Scale | Area of whitish exfoliating flakes on a thickened stratum corneum. Seen in psoriasis and fungal skin infections. |
| Spongiosis | Epidermal edema that results in vesicle or bullae formation. |
| Ulceration | Deep wound with loss of entire epidermis and part or all of the dermis. |
| Verrucae or Wart | Small nodular skin growth with a rough surface, often caused by viruses. |
| Wheal | Itchy, red, and indurated plaque, commonly seen in hives. Dermal process. |

# I. Rashes

## IMMUNE-MEDIATED RASHES

| Disease | Description | Pathology |
|---|---|---|
| **Acute Rashes** | | |
| Urticaria | Also known as hives. Presents within minutes of contact with the responsible allergen. Pruritic wheal and flare (central clearing) reaction that resolves within 24 hours. Associated with anaphylaxis (see Chapter 3), asthma, and hay fever. | IgE-mediated mast cell degranulation with histamine release. Results in dermal edema. |
| Acute Allergic Contact Dermatitis | After antigen sensitization, reexposure causes pruritic, vesicular, oozing, erythematous skin patch(es), with later crusting. Linear patches are commonly seen with poison ivy. In recent years, latex has been known to cause this reaction. | Cell-mediated type IV hypersensitivity. Dermal and epidermal involvement; spongiosis. |
| **Chronic Rashes** | | |
| Chronic Allergic Contact Dermatitis | Constant exposure results in well-demarcated patches of lichenification. Shape of the patch resembles the area of chronic contact (eg, watchband, ring, necklace, or bracelet). | Type IV hypersensitivity. Dermal edema and epidermal skin changes. |
| Atopic Dermatitis | Associated with a family history of allergies, asthma, or hay fever. Erythematous pruritic plaques appear in a characteristic distribution, commonly on the flexor surfaces of the elbows and knees. | Spongiosis. |
| Psoriasis | Affects up to 1% of the population. Recurrent disease of nonpruritic red papules or plaques covered by silvery scales. Involves the elbows, knees, scalp, and nails. Auspitz sign is pinpoint bleeding when a scale is removed. | Increased rate of cell turnover. May see acanthosis, hyperkeratosis, and parakeratosis. |
| Lupus | Immune complex deposition limited to skin lesions in discoid lupus erythematosus. Skin component in systemic lupus erythematosus is a characteristic malar rash on the face that resembles a butterfly. Also see Chapter 3. | Granular immunofluorescence pattern along the dermal–epidermal junction. Dermal perivascular lymphocytic infiltrate. |

| | | |
|---|---|---|
| **Pemphigus Vulgaris** | Affects the skin and oral mucosa in patients in their 30s to 60s. IgG antibodies against intercellular cement substance of the keratinocytes are found in the serum. Large bullae easily burst, leaving raw, tender, eroded skin. Positive Nikolsky's sign (skin moves with lateral traction). Fatal within a year without treatment. | Linear immunofluorescence around epidermal cells. Acantholysis is seen within the epidermis. Separation occurs within the epidermis. |
| **Bullous Pemphigoid** | Benign disorder affecting the skin in patients in their 60s to 80s. Large, tense bullae and negative Nikolsky's sign. IgG antibodies against the basement membrane are present. Separation of the basal cells from the dermis. | Linear immunofluorescence in basement membrane. Large subepidermal bullae are found with fluid rich in eosinophils. |
| **Dermatitis Herpetiformis** | Patients are in their 20s to 40s. Recurrent pruritic vesicles on the elbows, knees, scalp, and upper back. Associated with a high-gluten diet and may be seen together with celiac disease. IgA deposits in dermal papillae of the dermal–epidermal junction are responsible for the separation. | Dermal papillary microabscesses with PMNs and nuclear dust (disintegrating PMN nuclear material). |

## RASHES OF UNCERTAIN PATHOGENESIS

| Disorder | Description | Causes | Pathology |
|---|---|---|---|
| **Erythema Multiforme** | Minor form—self-limited, benign disorder that presents with macules, papules, vesicles, or characteristic target lesions (red papule with a central clearing)<br><br>Major form (Stevens-Johnson syndrome)—high fever, bullae, rash, skin and mucosal ulceration. May cause target lesions. May be fatal (15%). | Drugs, infections, or connective tissue disorders | Subepidermal bullae due to epidermal necrosis. Dermal edema and vasculitis may also be seen. |
| **Erythema Nodosum** | Most common type of panniculitis (fat inflammation). Painful subcutaneous red nodules, most commonly on the anterior tibial region. Remits in 3–4 weeks without scarring. | Idiopathic (most common), drugs, infections such as tuberculosis, fungi, leprosy, streptococci, sarcoidosis, acute rheumatic fever, and certain cancers | Early, edema and PMNs; then lymphocytic infiltration of the septa between subcutaneous fat lobules. |

## PIGMENTED LESIONS

| Disease | Description | Pathology |
|---------|-------------|-----------|
| Albinism | Complete absence of pigmentation in the skin and eyes. May be X-linked or autosomal recessive. | No melanin production by melanocytes. May be related to inability to convert tyrosine to dihydroxyphenylalanine (precursor to melanin). |
| Vitiligo | Loss of pigmentation in irregularly shaped macules or patches, particularly evident in dark-skinned individuals. Associated with Graves disease and Addison disease. | Loss of melanocytes in affected areas. Melanin production is normal. Mechanism is either autoimmune destruction by antibodies or melanocyte destruction by toxic metabolites. |
| Freckles | Also known as ephelis (plural: ephelides). Brown hyperpigmentation macules associated with sun exposure. Fade in winter and with puberty. Melasma (chloasma or facial hyperpigmentation) is associated with pregnancy and fades postpartum. | Normal melanocyte number. Increased melanin pigment in basal keratinocytes. |
| Lentigo | Common in infancy. In the geriatric population, also known as liver spots. Pigmented macules in the skin and mucosa that do not darken with sun exposure. | Linear hyperplasia of melanocytes in the basal cell layer of the skin. |
| Other Lesions | Also see Chapter 15, Rashes and Skin Lesions, for nevus; and Premalignant and Malignant Skin Tumors below for melanoma. | |

## SUNLIGHT-CAUSED LESIONS

| | | |
|---|---|---|
| Freckles | Melasma | Squamous cell carcinoma |
| Actinic keratosis | Basal cell carcinoma | Malignant melanoma |

# II. Skin Infections

## BACTERIAL SKIN INFECTIONS

| Disease | Description | Cause(s) | Pathology |
|---------|-------------|----------|-----------|
| Folliculitis | Usually appears on the face and trunk. Causes pain, swelling, and erythema around the hair shaft. Furuncle ("boil") is a small abscess around the hair shaft. Around the eyelash, it is known as a sty (hordeolum). In diabetes mellitus, furuncle may progress to a carbuncle (deeper abscess). | *Staphylococcus aureus* | Acute inflammation with PMNs. |
| Acne Vulgaris | Affects adolescents. Comedones are open ("blackhead") or closed ("whitehead"). Blackheads appear black because of oxidized keratin. Whiteheads can become inflammatory if they rupture, resulting in painful, swollen, red pustules. | *Propionibacterium acnes* | Plugged-up hair shaft with debris (keratin and sebaceous materials). Degraded debris eventually causes local inflammation. |
| Cellulitis | Irregular shaped, painful, swollen, hot patch with indurated borders. May be accompanied by fever and positive blood cultures. Acquired from minor skin trauma or lymphedema (damaged lymphatics). | Group A streptococcus (*S. pyogenes*) or *S. aureus*. *Haemophilus influenzae* seen in unimmunized children. | Subcutaneous infection with acute inflammation. |
| | Necrotizing cellulitis—severe cellulitis that can present as either Ludwig angina (soft neck tissue) or Fournier gangrene (scrotum). | Anaerobes | |
| | Erysipelas—cellulitis of the face or scalp. Well-demarcated, swollen, hot, red rash with a fever. | *S. pyogenes* | |
| | Infectious gangrene—cellulitis with extensive necrosis of the skin and underlying subcutaneous tissues. | *Clostridium perfringens*, *S. aureus*, and *S. pyogenes* | |
| Necrotizing Fasciitis | Deep infection in subcutaneous tissue with destruction of fascia, nerves, and muscle. Fever, toxic and hemorrhagic bullous rash, anesthesia (areas of numbness), and crepitus (gas in tissue). Usually seen in the setting of diabetes mellitus. | *C. perfringens* and group A β-hemolytic streptococci | Coagulative necrosis of nerves, fascia, and muscles, called myonecrosis. |
| Leprosy | Anesthetic depigmented macules in tuberculoid leprosy. Anesthetic skin nodules in lepromatous leprosy (widespread disease). Also see Chapter 13, Peripheral Neuropathies. | *Mycobacterium leprae* | In tuberculoid form, macules contain sparse bacteria. In lepromatous form, nodules are filled with bacteria. |
| Syphilis | Sexually transmitted infection with skin lesions. See Chapter 15, Congenital Infections; and Chapter 7, Comparison of Sexually Transmitted Infections. | *Treponema pallidum* | See Chapter 7. |

## VIRAL SKIN INFECTIONS

| Disease | Description | Cause | Pathology |
|---|---|---|---|
| Verrucae Vulgaris | Common wart, frequently occurring on the palm. Gray-white to brown papular growth with a rough surface. Transmitted by direct skin contact. Also see Chapter 7, Comparison of Sexually Transmitted Infections—Human Papillomavirus, for condyloma acuminatum (genital warts). | Human papillomavirus | Benign squamous papilloma that contains koilocytes (infected, vacuolated stratum granulosum cells) |
| Molluscum Contagiosum | Seen in children. Umbilicated, dome-shaped papules that heal spontaneously. Transmitted by direct skin contact. | Poxvirus | Epidermis dips into the dermis. Epidermal cells contain inclusion bodies (molluscum bodies). |
| Herpes Zoster (Shingles) | For primary infection, see Chapter 15, Rashes and Skin Lesions. Reactivates in patients in their 50s or if immuno-compromised. Herpes zoster is reactivation of varicella zoster virus. Causes painful vesicular lesions along a skin dermatome(s) supplied by the infected ganglion. Vesicular fluid contains the virus. | Varicella zoster virus | Epidermal cells contain inclusion bodies. May see giant cells. Vesicle undergoes necrosis and ulceration. |
| Herpes Labialis and Genital Herpes | Type 1 infects the oral mucosa. Type 2 infects the genital mucosa (sexually transmitted). Primary lesions are self-limited, severely ulcerative lesions. Recurrences: for HSV 1, see Chapter 9, Oral Cavity Lesions; for HSV 2, see Chapter 7, Comparison of Sexually Transmitted Infections. | HSV I and HSV II | |

See Chapter 15, Skin Infections, for pediatric rashes associated with measles, rubella, roseola, and hand-foot-mouth disease.

## SUPERFICIAL FUNGAL SKIN INFECTIONS

| Disease | Symptoms and Area Affected | Cause or Pathology |
|---|---|---|
| Tinea | Tinea (ringworm) is caused by dermatophytic fungi that infect the keratin of the stratum corneum, hair, and nails. All lesions appear as pruritic or painful, red, crusting, well-circumscribed plaques. | *Trichophyton*, *Epidermophyton*, and *Microsporum* are involved. |
| Tinea Capitis | Infects the scalp and causes balding patches with red, crusting scales. | Lesions are infected with fungus. Potassium hydroxide preparation reveals the hyphae. Fungi infect only the superficial layers of the skin (stratum corneum). |
| Tinea Corporis | Found on the body over moist areas, such as the axilla and under pendulous breasts. | |
| Tinea Cruris | Also known as "jock itch"; may be found in the inguinal region of obese patients. | |
| Tinea Pedis | Also known as "athlete's foot." Affects the areas between the toes. | |
| Tinea Versicolor | Causes asymptomatic macules that are red, brown, or white. Macules become hypopigmented in the summer. | Caused by *Pityrosporum orbiculare* (*Malassezia furfur*). Potassium hydroxide preparation reveals mycelia and round spores, often described as "spaghetti and meatballs." |

## ARTHROPOD-CAUSED SKIN INFECTIONS

| Condition | Description | Pathology |
|---|---|---|
| Scabies | Intensely pruritic inflamed papules, nodules, or red plaques. Skin is often excoriated from scratching. Secondary bacterial infection is common. | Caused by a mite. The female burrows beneath the stratum corneum to lay eggs. Commonly seen on the palms, webs of the fingers, and wrists. |
| Pediculosis or Lice | Pubic area, head, or trunk involvement depending on the type of louse. Causes severe pruritus and excoriation secondary to scratching. With head and pubic lice, white eggs can be found attached to the hair shafts. Body lice infest clothing. | Dermal eosinophilia at bite sites. |
| Other Insect Bites | Bites from ticks produce variable lesions and can transmit Rocky Mountain spotted fever, Lyme disease, and relapsing fever. Bites from mosquitoes or fleas produce pruritic papules. Pruritus occurs from the reaction to the insect's saliva. | |

## DESQUAMATION SYNDROMES

| Disease | Description | Cause and Pathology |
|---|---|---|
| Scarlet Fever | Common in children. Fever; sore throat; blanching, sand-paperlike, fine papular rash on the body, sparing the palms and soles; and strawberry tongue. Rash becomes desquamated in about 1 week. | Caused by group A streptococci (*S. pyogenes*) with bacterio-phage-derived toxin (erythrogenic toxin). May be complicated by poststreptococcal glomerulonephritis and rheumatic fever. |
| Toxic Shock Syndrome | Seen in adults, especially women of childbearing age. High fever, vomiting, diarrhea, headache, sore throat, and a sunburnlike rash (diffuse red macular rash). Desquamation, including the palms and soles, occurs during recovery. Has been associated with menses and the use of superabsorbent tampons. | Toxin-mediated reaction in which massive quantities of inflammatory cytokines are released. Caused by *S. aureus* with toxic shock syndrome toxin type 1. |
| Scalded Skin Syndrome | Occurs in children aged < 5 years. Causes fever and diffuse tender erythema. Progresses to bullous rash that ruptures, leaving a red eroded surface. Exfoliation may affect the entire body. Nikolsky's sign is present. | Caused by *S. aureus* with exfoliating toxin. May be differentiated from Stevens-Johnson syndrome by lack of mucous membrane involvement. |
| Toxic Epidermal Necrolysis | Variant of Stevens-Johnson syndrome. Most severe desquamation syndrome, with a 30% mortality rate. High fever, oral and conjunctival erosions, and a bullous rash resembling scalded skin syndrome. Epidermis is shed and Nikolsky's sign is present. | Unknown cause, but may be precipitated by sulfa drugs or anti-convulsants. |
| Kawasaki Disease | Multisystem disease that occurs in children. Diffuse erythematous mucocutaneous rash and strawberry tongue. Skin becomes desquamated, including the palms and soles. See Chapter 2, Types of Vasculitides (Vasculitis). | Unknown. |

# III. Skin Growths

## SKIN CYSTS

| Type of Cyst | Description | Pathology |
|---|---|---|
| Epidermal Inclusion Cyst | Thin-walled cyst filled with thick yellow material | Cyst is lined by keratinized squamous epithelium and filled with loose, laminated keratin. |
| Trichilemmal Cyst | Also called pilar or sebaceous cyst. Thick-walled cyst is not connected to the epidermis and is filled with thick yellow material. | Cyst is lined by keratinized squamous epithelium that lacks a granular layer and is filled with compact, amorphous keratin. |

## BENIGN SKIN TUMORS

| Disease | Description | Pathology |
|---|---|---|
| **Epidermal Tumors** | | |
| Fibroepithelial Polyp | Also called an acrochordon (squamous papilloma, or common skin tag). Soft, flesh-colored papule attached by a slender stalk of skin. Very common in middle-aged adults. Found on the face, eyelids, neck, trunk, and axilla. Associated with pregnancy, diabetes, or intestinal polyposis. | Central connective tissue core is covered by stratified squamous epithelium. |
| Seborrheic Keratosis | Occurs in older individuals. Raised, circumscribed brown papules or plaques on the head, trunk, and extremities. Appear "painted on." | Squamous epithelial proliferation with keratin-filled cysts. |
| Keratoacanthoma | Rapidly growing, flesh-colored, cup-shaped lesion often found on sun-exposed areas (face and extremities). Lesion regresses within a year. Frequently confused with squamous cell carcinoma of the skin. | Center of the cup is filled with keratin. Base of the lesion is smooth and remains at the level of the hair follicles. Cells may show mild atypia and mitotic activity. |

*Continued*

## BENIGN SKIN TUMORS (Continued)

| Disease | Description | Pathology |
| --- | --- | --- |
| **Dermal Tumors** | | |
| Dermatofibroma | Pigmented firm nodule | Consists of collagen and fibroblasts. A type of fibrous histiocytoma. |
| Xanthoma | Yellow papules or nodules. Common on extremities, trunk, and eyelids. | Consists of lipid-filled histiocytes |
| Vascular Tumors | Hemangioma and Kaposi sarcoma can also be found in the dermis. See Chapter 2, Vascular Diseases. | |
| **Miscellaneous Lesions in the Skin** | | |
| Keloid | Abnormally thickened deposition of collagen that occurs during scar formation and wound healing. Unlike a hypertrophic scar, a keloid can grow beyond the boundaries of the wound. Very common in blacks. | Composed of excess amounts of thick bands of hyalinized collagen |

# PREMALIGNANT AND MALIGNANT SKIN TUMORS

| Disease | Description | Pathology |
|---|---|---|
| Actinic Keratosis | Also known as solar keratosis. Occurs predominantly in fair-skinned individuals on areas chronically exposed to the sun. A premalignant epidermal lesion, with poorly circumscribed, small, rough, scaling, brown or red papules on the face, trunk, or extremities. | Dysplasia of the epidermis and solar elastosis in the dermis. Risk of squamous cell carcinoma is proportional to the degree of epithelial dysplasia. |
| Basal Cell Carcinoma | Most common cancer (> 400,000 cases per year in the United States). Occurs in chronically sun-exposed areas in patients over 40 years. A malignant lesion causing a pearly or waxy papule with small telangiectatic vessels on its surface, commonly found on the head, nose, cheeks, ears, or neck. Locally aggressive, but does not metastasize. | Resembles basal cells. Tumor invades the dermis and possibly bone and muscle. Peripheral palisading of cells in nests. Possible central necrosis of the lesion. |
| Squamous Cell Carcinoma | Occurs in chronically sun-exposed areas in patients over 60 years. A malignant lesion causing a shallow ulcer with a raised, everted border. Associated with previous burn scars, actinic keratosis, and arsenic or radiation exposure. Locally invasive with rare metastasis. | Composed of large polygonal cells with pink cytoplasm. Keratin pearls (whorls of pink-staining keratin) are evident. Atypia of the cells determines aggressiveness of the tumor. |
| **Pigmented Tumors** | See Terms to Learn—Melanoma above for growth phases. Also see Chapter 15, Rashes and Skin Lesions, for nevus. | |
| Acanthosis Nigricans | Verrucous pigmented lesion occurring on the axilla, antecubital area, neck, or groin region. Associated with benign conditions (80%) and malignant tumors (20%). Benign type is inherited and associated with endocrine abnormalities (obesity, diabetes, and pituitary tumors). Malignant type is not inherited and arises in older individuals with occult malignancies. | Hyperkeratosis with prominent rete ridges and basal hyperpigmentation. |
| Lentigo Maligna Melanoma | Also called a Hutchinson freckle. A type of malignant melanoma in situ. Occurs in chronically sun-exposed areas of the skin in patients over 50 years. Appears as an unevenly pigmented macule that grows over time. Can remain in situ, growing radially, for 10–15 years before invading the dermis. | Increased number of atypical melanocytes in the basal layer. |
| Superficial Spreading Melanoma In Situ | Small, raised, irregularly pigmented lesion on the trunk or extremities. May remain in situ for a few months, then invades. Invasion leads to ulceration and bleeding. Growth is predominantly radial, but may become vertical with time. | Nests of large, atypical melanocytes in the epidermis. |

*Continued*

## PREMALIGNANT AND MALIGNANT SKIN TUMORS (Continued)

| Disease | Description | Pathology |
|---|---|---|
| Malignant Melanoma | Responsible for 44,200 cases and 7300 deaths per year in the United States. It is the sixth and seventh most common cancer in men and women, respectively. More common in fair-skinned individuals. May occur de novo or from nevi, lentigo maligna, or superficially spreading melanoma in situ. | Melanocytes in the basal layer are pleomorphic and show increased mitotic activity. Tumor may contain melanin or not (amelanotic). |
| | Nodular type is invasive. Vertical phase predominates early. Pigmented nodule ulcerates and bleeds. Early metastasis occurs via the lymphatics and hematogenously. | |
| **Miscellaneous Tumors** | | |
| Mycosis Fungoides | Cutaneous T-cell–derived malignant lymphoma. Affects the skin, lymph nodes, and viscera. See Chapter 4 for lymphomas. | Sezary syndrome is a variant of cutaneous T-cell lymphoma with seeding of tumor cells in the blood. |
| | First stage (lasts for years) involves scaling, red, pruritic patches. | Infiltration of the epidermis by atypical lymphoid cells with perivascular dermal infiltration. |
| | Second stage is marked by well-demarcated, raised red plaques. | Epidermal infiltrates form Pautrier microabscesses. |
| | Third stage shows reddish-brown nodules that ulcerate. | Resembles other lymphomas. |
| Langerhans Cell Histiocytosis | Letterer-Siwe disease, Hand-Schüller-Christian disease (on the head), and eosinophilic granuloma disease may present as red scaly nodules or papules resembling seborrheic dermatitis. | Histiocytic infiltration. See Chapter 4, Langerhans Cell Histiocytosis. |
| Dermatofibrosarcoma Protuberans | Slowly growing malignant sarcoma that rarely metastasizes. Appears as ulcerated plaques on the trunk. | Composed of neoplastic fibroblasts. |

# CHAPTER 12
# MUSCULOSKELETAL SYSTEM AND SOFT TISSUE TUMORS

**I. MUSCULAR DISEASES**

Myopathies

Neuromuscular Disorders

**II. BONE DISEASES**

Bone Architecture

Bone Metabolism

Differential Diagnosis of Metabolic Bone Diseases

Metabolic Bone Diseases

Pyogenic Osteomyelitis

Mechanisms of Osteomyelitis

Primary Bone Tumors

Other Bone Diseases

**III. JOINT DISEASES**

Types of Joint Diseases

Comparison of Gonococcal and Nongonococcal Bacterial Arthritis

Joint Fluid Analysis

SoftTissue Tumors

**ABBREVIATIONS**

**DIP** = distal interphalangeal
**HLA** = human leukocyte antigen
**Ig** = immunoglobulin
**MCP** = metacarpophalangeal

**MTP** = metatarsophalangeal
**PIP** = proximal interphalangeal
**PMN** = polymorphonuclear leukocyte
**PTH** = parathyroid hormone

## MOST COMMON Causes and Types

| Disorder | Common Cause |
| --- | --- |
| Arthritis | Osteoarthritis (really an arthrosis) |

| Disorder | Common Type |
| --- | --- |
| Inherited myopathy | Duchenne muscular dystrophy |
| Primary benign tumor of soft tissue | Lipoma |
| Primary benign tumor of bone | Osteochondroma |
| Primary malignant tumor of bone | Osteosarcoma |

| Arthralgia | Joint pain, usually without swelling or warmth. Common with many viral illnesses. |
| --- | --- |
| Arthritis | Inflammation of the joints, characterized by pain, warmth, redness of the overlying skin, and decreased range of motion. Types of arthritis include rheumatoid arthritis, gouty arthritis, and septic arthritis. Arthritis caused by viruses is mild and self-limited (weeks). Do not confuse arthritis with arteritis (inflammation of the arteries). |
| Arthrosis or Arthropathy | Any joint disease. |
| Bursitis | Inflammation of the bursal sac resulting from infection, trauma, or a rheumatoid process. Bursae are synovia-lined, fluid-filled sacs that surround tendons, joints, and ligaments and serve to decrease friction between moving parts. |
| Ganglion and Synovial Cyst | Cyst that arises from myxoid degeneration of connective tissue. Mass occurs in a tendon or joint capsule from herniation of synovium through the capsule. Baker cysts (the most common synovial cyst) occur at the knee joints. |
| Myopathy | Any muscular disease. Acquired inflammatory myopathies exhibit symmetric proximal muscle weakness (hip and shoulder) with pain in muscle groups surrounding those joints. Inherited myopathies often present with progressive muscle weakness. Serum creatine kinase is elevated. |
| Myositis | Degenerative and inflammatory muscular disease. The best known is polymyositis. |
| Osteomyelitis | Inflammation of the bone and bone marrow as a result of infection. |
| Osteopenia | Decreased bone mass secondary to reduced osteoid matrix. Mineralization of the remaining bone is not affected. One of the most common causes is osteoporosis. Other common causes include corticosteroid excess, hyperthyroidism, and hypoparathyroidism. Osteopenia may also be caused by lytic bone lesions as in osteomyelitis, multiple myeloma, Langerhans histiocytosis, Paget disease, lymphomas, and metastases from solid tumors. |
| Proteins Associated with Muscle | All of the following proteins may be released with myocyte damage (crush injuries):<br><br>• Myoglobin—oxygen-storing protein of muscle fibers. Excess can cause renal failure (too much to filter).<br><br>• Creatine kinase—enzyme present in the heart and skeletal muscle.<br><br>• Aldolase—nonspecific but very sensitive enzyme for myocyte damage.<br><br>• Lactate dehydrogenase—elevated with muscle damage. |
| Soft Tissues | Include fibrous connective tissue, adipose tissue, skeletal muscle, joints, and nerve tissue. |
| Synovitis | Inflammation of the synovial membrane lining the joints. Seen in inflammatory arthritides such as rheumatoid arthritis. |

# I. Muscular Diseases

## MYOPATHIES

| Disease | Description | Cause or Pathogenesis | Pathologic Findings |
|---|---|---|---|
| Inherited Inflammatory Myopathies | Duchenne muscular dystrophy—The most common inherited myopathy (1 in 3300 male births). Infant is normal at birth but by the time the child starts to ambulate, delays in gross movement (climbing stairs and running) are apparent. Calf thickening is called pseudohypertrophy. By their teens, patients cannot ambulate. Patients die from respiratory failure by their 20s. | X-linked. Defective dystrophin gene. | Necrosis of individual muscle fibers and replacement by fibrous-fatty tissue. |
| | Becker muscular dystrophy—Milder than Duchenne muscular dystrophy. Similar symptoms but disease is drawn out, with onset in the teens and loss of ambulation by the 30s. | Abnormal dystrophin and normal dystrophin are produced. | Necrosis of individual muscle fibers and replacement by fibrous-fatty tissue. |
| | Mitochondrial—Kearns-Sayre syndrome—Patients may have ophthalmoplegia, pigment retinopathy, heart block, and cerebellar ataxia. | Non-mendelian maternal mode of transmission. | Ragged red muscle fibers may be seen. |
| | Myotonic dystrophy—Onset is in teens with muscle weakness, followed by myotonic contractures later in life. | Autosomal dominant. | Large muscle fibers with numerous central nuclei. Few to no necrotic fibers. |

| Acquired Inflammatory Myopathies | Dermatomyositis—Occurs at any age with progressive weakness of the proximal limb muscles, usually without pain (90%). Also, heliotrope rash on the eyelids with periorbital edema and rash on the cheeks, bridge of the nose, and over hand and knee joints. If onset is at > 40 years, an underlying malignancy must be suspected. | Autoimmune origin suspected. Antibody damage to vasculature in perimysium of the muscle. | Inflammatory infiltration in muscle around vessels and in perimysium. |
|---|---|---|---|
| | Polymyositis—Identical to the above except without skin manifestations. | Autoimmune origin suspected. | CD8-positive T cells are found around damaged muscle fibers. Necrosis and regeneration are seen. |
| | Inclusion body myositis—Patients present in their 50s. The distal muscles are affected asymmetrically. Creatine kinase level is normal to mildly elevated. | Autoimmune origin suspected. | Exudate rich in CD8-positive T cells. Myocytic vacuoles rimmed by purple granules. |
| | Toxic myopathies—These can be due to alcohol abuse (most common), hypothyroidism or hyperthyroidism, corticosteroid excess, and hypokalemia or hyperkalemia. | Toxin mediated. | Acute alcohol myopathy may show necrotic or regenerating myofibers, especially type 1. Chronic alcohol myopathy shows type 2 myofiber atrophy. |

## NEUROMUSCULAR DISORDERS

| Disease | Description | Pathogenesis |
|---|---|---|
| Myasthenia Gravis | Occurs at any age with slowly progressive onset of ptosis; diplopia; difficulty chewing, speaking, and swallowing; limb weakness; and respiratory difficulty. Weakness becomes worse with muscle use and recovers with rest. The extraocular and facial muscles and extremities are most affected. | Autoimmune antibody to acetylcholine receptors. Occurs most frequently in women with HLA-DR3. |
| Lambert-Eaton Syndrome | Also known as myasthenic syndrome. Initial muscle weakness but increased power with use (acetylcholine accumulates in the synaptic cleft with each muscle contraction). Strongly associated with small cell carcinoma of the lung. | Defective acetylcholine release from presynaptic neurons. |
| Botulism | Occurs about 3 days after ingestion of botulinum toxin (produced by *Clostridium botulinum*), which may be found in contaminated home-canned food. Presents with sudden weakness, ptosis, diplopia with blurry vision, dysphagia, and facial weakness, followed by respiratory difficulty. Treatment is an antitoxin. | Toxin prevents presynaptic acetylcholine release. |

# II. Bone Diseases

## BONE ARCHITECTURE

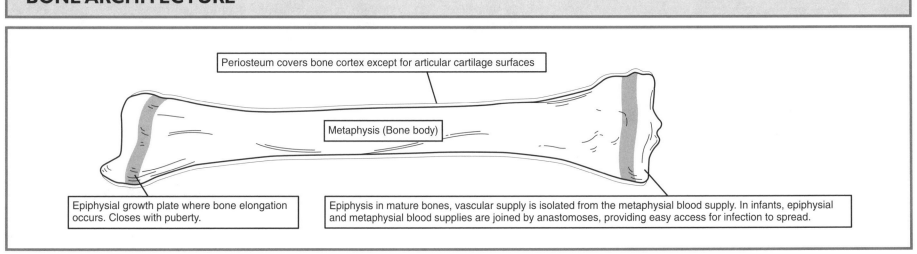

Periosteum covers bone cortex except for articular cartilage surfaces

Metaphysis (Bone body)

Epiphysial growth plate where bone elongation occurs. Closes with puberty.

Epiphysis in mature bones, vascular supply is isolated from the metaphysial blood supply. In infants, epiphysial and metaphysial blood supplies are joined by anastomoses, providing easy access for infection to spread.

## BONE METABOLISM

| Hormone | Function in Bone Metabolism | Action on Serum Mineral Levels | Action on Bone | Action on Intestine | Action on Kidney |
|---|---|---|---|---|---|
| Parathyroid Hormone | Increases serum calcium | ↑ Calcium; ↑ phosphate | ↑ Calcium and phosphate resorption | ↑ Calcium and phosphate absorption indirectly (through ↑ vitamin $D_3$) | ↓ Calcium excretion; ↑ phosphate excretion. Increases vitamin $D_3$ production. |
| Vitamin $D_3$, Calcitriol, or 1,25 $(OH)_2$ | Mineralizes the bone matrix with calcium and phosphate by maintaining adequate serum calcium levels | ↑ Calcium; ↑ phosphate | Vitamin $D_3$ causes bone resorption | Vitamin $D_3$ acts to increase calcium and phosphate absorption | ↓ Calcium excretion |
| Calcitonin | Decreases serum calcium and phosphate | ↓ Calcium; ↓ phosphate | ↓ Bone resorption due to decreased osteoclast activity | No effect | ↑ Calcium and phosphate excretion |
| Estrogen (Women) | No effect on calcium or phosphate levels | | ↓ Bone resorption due to increased osteoblast activity | No effect | No effect |
| Androgens (Men) | | | ↑ Bone matrix | | |

## DIFFERENTIAL DIAGNOSIS OF METABOLIC BONE DISEASES

| Disease | Calcium | Phosphate | Alkaline Phosphatase | Vitamin D Activity | Parathyroid Hormone | Bone Mineralization | Bone Trabeculae |
|---|---|---|---|---|---|---|---|
| Osteoporosis | Normal | Normal | Normal | Normal | Normal | Normal | Thin |
| Osteomalacia or Rickets | ↓ or Normal | ↓ or Normal | ↑ | ↓ or normal if ↑ PTH | Normal or ↑ | ↓ | Thick |
| Paget Disease of Bone | Normal | ↑ or Normal | ↑ | ↓ | Normal | Normal or ↓ | Thick, but irregular |
| Primary Hyperparathyroidism | ↑ | ↓ | ↑ | Normal or ↑ | ↑ | Normal or ↓ | Thin |
| Secondary Hyperparathyroidism | Normal, ↑, or ↓ | Normal, ↑, or ↓ | Normal or ↑ | ↑ | ↑ | Normal or ↓ | Thin |
| Lytic Bone Lesions | Normal or ↑ | Normal or ↑ | Normal or ↑ | ↓ | Normal | ↓, ↑, or normal | Thin |

## METABOLIC BONE DISEASES

| Syndrome | Description | Cause(s) | Pathology |
|---|---|---|---|
| Osteoporosis | Most common metabolic bone disease in the United States. Often called postmenopausal osteoporosis. Causes spontaneous crush vertebral fractures, femoral head fractures, and fractures of the distal ends of the radius. | Menopause, due to estrogen deficiency (most common), prolonged inactivity, Cushing syndrome, hyperparathyroidism, hyperthyroidism, and multiple myeloma. | Called "bone atrophy." Trabecular bone is lost. Bone formation is normal, but bone resorption is increased. Mineralization is also normal, but mineral density is decreased. |
| | Osteogenesis imperfecta—a genetic cause of severe osteoporosis. Spontaneous fractures start during the neonatal period. Other features include problems with teeth, eyes (blue sclerae), and skin. | Autosomal dominant inheritance of a defective collagen I gene, resulting in defective collagen synthesis. | |
| | Other genetic causes of osteoporosis include Ehlers-Danlos syndrome and Marfan syndrome. | | |
| Osteomalacia | Affects adults. Patients are asymptomatic at first, then develop proximal muscle weakness and bone pain. If condition is caused by renal disease, it is called renal osteodystrophy. | Vitamin D deficiency, malnutrition, or malabsorption. Can also occur from defective calcium and phosphate homeostasis from renal tubular defect, alcoholism, poor nutrition, or aluminum antacid abuse. | Called "bone softening." Defective mineralization of the osteoid bone matrix. |
| | Rickets—children's form of osteomalacia. Manifestations include craniotabes (thinning of the occipital and parietal bones), late fontanelle closure, Harrison's groove (where diaphragm inserts), decreased height (spinal deformation), and pigeon breast (protrusion of the sternum). | | Lack of mineralization. Increased thickness of the epiphysial growth plate. |

*Continued*

## METABOLIC BONE DISEASES (Continued)

| Syndrome | Description | Cause(s) | Pathology |
|---|---|---|---|
| Paget Disease | Also called osteitis deformans. Causes deep bone pain. Bones become soft, leading to tibial bowing, kyphosis, and fractures. May involve the skull, causing an increase in head diameter and deafness. | Unknown. | Thickened bones with irregular trabecular patterns. Three stages: osteoclastic resorption, osteoblastic compensation (balances the resorption), and increased osteoblastic activity with sclerosis. New bone is highly vascular. |
| Hyper-parathyroidism | Also called osteitis fibrosa cystica. PTH increases because of primary or secondary hyperparathyroidism. Patients are often asymptomatic, but occasionally present with bone pain, fractures, and bone cysts. Clinically may be mistaken for giant cell bone tumor. | Primary: parathyroid adenoma and diffuse hyperplasia. Secondary: chronic renal failure and vitamin D deficiency. | Osteolytic lesions and brown tumors (cystic spaces that may display hemorrhage and later fibrosis). Marked osteoclastic activity (osteoclastic giant cells). |
| Scurvy | Mainly affects chronic alcoholics, infants < 1 year, and smokers with chronic renal failure or cancer. Causes weakness, then painful subperiosteal hemorrhages, purpura, bleeding gums, and anemia. | Vitamin C deficiency impairs synthesis of osteoid matrix. Lysine and proline are not hydroxylated. | Epiphysial cartilage is not replaced by osteoid matrix. Wound healing is impaired. |

# PYOGENIC OSTEOMYELITIS

| Disease | Description and Causation | Pathology |
|---------|---------------------------|-----------|
| Acute Osteomyelitis | In healthy children, disease is due to *Staphylococcus aureus* (most commonly) or group A streptococcus. Neonates are at risk with group B streptococcus. If patients have sickle cell disease, they are at risk for *Salmonella* osteomyelitis (*S. aureus* is still the most common cause). *Pseudomonas* may be causative (wounds made by piercing the rubber sole of a shoe). Drug abusers mainly develop disease from *S. aureus* and *Escherichia coli*. Disease causes high fever, severe pain over the infected bone, swelling, and warmth over the skin. | Process starts in the metaphysis. Inflammation leads to increased bone tension and bone necrosis. Radiographs are normal for the first week. |
| Chronic Osteomyelitis | A complication of acute osteomyelitis. Poor circulation (e.g., in diabetic patients and those with peripheral vascular disease) can predispose. Sinus tracts to the skin surface are common. Chronic skin inflammation overlying the bone causes epithelial hyperplasia. Potential site for later squamous carcinoma. | Sequestrum (dead, infected, necrotic bone) becomes covered by reactive, disorganized new bone formation (involucrum). Brodie's abscess may form in a lytic area of infected bone. Reactive amyloidosis (AA type) may be present. |
| | Tuberculosis of the bones may mimic chronic osteomyelitis. Affects children, the elderly, and immunocompromised patients. Infection may spread hematogenously from a site of active disease (lungs). Pain over the bone, warmth, and swelling may be seen. Bone is progressively destroyed if not treated. Infection of the spinal vertebrae is called Pott disease. | Acid-fast stained organisms are found on bone biopsy. Radiographs usually show bone destruction at the time of presentation. |

## MECHANISMS OF OSTEOMYELITIS

| Characteristic | Hematogenous Spread | Contiguous Spread |
|---|---|---|
| Fever, Pain, and Warmth | Often present. | Occasionally present. |
| Causative Organism(s) | S. *aureus* or group A streptococcus. | Polymicrobial. Can involve S. *aureus* and gram-negative rods. |
| Bones Affected | In children, usually the long bones. In the elderly, usually the vertebral bones. | Skull, leg bones, and mandible. |
| Chronic Phase | Rare. | Occasionally. |
| Mechanism | Bacteremia seeds the bone. | Spreads from infected teeth, animal bites, fractures or penetrating injuries, or soft-tissue infections. |

## PRIMARY BONE TUMORS

| Disease | Description | Age Involved | Histopathology |
|---|---|---|---|
| **Benign Tumors** | | | |
| Osteochondroma | Also known as osteocartilaginous exostosis. The most common benign primary bone tumor in children. Occurs in the lower extremities including the femur, tibia, and pelvis. | 10–30 years | Most tumors are solitary. Mature bony mass with a cap of hyaline cartilage projecting from the bone surface. |
| Chondroma | Occurs in the medulla of the bone diaphysis (enchondroma) in the small bones of the hand and feet. | 10–40 years | Two-thirds of tumors are solitary. Appears as a firm, well-circumscribed mass of well-differentiated hyaline cartilage that grows from the bony center outward, often thinning the cortex. |

| Giant Cell Tumor | Occurs around the knee (femur and tibia) and may extend into the soft tissues. Locally aggressive and 50% of cases recur; 10% can metastasize. | 20–40 years | Cysts with hemorrhage, leading to the "soap bubble" appearance on X-ray. Numerous osteoclastlike multinuclear giant cells and small neoplastic spindle cells. |
| --- | --- | --- | --- |
| Uncommon Benign Tumors | Four other benign primary bone tumors include: osteoma (in skull and facial bones), osteoid osteoma, chondroblastoma, and osteoblastoma (in the vertebrae). Osteomas are associated with Gardner syndrome (see Chapter 9, Intestinal Tumors). | | |
| Malignant Tumors | Responsible for 2600 cases and 1400 deaths per year in the United States. | | |
| Osteosarcoma | Also called osteogenic sarcoma. The most common primary malignant tumor in children and adults. Found in the metaphysial medulla of the long bones of the upper and lower extremities (femur, tibia, and humerus). Very aggressive and metastasizes early. Causes a bone mass with pain and swelling. Associated with familial retinoblastoma. | Bimodal, at 10–25 years and 60 years | Fleshy mass with bone and cartilage and areas of necrosis and hemorrhage. Anaplastic osteoblasts may be seen. Calcified osteoid of tumor (bone tumor) is diagnostic of this tumor. |
| Chondrosarcoma | The most common malignant primary bone tumor in this age group. Involves the pelvis, ribs, shoulder girdle, long bones, and the vertebrae. Causes a bony mass or a fracture. | 30–60 years; males | Most tumors are solitary. Destructive white mass that expands the bone. Consists of malignant chondrocytes in a chondroid matrix. |
| Ewing Sarcoma | Although uncommon, it is the second leading cause of malignant primary bone tumor in children. Arises in the long bones, ribs, pelvis, and vertebrae. Grows within the medulla of the diaphysis. Very aggressive and metastasizes early. Associated with 11:22 translocation. | 5–30 years; more common in males | Soft tumor with areas of necrosis and hemorrhage. Sheets of small round and oval cells with large nuclei and scant cytoplasm. May resemble malignant lymphoma. |
| Metastatic Tumors | Many tumors metastasize to bone. Lung, prostate, breast, thyroid, kidney, and colon are the most common. Other metastatic bone tumors include multiple myeloma, lymphomas, and Langerhans cell histiocytosis. | | |

## OTHER BONE DISEASES

| Disease | Description | Cause(s) |
|---|---|---|
| Aseptic Necrosis | Also known as avascular necrosis (osteonecrosis). Bone undergoes infarction from loss of the blood supply. Most commonly affected site is the femoral head, leading to hip disease. | Idiopathic or secondary to corticosteroid use, trauma, gout, sickle cell disease, lupus, and infiltrative storage diseases |
| Fibrous Dysplasia | May present with bone pain, bone deformity, or pathologic bone fracture. May cause lytic lesions.<br><br>• Monostotic—lesion affecting 1 bone. Usually asymptomatic.<br><br>• Polyostotic—rare condition in which multiple bones are affected, causing deformity and fractures. May be associated with Albright syndrome (disorder of endocrine abnormalities and café-au-lait spots). | Unknown |

## III. Joint Diseases

### TYPES OF JOINT DISEASES

| Disease | Description | Joint(s) Involved | Pathology or Organism Involved |
|---|---|---|---|
| Osteoarthritis | The most common arthritis (arthrosis). Affects all ages (most common at > 50 years). Primary type is the most common. Slow onset, with transient joint stiffness progressing to pain with motion or weight bearing. Relieved by rest. Patients experience crepitus (grinding sensation between the bones) and limited joint motion. | Asymmetric and poly-articular. Heberden's nodes (osteophytes in DIP joint). Bouchard's nodes (osteophytes in PIP joint). Also hips, knees, and spine. | Chronic noninflammatory degeneration of articular cartilage and distortion by new osteophyte formation at articular edges. Loss of articular cartilage exposes "polished" subchondral bone (eburnation). |
| | Secondary type is found in younger patients with damaged joints, overuse injuries, or rheumatoid arthritis. Chronic "wear and tear" and the loosening of collagen matrix decrease the cushioning barrier to stress. | Involves any joint. | |
| Rheumatoid Arthritis | Chronic, recurrent, systemic inflammatory disease occurring in patients in their 20s to 40s (women > men). Causes fever, weight loss, malaise, and joint swelling with stiffness (worst in the morning), warmth, and pain. Swan-neck (DIP hyperextension) and boutonniere deformities (DIP flexion) occur if not treated. Still disease (juvenile rheumatoid arthritis) in children presents with high fevers, rash, sple- nomegaly, and arthritis. | Polyarticular and sym- metric, affecting the distal joints: MCP, PIP, wrists, knees, and elbows. Spinal sublux- ation can occur from loosening of the joints between C1 and C2. | Pannus (proliferating hyper- plastic synovial membrane) is infiltrated with lymphocytes, plasma cells, and PMNs. Ero- sion of bone, cartilage, liga- ments, and tendons. Eventual fibrosis and joint deformity. Ele- vated rheumatoid factor (anti- IgG Fc antibody) in 90%. |

Continued

## TYPES OF JOINT DISEASES (Continued)

| Disease | Description | Joint(s) Involved | Pathology or Organism Involved |
|---|---|---|---|
| Gouty Arthritis | Recurrent, acute inflammatory monoarticular arthritis. Causes sudden attacks of intense joint pain with swelling and high fever. Asymptomatic between attacks. After multiple attacks, tophi (crystal deposits) are evident in bursae of the involved joints. High serum uric acid level. Attacks may be precipitated by alcohol use, eating, surgery, infections, or diuretics. | Most often in the MTP joint of the great toe (podagra). Also may occur in feet, ankles, and knees. | Severe inflammatory reaction. Crystals engulfed in PMNs are diagnostic. Sodium urate crystals precipitating in the kidneys lead to tubular damage and stone formation (urolithiasis). Crystals are thin and needle shaped. |
| | Primary gout is familial in origin and the most common type. Occurs in men > 30 years. | | |
| | Secondary gout is due to hyperuricemia from myeloproliferative syndromes, leukemia, multiple myeloma, hemoglobinopathies, chronic renal disease (decreased urate excretion), hypothyroidism, and lead poisoning. | | |
| Pseudogout | Also known as chondrocalcinosis (calcium pyrophosphate deposition disease). Patients present in their 60s or older. Self-limited inflammatory acute arthritis. Associated with hemochromatosis, diabetes mellitus, thyroid disorders, Wilson disease, and gout. | Knees and wrists. | Synovial fluid is full of crystals and leukocytes. Rhomboid-shaped crystals. |
| Seronegative Spondyloarthropathies | Inflammatory arthritis associated with HLA-B27. Usually affects patients < 40 years old. Seronegative = rheumatoid factor–negative. | | |
| | Ankylosing spondylitis—slowly progressive disease in patients < 20 years old. Higher incidence in males. Causes low back pain and stiffness with eventual fusion of the spine (ankylosis). Radiographs show a rigid, calcified spine, resembling a bamboo stick. | Symmetric involvement of the sacroiliac joints. | Chronic inflammation with fibrosis and calcification of the spinal joints. |
| | Reiter syndrome (reactive arthritis)—triad of urethritis, conjunctivitis or uveitis, and arthritis (males > females). Follows diarrhea caused by *Shigella, Salmonella, Yersinia,* or *Campylobacter,* or a sexually transmitted infection with *Chlamydia trachomatis.* Self-limited, with recurrences. | Asymmetric involvement of the knees, ankles, and sacroiliac joints. | Synovitis. |
| | Enteropathic arthropathy—associated with Crohn disease and ulcerative colitis. | Hips and knees or sacroiliac, depending on the form. | Inflammatory cells and bacterial components in the joints. |

| Infectious Arthritis | Gonococcal arthritis is the most common cause of bacterial arthritis and occurs in healthy adults (females > males). Disseminated gonococci are the primary cause. First symptoms are fever, rash, and arthralgias. Then, tenosynovitis or purulent monoarthritis. Genitourinary symptoms may be present. Radiographs show only tissue swelling. | Monoarticular, oligoarticular, or polyarticular. Knee is the most common location. | *Neisseria gonorrhoeae*. |
|---|---|---|---|
| | Nongonococcal septic arthritis results from persistent bacteremia. Infection occurs with impaired immunity or in previously damaged joints. Causes fever, chills, and sudden joint swelling, pain, and warmth. Radiographs can be negative in the first week (bone erosion occurs later). If not treated, may cause articular destruction. | Monoarticular process in the knee, hip, wrist, ankle, or shoulder. | *S. aureus* (most common), group A and group B streptococci. Gram-negative arthritis: *E. coli* and *Pseudomonas* are most common. |
| | Chronic arthritis causes chronic swelling, warmth, and pain, progressing to joint destruction and muscle atrophy if not treated. Spreads hematogenously from an active lesion. | Any. | *Mycobacterium tuberculosis* and *Coccidioides*. |
| | Lyme disease:<br><br>• First stage—distinctive bull's-eye rash (erythema chronicum migrans) and flulike symptoms<br><br>• Second stage—systemic manifestations (migratory acute arthritis, myocarditis, aseptic meningitis, or peripheral neuropathy)<br><br>• Third stage (years from initial infection)—chronic arthritis, chronic synovitis, and encephalopathy | Large joints, such as the knees. | *Borrelia burgdorferi*. |
| | Viral arthritis—mild, self-limited arthritis without joint destruction. | Any joint. | Rubella virus and postvaccination in adults. Mumps virus, hepatitis B, and parvovirus B19. |

## COMPARISON OF GONOCOCCAL AND NONGONOCOCCAL BACTERIAL ARTHRITIS

| Arthritis Type | Population Affected | Number of Joints Involved | Blood Culture | Synovial Fluid Culture | Therapeutic Response |
|---|---|---|---|---|---|
| Gonococcal | Sexually active adults (females > males) < 40 years | Monoarticular, oligoarticular, or polyarticular | Early: positive (40%). Late: negative. | Early: negative. Late: positive. | Rapid (3 days) |
| Nongonococcal | Infants, children, and immunocompromised adults | Monoarticular | Positive 50% of the time. | Positive 75% of the time. | Slow (4–6 weeks) |

## JOINT FLUID ANALYSIS

| Characteristic | Normal | Noninflammatory | Inflammatory | Septic |
|---|---|---|---|---|
| Fluid Clarity and Color | Transparent and clear | Transparent and yellow | Translucent to opaque and yellow | Opaque yellow to green |
| White Blood Cells (cells/µL) | < 200 | 200–300 | 3000–50,000 | > 50,000 |
| PMNs | < 25% | < 25% | ≥ 50% | ≥ 75% |
| Bacterial Culture | Negative | Negative | Negative | Usually positive |
| Glucose | Nearly equal to serum | Nearly equal to serum | > 25 mg/dL but lower than serum | < 25 mg/dL, much lower than serum |
| Representative Diseases | | Osteoarthritis or trauma | Rheumatoid arthritis, gout, pseudogout, Reiter syndrome, ankylosing spondylopathy, enteropathic arthropathy, or chronic infectious arthritis including tuberculosis and fungi | Pyogenic bacterial infections |

Adapted from Tierney LM, Jr., McPhee SJ, Papadakis MA: *Current Medical Diagnosis and Treatment*, 39th ed. New York: McGraw-Hill, 2000.

## SOFT TISSUE TUMORS

| Disease | Description | Pathology |
|---|---|---|
| **Benign Tumors** | | |
| Lipoma | The most common soft tissue tumor. Tumor of mature adipose tissue. | Circumscribed mass that resembles the tissue of origin. Local excision is often curative. |
| Hemangioma | Vascular tumor. Another very common soft tissue tumor. | |
| Leiomyoma | Smooth-muscle tumor common in the uterus. | |
| Fibrous Histiocytoma | Tumor of fibroblasts and histiocytes. | |
| Fibroma | A soft gray-white tumor usually found in the ovary. | |
| **Malignant Tumors**—responsible for **7800 cases** and **4400 deaths per year in the United States.** Mesenchymal origin may be obscured when cells are anaplastic. | | |
| Malignant Fibrous Histiocytoma | The most common soft tissue sarcoma of late middle age. | Tumor is soft and large, commonly in the retroperitoneum. |
| Liposarcoma | The second most common soft tissue sarcoma of adult life. | As above. Also may see lipoblasts. |
| Rare Tumors | Include rhabdomyosarcoma, synovial sarcoma, leiomyosarcoma, fibrosarcoma, and angiosarcoma. | As above. Remnants of striations and vascular channels may be seen in rhabdomyosarcoma and angiosarcoma, respectively. |

# CHAPTER 13
# NERVOUS SYSTEM

I. PERIPHERAL NERVOUS SYSTEM DISEASES

Peripheral Nerve Tumors

Peripheral Neuropathies

II. CENTRAL NERVOUS SYSTEM DISEASES

Cerebral Trauma

Cerebrovascular Diseases

Hydrocephalus

Cytologic Analysis of Cerebrospinal Fluid

Infections of the Central Nervous System

Viral Encephalitis

Slow Viral Encephalitis/ Encephalopathies

III. DEGENERATIVE DISEASES

Demyelinating Diseases

Areas of Brain Affected in Dementia

Incurable Dementias

Treatable/Curable Dementias

Other Degenerative Diseases

Distribution of Common Intracranial Tumors

Adult Central Nervous System Tumors

**ABBREVIATIONS**

**CSF** = cerebrospinal fluid

**GABA** = gamma-aminobutyric acid

**HIV** = human immunodeficiency virus

**HLA** = human leukocyte antigen

**PMN** = polymorphonuclear leukocyte

# MOST COMMON Causes and Types

| Disorder | Common Cause |
|----------|--------------|
| Encephalitis | Herpes simplex virus type 1 |
| Demyelinating disease | Multiple sclerosis |
| Dementia | Alzheimer disease |

| Disorder | Common Type |
|----------|-------------|
| Intracranial tumor | Metastatic tumor |
| Primary intracranial tumor | Astrocytomas, including glioblastoma multiforme (grade IV) |

| | |
|---|---|
| Encephalitis | Inflammation of the brain, usually due to bacterial or viral infection. |
| Intracranial Tumors | Pathology (atrophy and hydrocephalus) caused by compression, direct infiltration, cerebral edema, and irritative focal effects (seizures). |
| Meningitis | Inflammation of the meninges due to an infection (e.g., bacteria, viruses, tuberculosis, fungi) or chemical toxicity. In aseptic meningitis, no organisms are found in the CSF. |
| Neuritis | Inflammatory peripheral nerve disease. Sometimes used interchangeably with neuropathy. |
| Neuropathy | Peripheral nerve disease with sensory, motor, or sensorimotor (mixed) loss. Mononeuropathy affects a single nerve. Includes Bell palsy (facial nerve) and carpal tunnel syndrome (median nerve). Polyneuropathy affects many nerves at once. Includes diabetic neuropathy, uremic neuropathy, Guillain-Barré syndrome, alcoholic neuropathy, and vitamin $B_{12}$-deficient neuropathy. |
| Slow Viruses | Viruses that cause no inflammation. They have a progressive, slow course and a long incubation period. |

# I. Peripheral Nervous System Diseases

## PERIPHERAL NERVE TUMORS

| Tumor | Description | Pathology |
|---|---|---|
| Schwannoma | Commonly involve cranial nerve VIII (acoustic neuroma). Patients may present with tinnitus followed by nerve deafness. Associated with neurofibromatosis. | Benign, slowly growing, and encapsulated. Compressive, but not infiltrating. Neural crest origin. Composed of Schwann cells in one of two patterns:<br><br>• Antoni A: cellular spindle cells shaped into interlacing bundles<br><br>• Antoni B: has fewer cells in a loose myxedematous stroma |
| Neurofibroma | Compresses the involved nerve and may be malignant (especially if associated with neurofibromatosis). | Benign and slowly growing firm, rubbery mass that invades the nerve. Cells appear spindlelike and can include Schwann and fibroblast cells. |

## PERIPHERAL NEUROPATHIES

| Syndrome | Causes and Symptoms | Pathologic Process |
|---|---|---|
| Sensory or Mixed Neuropathies | Diabetic neuropathy produces symmetric "glove and stocking" sensory loss. Autonomic neuropathy may also occur. | Symmetric sensory and sensorimotor axonal degeneration. |
| | Alcoholic polyneuropathy is a sensorimotor and autonomic neuropathy. Decreased sensation and painful paresthesias in the legs. | Axonal degeneration of the neurons directly from the toxic effects of alcohol and from nutritional deficiency of B vitamins. |
| | Vitamin $B_1$, vitamin $B_6$, and vitamin $B_{12}$ deficiency neuropathies cause sensory loss in the legs. In thiamine ($B_1$) and cobalamin ($B_{12}$) deficiency, there are also central nervous system signs. | Axonal degeneration of the neurons. |
| | Lyme disease neuropathy is a mixed sensorimotor neuropathy. Occurs during the second and third stages of the disease. May have an associated encephalopathy. | Axonal degeneration of the neurons. |
| | Uremic neuropathy is a symmetric sensorimotor neuropathy that affects the legs > arms. May mimic painful paresthesias of alcoholic polyneuropathy. | Axonal degeneration of the neurons. Urea is toxic to neurons. |
| | Leprosy (*Mycobacterium leprae*) causes a sensory polyneuropathy. Slow, chronic course. Pale, anesthetic macules appear usually over cooler areas of the skin (earlobes and nose). | |
| | • Tuberculoid neuropathy occurs in patients with normal cell-mediated immunity and manifests itself as macular skin lesions with asymmetric nerve involvement. | Granulomas in nerve sheaths damage the nerves. Granulomas contain few mycobacteria (paucibacillary). Lepromin skin test is positive. |
| | • Lepromatous neuropathy occurs in patients with cell-mediated immunocompromise and presents as bacteria-laden, anesthetic nodular skin lesions with symmetric nerve involvement. | Granulomas have many mycobacteria (multibacillary). Lepromin skin test is negative. |
| | In diphtheric neuropathy (due to *Corynebacterium diphtheriae*), exotoxin damages the peripheral nerves, leading to loss of sensation and weakness. | Demyelination of the nerves. |
| | Malignancy-related neuropathy can occur from neuron compression, amyloid deposition into neurons, or as part of paraneoplastic effects. | Amyloid deposition by multiple myeloma and other plasma cell dyscrasias. Solid tumors can be compressive. |

*Continued*

## PERIPHERAL NEUROPATHIES (Continued)

| Syndrome | Causes and Symptoms | Pathologic Process |
|---|---|---|
| Pure Motor Neuropathies | Guillain-Barré syndrome is also known as acute inflammatory demyelinating polyradiculoneuropathy. Symmetric polyneuropathy with ascending paralysis, beginning in the legs. Follows a viral illness, Lyme disease, or *Campylobacter* infection. Patients often recover completely after several months. Severe cases may involve sensory loss as well. | Probably an autoimmune mechanism. Segmental demyelination by lymphocytic infiltrate of the nerve roots. CSF usually contains high protein level, without cells. |
| | Lead neuropathy causes wrist and foot drop. See Chapter 14 for more on lead. | Demyelination of the nerves. |
| Carpal Tunnel Syndrome | Median nerve entrapment in the transverse carpal ligament compartment results in tingling and numbness of the hand supplied by the median nerve. Caused by tissue edema from pregnancy, hypothyroidism, compression from arthritis, and inflammation from repetitive hand movements. | Axonal degeneration of the neurons. |

# II. Central Nervous System Diseases

## CEREBRAL TRAUMA

| Disorder | Description | Pathology |
|---|---|---|
| Concussion | Transient loss of consciousness from a blunt, nonpenetrating head injury. | No visible gross or histologic pathology. |
| Contusion | Causes a hematoma (blood pooling) in the brain. Forms when capillaries rupture from brain movement during blunt trauma. Coup is a brain injury on the same side as the impact. Contrecoup is a brain injury on the opposite side of impact. | Significance is that a hematoma can be a space-occupying lesion and can be compressive. Injury may also cause diffuse axonal damage. |
| Penetrating Injuries | May be caused by bullets, knives, or severe blunt trauma. Laceration of brain tissue may result in an acute subarachnoid or subdural bleed. | Severe neuronal and axonal damage from trauma or infection. |
| Epidural Hematoma | Also known as extradural hematoma. Usually associated with a skull fracture and laceration of the middle meningeal artery and caused by arterial bleeding. Blood pools between the skull and the dura, forming a convex hematoma resembling a walnut. A period of lucidity is followed by progressive deterioration. Signs of compression and increased intracranial pressure are evident. Immediate evacuation of the hematoma is necessary. | Hematoma compresses the brain tissue and increases intracranial pressure as blood accumulates. It is limited by dural attachments to the skull. |
| Subdural Hematoma | Usually caused by tearing of the bridging veins, with subsequent venous bleeding. Signs of cerebral compression occur as with an epidural hematoma. <br>• Acute type is due to severe head trauma. May result in rapid deterioration in mental status and death if not evacuated. <br>• Chronic type is due to minor head trauma. Patients may be asymptomatic or display progressive deterioration of mental status over days to weeks. | Hematoma compresses the brain tissue as above. Unlike the epidural hematoma, which is limited by dural attachments, a subdural hematoma continues to expand. |

## CEREBROVASCULAR DISEASES

| Disease | Description | Risk Factors and Pathology |
|---|---|---|
| Stroke | Third most frequent cause of death in the United States. Two kinds of strokes exist: thrombotic (most common) and hemorrhagic. Also see Chapter 1, Types of Thrombosis and Types of Embolism; and Chapter 2, Arteriosclerotic Disorders—Atherosclerosis. | Hypertension, diabetes, hyperlipidemia, smoking, heavy alcohol use, and a family history of stroke. |
| | Transient ischemic attack is caused by a transient loss of blood supply with a temporary loss of central nervous system function (no permanent damage). | Ischemia, but no damage. |
| | Lacunar infarction (minor thrombotic stroke) is caused by a small artery or arteriolar occlusion. Often involves the internal capsule, pons, cerebellum, or basal ganglia and produces a contralateral pure motor or sensory deficit. Most patients recover completely. | Small association with hypertension and diabetes. Ischemic necrosis with edema as below, except that area involved is much smaller. |
| | Cerebral infarction (major thrombotic stroke) is caused by thrombotic atherosclerosis or embolization from large arteries or mural thrombus. Often involves the middle cerebral artery. Presents in patients < 60 years old with an abrupt and progressive contralateral sensory and motor paralysis, aphasia, and disruption of the visual fields (on the same side as the infarct). | Risk factors are as above. Process involves cerebral ischemia, with liquefactive necrosis and edema. Infarct may be hemorrhagic or pale. |
| | Hemorrhagic stroke is also known as intracerebral hemorrhage. Bleeding may occur in the basal ganglia (most commonly), pons, frontal lobe, or cerebellum. Abrupt headache, papilledema, focal neurologic deficits, and loss of consciousness occur. When untreated, many patients die. | Risks include hypertension, bleeding disorders, trauma, arteriovenous malformation, or microaneurysm. Rapidly expanding hematoma dissects through brain tissue. |
| Subarachnoid Hemorrhage | Causes sudden severe headache with nausea, vomiting, and loss of consciousness. May have nuchal rigidity and altered mental status if the patient regains consciousness. | Risks include berry aneurysm of the circle of Willis, trauma, and arteriovenous malformation. Bleeding occurs into the subarachnoid space. |
| Hypertensive Encephalopathy | Acute and transient onset of neurologic dysfunction, convulsions, and increased intracranial pressure. Most patients recover with immediate treatment. | Malignant hypertension increases the risk. Cerebral edema and ischemia are present. Little or no necrosis. |

## HYDROCEPHALUS

| Disease | Description | Cause |
|---|---|---|
| High-Pressure Hydrocephalus | Communicating hydrocephalus occurs when there is reduced absorption of the CSF or there is an obstruction in the subarachnoid space. Noncommunicating hydrocephalus occurs when the flow is obstructed within the ventricles. Also see Chapter 15, Congenital Neurologic Diseases—Hydrocephalus. | Obstruction of CSF flow |
| Normal-Pressure Hydrocephalus | Slowly evolving hydrocephalus in the elderly. Causes mental slowness, incontinence, and gait disturbances. | Cause is often unknown, but it can follow head trauma, subarachnoid hemorrhage, or meningoencephalitis |

## CYTOLOGIC ANALYSIS OF CEREBROSPINAL FLUID

| Characteristic | Encephalitis | Bacterial Meningitis | Viral Meningitis | Chronic Meningitis | Brain Abscess |
|---|---|---|---|---|---|
| Pressure | Raised | Raised | Raised | Raised | Very high |
| Gross Appearance | Clear | Turbid | Clear | Clear | Clear |
| Protein | Slightly elevated | High | Slightly elevated | Very high | Elevated |
| Glucose | Normal | Very low | Normal | Low | Normal |
| Cells | Lymphocytes or none | PMNs | Lymphocytes | Pleocytosis and PMNs | Pleocytosis (abnormally high number of lymphocytes in CSF) |
| Gram Stain or Acid-Fast | Negative | Positive (90%) | Negative | Rarely positive | Occasionally positive |
| Culture | Viral positive ($\leq$ 30%) | Bacterial positive (90%) | Viral positive (70%) | Mycobacteria positive | Occasionally positive bacterial culture |

Adapted from Chandrasoma P, Taylor CR (editors): *Concise Pathology*, 3rd ed, p 915. Originally published by Appleton & Lange. © 1998 by the McGraw-Hill Companies, Inc.

## INFECTIONS OF THE CENTRAL NERVOUS SYSTEM

| Disease | Description | Cause | Pathology |
|---|---|---|---|
| Meningitis | Bacterial meningitis—Most common in patients < 5 years. Acquired from respiratory tract or from direct spread (sinuses or skull fracture). Acute onset of high fever, headache, and nuchal rigidity (stiff neck). | Neonates: *Escherichia coli*, *Listeria*, and β-hemolytic streptococci. Children: *Haemophilus influenzae*. Adolescents and young adults: meningococci. Elderly: pneumococci. | Meninges are opaque and edematous, with purulent exudate. PMNs predominate. |
| | Viral meningitis—mild, self-limited illness consisting of fever, headache, and nuchal rigidity. | Coxsackievirus, herpesvirus, ECHO virus, HIV, and mumps virus. | Meninges are opaque and edematous, with an exudate. Lymphocytes predominate. |
| | Meningitis can also be due to immunocompromise, skull trauma, or spread of infection from prosthetic valves. | Immunocompromise: gram-negative bacteria, *Listeria*, and fungi. Trauma: coagulase-positive and -negative staphylococci and gram-negative bacteria. Prosthetic valves: coagulase-positive and -negative staphylococci. | Meninges are opaque and edematous, with an exudate. |
| | Other types:<br><br>• Chronic meningitis—slow personality change and poor concentration<br><br>• Neurosyphilis (*Treponema pallidum*, tertiary stage)<br><br>• Lyme disease (*Borrelia burgdorferi*)—aseptic meningitis | *Mycobacterium tuberculosis*, *Mycobacterium avium-intracellulare*, *Cryptococcus*, *Coccidioides*, *Histoplasma*, *T. pallidum*, and *B. burgdorferi*. | Depending on the cause, brain surface may be covered with granulomas, fibrosis, vasculitis, or plasma cell infiltrates. |
| Encephalitis | Presents the same as meningitis but causes rapidly progressive alteration of consciousness, seizures, and coma. | Herpes simplex virus type 1 (most common), cytomegalovirus, rabies, eastern equine encephalitis, western equine encephalitis, and HIV. | Necrosis of infected brain tissue and edema. May see perivascular lymphocytic cuffing, inclusion bodies in neurons, or glial nodules, depending on the cause. |

| | | | |
|---|---|---|---|
| **Cerebral Abscess** | Space-occupying lesion (also see Cerebral Trauma—Epidural Hematoma and Subdural Hematoma above; and Adult Central Nervous System Tumors below). Causes headache, vomiting, and papilledema. Infections occur after penetrating skull injuries and middle-ear or sinus infections. Hematogenous spread occurs. | Anaerobic streptococci, *Bacteroides*, *Nocardia*, *Staphylococcus aureus*, and gram-negative bacteria. In diabetes, may see *Mucor*. | Pus-filled cavity containing liquefactive necrosis of brain tissue and PMNs. |
| **Toxoplasmosis** | In an immunocompetent host, resembles infectious mononucleosis with arthralgias, fever, sore throat, myalgias, and a rash. In an immunocompromised host, it is an opportunistic infection with disseminated disease. Neurologic symptoms include headache, fever, altered mental status, seizures, and focal neurologic signs. | *Toxoplasma gondii.* | Multiple necrotic lesions in the brain. Pseudocysts containing the organism may be retrieved with a brain biopsy. |
| **Tetanus** | Occurs in unvaccinated individuals. Increased risk with deep puncture wounds, in newborns and the elderly, and in intravenous drug users. Spreading muscular spasms, eventually involving the neck, jaw (trismus, or lockjaw), back, and abdomen. | *Clostridium tetani.* | Neurotoxin inhibits neurotransmission at the inhibitory neurons of the spinal cord. Inhibits GABA and glycine. |
| **Myelitis (Poliomyelitis)** | Rare in the United States because of vaccination. Most patients are asymptomatic. Can cause meningitis and long-term flaccid paralysis. | Polio virus. | Destruction of the anterior horn motor neurons and infection of the meninges. |

## VIRAL ENCEPHALITIS

| Organism | Description | Population Affected | Pathology |
|---|---|---|---|
| **Herpes Simplex Virus Types 1 and 2** | The most common cause of encephalitis. Temporal and frontal lobes are affected. Fatal if not treated. Xanthochromia is present (red blood cell lysis in the CSF). | Neonates (see Chapter 15), recurrence of HSV in healthy adults, and immunocompromised patients | Necrotizing hemorrhagic encephalitis. Cerebral edema with lymphocytic infiltration and inclusion bodies in the infected cells. |
| **Rabies Virus** | Causes severe encephalitis. Transmitted by bite of an infected animal (carried by dogs, raccoons, foxes, squirrels, skunks, and bats). Untreatable and fatal once symptoms begin. Violent muscle contractions and convulsions occur to minor stimuli. | Anyone | Edema and degeneration of nerve cells in the basal ganglia, hippocampus, and brainstem. May see characteristic Negri bodies, eosinophilic inclusions in infected cells. |
| Cytomegalovirus | The most common opportunistic viral agent in AIDS. | Neonates (see Chapter 15) and immunosuppressed patients | Microglial nodules of necrotizing encephalitis with cytomegalic inclusions. |
| **Human Immunodeficiency Virus** | Directly infects the brain and spinal cord. Causes difficulty concentrating, memory impairment, slow thinking, depression, and difficulty with coordination and motor function. | Gay men (although heterosexual transmission is just as common), intravenous drug use, multiple blood transfusions | Small microglial nodules associated with multinucleated giant cells, tissue necrosis, and reactive gliosis. |
| **Arthropod-Borne Viral Encephalitis** | Includes western equine encephalitis, eastern equine encephalitis, and St. Louis encephalitis. Causes seizures, confusion, stupor, or coma. Transmitted by mosquito or tick vector. | Anyone exposed to infected mosquitoes and ticks | Cerebral edema, lymphocytic infiltration, and focal necrosis. |

## SLOW VIRAL ENCEPHALITIS/ENCEPHALOPATHIES

| Disease | Description | Cause | Pathology |
|---|---|---|---|
| Creutzfeldt-Jakob Disease | Mainly affects patients in their 50s and older. Causes progressive dementia and confusion followed by ataxia and death. | Prion, an infective protein | Slowly progressive neuronal loss, demyelination, and spongiosis of the white matter. No inflammation. |
| Kuru | Was found among New Guinea cannibals who ate human brains. Kuru affects mostly the cerebellum. Symptoms are similar to above. | Prion | Same as above plus kuru plaques (deposits of prion protein). |
| Subacute Sclerosing Panencephalitis | Previous measles infection manifests years later as a slowly progressive and fatal encephalitis. Mechanism is unknown. Causes personality changes and involuntary myoclonic movements. Death occurs within 2 years of onset. | Chronic measles viral infection | Gray matter and basal ganglia neurons degenerate. Intranuclear inclusions in infected cells. Demyelination of white matter with perivascular cuffing. |
| Progressive Multifocal Leukoencephalopathy | Acute-onset, rapidly progressing encephalitis. Often found in patients with leukemia, lymphoma, or immunodeficiency. | JC virus (papovavirus) | Focal demyelination and abnormal giant oligodendrocytes and astrocytes. |

# III. Degenerative Diseases

## DEMYELINATING DISEASES

| Disease | Description | Predisposing Factors | Pathology |
|---|---|---|---|
| Multiple Sclerosis | Most common central nervous system demyelinating disease. Onset in the 20s to 40s (females > males). Chronic disease with relapses. Common presentation includes weakness of the lower extremities, visual disturbances, sensory disturbances, loss of bladder control, and ataxia. | May have an autoimmune mechanism. Associated with HLA-DR2. | Multiple focal areas of demyelination scattered in the white matter of the brain (plaques), spinal cord, optic nerve, and paraventricular regions. Plaques are infiltrated by T cells. Reactive gliosis is present. |
| Acute Disseminated Encephalomyelitis | Causes headache, lethargy, and coma. | Follows measles (most commonly), mumps, rubella, and varicella zoster virus. Also seen after vaccination with pertussis. | Cell-mediated autoimmunity to myelin proteins shown in vitro. Patchy areas of white matter demyelination in brain and spinal cord associated with lymphocytic infiltration. |

Also see Slow Viral Encephalitis/Encephalopathies—Subacute Sclerosing Panencephalitis and Progressive Multifocal Leukoencephalopathy; Chapter 15, Congenital Neurologic Diseases—Phenylketonuria; and Other Degenerative Diseases—Subacute Combined Degeneration of the Spinal Cord, below, for vitamin B$_{12}$ deficiency.

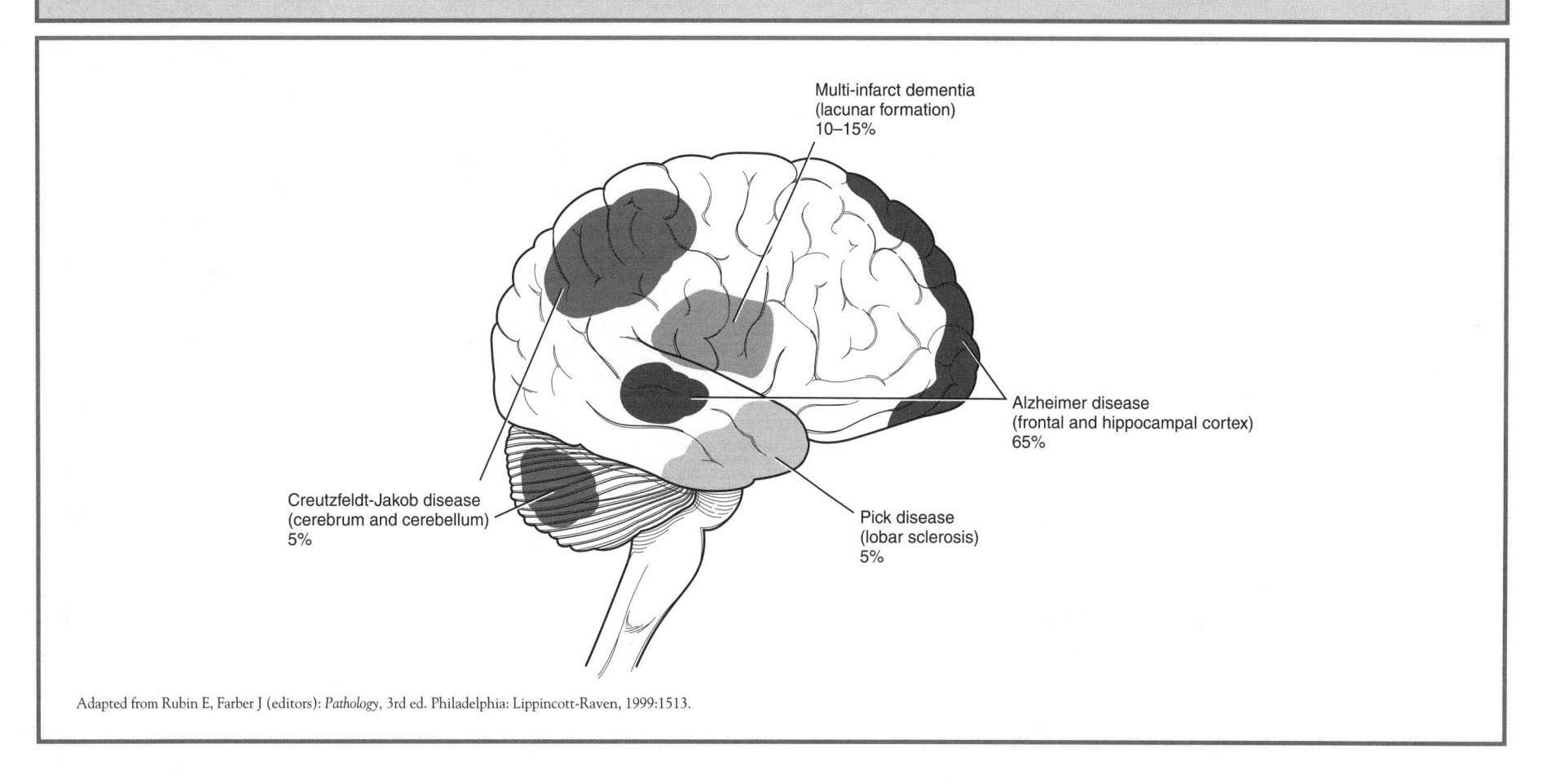

Multi-infarct dementia
(lacunar formation)
10–15%

Alzheimer disease
(frontal and hippocampal cortex)
65%

Creutzfeldt-Jakob disease
(cerebrum and cerebellum)
5%

Pick disease
(lobar sclerosis)
5%

Adapted from Rubin E, Farber J (editors): *Pathology*, 3rd ed. Philadelphia: Lippincott-Raven, 1999:1513.

## INCURABLE DEMENTIAS

| Disease | Description | Cause(s) | Pathology |
|---|---|---|---|
| Alzheimer Disease | The most common dementia (50% of all dementias). Occurs in patients aged > 50 years. Causes slowly progressive mental deterioration, including inability to solve complex problems, emotional lability, and loss of long-term memory and intellectual functions (reading or speaking). Associated with Down syndrome. | Apoprotein E4 gene expression and chromosome 14, 19, and 21 abnormalities | Global atrophy of the cerebral cortex in the frontal lobes and hippocampus. Neurofibrillary tangles (on silver stain) are intracytoplasmic bundles of microtubular filaments in neurons. Neuritic plaques (on silver stain) are degenerated nerve cell processes surrounding an amyloid core (in the hippocampus and amygdala). Cerebral amyloid angiopathy is amyloid material in small cerebral arteries. Hirano bodies are pink inclusions containing actin, found in dendrites. |
| Pick Disease | Uncommon. Occurs at 40–65 years. Resembles Alzheimer disease except that personality is more affected than memory. | Unknown | Cortical atrophy of the temporal and frontal lobes. Pick bodies (round eosinophilic inclusions) are found in surviving neurons. |
| Huntington Disease | Occurs in the 30s to 50s. Causes involuntary choreiform movements, progressing to dementia and death by 10–20 years from onset. | Autosomal dominant | Degeneration of the caudate nucleus, putamen, and frontal cortex. Destruction of the GABA and cholinergic neurons. |
| Parkinson Disease | Occurs in patients aged > 50 years. Slowly progressive disease with increased rigidity, resting tremor (pill-rolling tremor), masklike expression, slow movements, and a shuffling gait. About 20% of patients develop dementia. Treatable, but not curable. | Unknown | Loss of pigmented neurons in the substantia nigra and the locus ceruleus. The remaining neurons contain pink intracytoplasmic inclusions (Lewy bodies). Parkinsonism may also be secondary to Wilson disease. |
| Multiple Infarct Dementia | Occurs in the 70s. Abrupt onset or worsening of emotional lability, memory loss, and personality change. Symptoms are progressive as more areas of the brain undergo infarction. Disease is preventable but is irreversible once the damage is done. | Untreated chronic hypertension | Cerebral infarcts secondary to atherosclerotic emboli. Also see Chapter 2, Arteriosclerotic Disorders—Atherosclerosis; and Chapter 1, Types of Thrombosis and Types of Embolism. |
| Normal-Pressure Hydrocephalus | See Hydrocephalus above. | Unknown | See Hydrocephalus above. |
| Other Causes | HIV and Creutzfeldt-Jakob disease | | |

## TREATABLE/CURABLE DEMENTIAS

| Dementia | Cause(s) | Description | Pathology |
|---|---|---|---|
| Cerebral Beriberi or Wernicke Encephalopathy | Thiamine (vitamin $B_1$) deficiency, often associated with chronic alcohol abuse | Patients present with confusion, nystagmus, and ocular muscle paralysis. Also see Chapter 14 for alcohol manifestations. | Atrophy and degeneration of the mamillary bodies and the periventricular area of the brainstem following petechial hemorrhages |
| Pellagra-Associated Dementia | Niacin (vitamin $B_3$) deficiency | Causes dementia, dermatitis, and diarrhea. Also see Chapter 14, Vitamin Deficiencies and Excesses—Water-Soluble Vitamins. | Neuronal degeneration of the cerebral cortex, pons, and anterior horn cells of the spinal cord |
| Infectious Causes of Dementia | Syphilis and chronic meningitis | Dementia is the end stage. For specifics, see each disease above. | See each specific disease above |

## OTHER DEGENERATIVE DISEASES

| Disease | Description | Pathology |
|---|---|---|
| Amyotrophic Lateral Sclerosis | Also known as Lou Gehrig's disease. The most common motor neuron disease. Muscles are denervated because of destruction of the lower motor neurons. Upper motor neuron signs include hyperreflexia and spasticity. | Degeneration of the upper and lower motor neurons. Atrophy of the lateral corticospinal tracts (lateral sclerosis) and anterior motor neurons of the spinal cord. |
| Subacute Combined Degeneration of the Spinal Cord | Caused by vitamin $B_{12}$ deficiency. Presents with or without anemia. Causes loss of vibratory and position sense and upper motor neuron paralysis with hyperreflexia. Treatment with vitamin $B_{12}$ stops progression of the disease. See also Peripheral Neuropathies above; Chapter 14, Vitamin Deficiencies and Excesses—Water-Soluble Vitamins; and Chapter 4 for pernicious anemia. | Demyelination of the posterior columns and the lateral columns of the spinal cord. |

## DISTRIBUTION OF COMMON INTRACRANIAL TUMORS

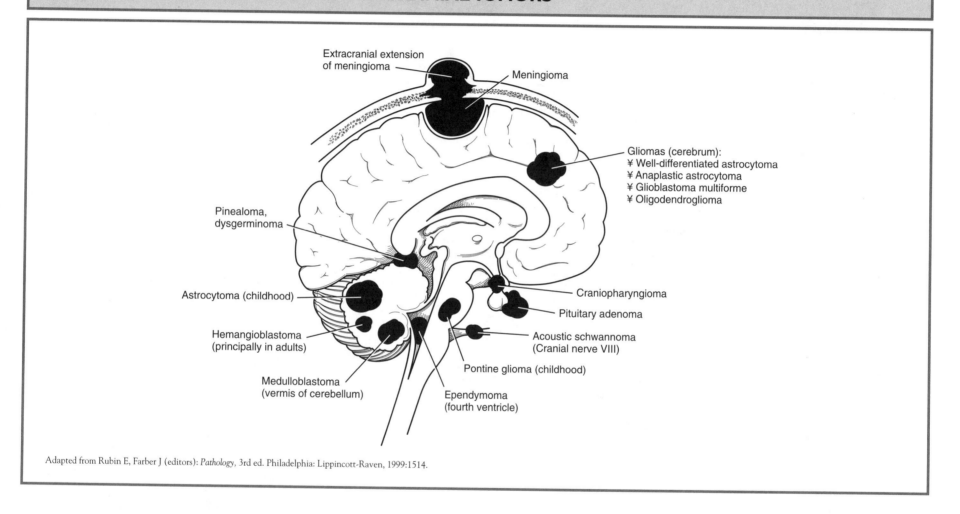

Extracranial extension of meningioma

Meningioma

Gliomas (cerebrum):
¥ Well-differentiated astrocytoma
¥ Anaplastic astrocytoma
¥ Glioblastoma multiforme
¥ Oligodendroglioma

Pinealoma, dysgerminoma

Astrocytoma (childhood)

Craniopharyngioma

Pituitary adenoma

Hemangioblastoma (principally in adults)

Acoustic schwannoma (Cranial nerve VIII)

Pontine glioma (childhood)

Medulloblastoma (vermis of cerebellum)

Ependymoma (fourth ventricle)

Adapted from Rubin E, Farber J (editors): *Pathology*, 3rd ed. Philadelphia: Lippincott-Raven, 1999:1514.

# ADULT CENTRAL NERVOUS SYSTEM TUMORS

| Tumor | Description | Pathology |
|---|---|---|
| Spinal cord tumors are mainly found in adults and are due to metastases (most commonly), neurofibromas, schwannomas, meningiomas, and astrocytomas. | | |
| **Benign Tumors** | | |
| Meningioma | Benign tumor that occurs in females > males. Tumor remains attached to the dura. 10% may recur after resection. All clinical features are due to compression of the brain or brainstem tissue. Malignant meningioma may arise with recurrence. | Neural crest origin. Firm, well-encapsulated mass. Whorled pattern of concentric spindle cells and laminated calcified psammoma bodies may be found. Mitoses are rare. |
| Hemangioblastoma | Cerebellar tumor. May cause cerebellar dysfunction, hydrocephalus, or polycythemia from erythropoietin production. May be part of von Hippel-Lindau disease. Surgical resection is curative. | Vascular cell origin. Well-circumscribed mass with solid and cystic components. Endothelium-lined spaces are separated by trabeculae. |
| **Malignant Tumors**—responsible for 16,800 cases and 13,100 deaths per year in the United States. | | Ninth most common cancer in women. |
| Astrocytoma | The most common primary brain tumor. Most common type is diffuse (fibrillary). The most malignant is glioblastoma multiforme. Involves the cerebral cortex. Poor prognosis, with a median of 1-year survival. | Glioma of glial cell origin. Infiltrating mass, often crossing the midline. May show necrosis and hemorrhage. Anaplasia, pleomorphism, and frequency of mitosis range from little or none to extensive and many. Neovascularization is common. |
| Oligodendroglioma | Slowly growing tumor of the cerebral cortex. Prognosis is good, but recurrences are common after resection. | Glioma of glial cell origin. Well-circumscribed and solid. Focal calcifications may be observed on X-ray. Cells are uniform with clear halo surrounding the nucleus, resembling a fried egg. |
| Primary Malignant Lymphoma of Brain | Malignant tumor seen with AIDS. Commonly has multiple foci and involves both cerebral hemispheres. | Most common type is B-cell immunoblastic lymphoma. See Chapter 4. |
| Metastatic Tumors | The most common intracranial tumors. Metastases are common from cancers in the lungs, breast, kidney, gastrointestinal tract, and thyroid, as well as melanoma. | |
| For pediatric neurologic tumors, see Chapter 15. | | |

# CHAPTER 14
# NUTRITIONAL AND ENVIRONMENTAL DISEASES

## I. CHEMICAL AND DRUG INJURY

Chemical Injuries

Therapeutic Drug Toxicity

Pathology of Smoking, Alcoholism, and Lead Intoxication

## II. ENVIRONMENTAL DISORDERS

Environmentally Caused Disorders

## III. NUTRITIONAL AND DIET-RELATED DISORDERS

Nutrition, Weight, and Diet Abnormalities

Vitamin Deficiencies and Excesses—Fat-Soluble Vitamins

Vitamin Deficiencies and Excesses—Water-Soluble Vitamins

Diet-Related Disorders

**ABBREVIATIONS**

**G6PD** = glucose-6-phosphate dehydrogenase

**HMG-CoA** = 3-hydroxy-3-methylglutaryl coenzyme A

**RBC** = red blood cell

# I. Chemical and Drug Injury

## CHEMICAL INJURIES

| Compound or Entity | Pathology |
| --- | --- |
| Aniline Dyes | Can cause transitional cell carcinoma of the bladder. |
| Arsenic | Acutely, can cause gastrointestinal symptoms such as nausea, vomiting, or diarrhea. If taken in large doses, can cause coma and death. Chronically, causes squamous cell and basal cell carcinomas of the skin. |
| Asbestos | Can cause pneumoconiosis, bronchogenic carcinoma, and mesothelioma of the lung. |
| Benzene | Can cause acute myelogenous leukemia (blood disorder). |
| Carbon Monoxide | Found in smoke (smoke inhalation) and in motor vehicle exhaust. Decreases the oxygen-carrying capacity of RBCs by combining with hemoglobin to form carboxyhemoglobin, which leads to hypoxia. |
| Carbon Tetrachloride | Found in dry-cleaning solution. Can lead to hepatic centrilobular necrosis, fatty change of the liver, and toxic nephrosis (kidney tubular necrosis). |
| Cyanide | Produces loss of cytochrome oxidation (mitochondrial malfunction), leading to immediate halting of cellular respiration and cellular death. Fatal in minutes if not treated. |
| Ethylene Glycol | Found in antifreeze. Calcium oxalate crystals in the kidneys cause toxic nephrosis (tubular necrosis). |
| Mercuric Chloride | Can cause gastrointestinal ulceration and necrosis of the renal convoluted tubules. |
| Methanol | Blindness can be caused by formaldehyde byproducts (formic acid). Coma or death results from respiratory failure. |
| Nickel, Chromium, and Uranium | Can cause lung carcinoma. |
| Polyvinyl Chloride | Can cause angiosarcoma (hemangiosarcoma) of the liver. |

## THERAPEUTIC DRUG TOXICITY

| Drug | Toxic Effect |
|------|--------------|
| **ANTIMICROBIAL, ANTIFUNGAL, and ANTIVIRAL AGENTS** | |
| Acyclovir | Nephrotoxicity (drug crystallizes in the nephrons). |
| Amphotericin B | Dose-dependent nephrotoxicity. |
| Chloroquine | Skin rash and peripheral neuropathy. |
| Penicillin | Urticaria is the most common. Anaphylactic shock also can occur. See Chapter 3, Hypersensitivity Diseases; and Chapter 11, Immune-Mediated Rashes—Urticaria. |
| Streptomycin | Prototype of aminoglycosides. Can cause ototoxicity and renal failure. |
| Sulfonamides | Drug-induced polyarteritis nodosa. Obstruction of the renal collecting system from crystals (tubular damage). Bone marrow failure (aplastic anemia). Self-limited hemolytic anemia (if G6PD deficient). |
| Tetracycline | Microvesicular fatty change of the liver. See Chapter 10, Fatty Liver. |
| **CHEMOTHERAPEUTIC AGENTS** | |
| In general, these drugs cause hair loss, gastrointestinal erosions and ulcers, and myelosuppression (all due to stem cell destruction). | |
| Bleomycin | Pulmonary fibrosis |
| Cyclophosphamide | Alopecia and hemorrhagic cystitis |
| Cyclosporine | Dose-dependent nephrotoxicity |
| Doxorubicin | Cardiotoxicity |
| **ANTIEPILEPTICS and ANTISEIZURE MEDICATIONS** | |
| Carbamazepine | Hematotoxic effects |
| Phenytoin | Gingival hyperplasia and hirsutism |
| Valproic Acid | Rare hepatic necrosis |

*Continued*

## THERAPEUTIC DRUG TOXICITY (Continued)

### NONSTEROIDAL ANTI-INFLAMMATORY DRUGS

In general, these drugs produce gastrointestinal bleeding (gastric or peptic ulcer) and renal damage from prolonged use.

| | |
|---|---|
| Acetaminophen | Fatty liver change and centrilobular necrosis of the liver. |
| Aspirin | Reye syndrome (associated with use during a viral illness). |
| Phenacetin | All kidney manifestations, including chronic analgesic nephritis and renal papillary necrosis from prolonged use. Increased risk of transitional cell carcinoma of the renal pelvis. Hepatic necrosis also can occur. |

### STEROIDS

| | |
|---|---|
| Corticosteroids | See Chapter 8 for Cushing syndrome. |
| Exogenous Estrogens | Endometrial carcinoma (risk is reduced if concurrently taking progesterone), venous thrombosis, vaginal adenosis, gallbladder disease, and cholestasis. Diethylstilbestrol (DES) has been found to cause clear cell adenocarcinoma and adenosis of the vagina in daughters of mothers who used it during pregnancy. |
| Exogenous Progestins | Suppression of insulin-mediated glucose uptake. |

### ANTILIPIDEMIC DRUGS

The statins are a class of HMG-CoA reductase inhibitors that reduce the amount of cholesterol manufactured by the liver.

| | |
|---|---|
| Lovastatin | Hepatitis and muscle damage |

### ANTIHYPERTENSIVE AGENTS

| | |
|---|---|
| Methyldopa | Positive Coombs test (autoimmune reaction to RBCs) and hemolysis |

# PATHOLOGY OF SMOKING, ALCOHOLISM, AND LEAD INTOXICATION

## ALCOHOL-RELATED DISORDERS

### Neurologic Changes

- Peripheral neuropathy caused by thiamine ($B_1$) deficiency
- Cerebral encephalopathy—Wernicke encephalopathy due to thiamine ($B_1$) deficiency. Without thiamine replacement, progresses to Korsakoff syndrome (memory loss).

### Neoplasms

- Hepatocellular carcinoma (hepatoma)
- Oral and esophageal squamous cell carcinoma

### Gastrointestinal Changes

- Alcoholic hepatitis and liver cirrhosis
- Pancreatitis
- Acute gastritis

### Other Changes

- Dilated cardiomyopathy
- Fetal alcohol syndrome
- Risk of aspiration pneumonia due to diminished gag reflex
- Trauma (motor vehicle accidents and falls)

## TOBACCO-RELATED DISORDERS

### Cardiovascular Injury

- Myocardial infarction
- Cerebral stroke
- Systemic atherosclerosis
- Peripheral vascular disease

### Neoplasms

- Bronchogenic carcinoma
- Renal cell carcinoma
- Lip, oral cavity, laryngeal, and esophageal squamous cell carcinomas
- Pancreatic adenocarcinoma
- Cervical carcinoma in situ

### Lung Changes

- Chronic bronchitis (chronic obstructive pulmonary disease)
- Emphysema

### Other Changes

- Macrophage dysfunction
- Acute gastritis
- Pregnancy problems (low birth weight, stillbirths, abortions, infant mortality)

## LEAD TOXICITY

### Blood Disorders

- Microcytic hypochromic anemia
- Basophilic stippling of RBCs

### Neurologic Disorders

- Brain damage in infants
- Peripheral neuropathy—demyelination of motor axons causes "wrist drop"

### Kidney Disorders

- Elevated urine coproporphyrins
- Fanconi syndrome—tubulointerstitial nephritis with acid-fast intranuclear inclusions

# II. Environmental Disorders

## ENVIRONMENTALLY CAUSED DISORDERS

| Injury | Causation and Description of Symptoms |
|---|---|
| Burns | Injury depends on the degree of burn. In first-degree burns, only the superficial epidermis is lost. In second-degree burns, the entire epidermis is lost. Third-degree burns involve the dermis. Plasma loss from damaged skin leads to hypoalbuminemia, edema, and hypovolemic shock. Burn areas are prone to infection with *Pseudomonas*, and patients are prone to developing septic shock. |
| Excessive Sun Exposure | Prolonged exposure to the sun and to ultraviolet light over the years can lead to actinic keratosis, squamous cell carcinoma, basal cell carcinoma, or melanoma (skin cancer). |
| Frostbite | Frostbite causes damage by three mechanisms: tissue freezing, in which ice crystals damage cell membranes; hypoxia, which results from local vasoconstriction; and release of inflammatory mediators, including thromboxane $A_2$ and prostaglandins, which promotes thrombosis and platelet aggregation. The last mechanism is the reason that frostbitten skin blisters. |
| Heatstroke | Heatstroke occurs when there is excessive air temperature (> 95°F or 35°C) or humidity (> 75%). Sweating after this point does not help body cooling. <br><br>• Classic (passive) heatstroke has a mortality rate as high as 70–80% and affects the elderly and the young. <br><br>• Exertional heatstroke has a mortality rate of about 20% and occurs in young active adults. |
| Radiation Exposure | Can cause dermatitis and skin malignancies, acute myelocytic anemia, lymphoid and hematopoietic germ cell destruction (in bone marrow), and adult respiratory distress syndrome (in the lungs). Mainly affects rapidly dividing cells. |

# III. Nutritional and Diet-Related Disorders

## NUTRITION, WEIGHT, AND DIET ABNORMALITIES

| Condition | Description | Population Affected | Pathologic Findings |
|---|---|---|---|
| Marasmus | All nutrients are deficient; patient "wastes away." | Children < 1 year old who are not being breast-fed or formula-fed. | ☞ Marasmus and malnutrition both start with "M". Growth is slowed and muscle and subcutaneous fat are lost. |
| Kwashiorkor | Diet is deficient only in protein. Calorie intake is normal. Causes retarded growth and muscle wasting, but subcutaneous fat is preserved. | Children > 6 months old or after breast-feeding is stopped. Mother may be feeding watered-down formula or sugar water. | Fatty liver, edema (hypoalbuminemia), anemia, and atrophy of the small intestinal villi. |
| Obesity | Results from excessive calorie intake. Can also be a sign of various endocrinologic disorders such as Cushing disease. | Any age. | Risk factor for insulin resistance, hypertension, heart disease, cholesterol gallstones, and endometrial uterine cancer. |

## VITAMIN DEFICIENCIES AND EXCESSES—FAT-SOLUBLE VITAMINS

☞ ADEK can be used to remember the fat-soluble vitamins, where each letter represents one of the vitamins.

| Vitamin | Symptoms of Vitamin Deficiency | Symptoms of Vitamin Excess | Notes and Findings |
|---|---|---|---|
| Vitamin A | Night blindness and dry, brittle skin. Squamous metaplasia in eyes and lungs. | Hepatocellular damage, bone changes, and alopecia | Found in animal products, especially milk, egg yolk, and the liver. |
| Vitamin D | Rickets in children, with failure of bone mineralization (leg bowing), and osteomalacia in adults. See Chapter 12, Bone Metabolism. | Growth retardation, hypercalciuria, neurocalcinosis (deposition of calcium in the brain), and kidney stones | Skin can manufacture enough vitamin D when there is sufficient contact with sunlight. |
| Vitamin E | Neurologic dysfunction (spinocerebellar degeneration). | None known | Abundant in staple foods such as eggs, cereals, and butter. Deficiencies are rare. |
| Vitamin K | Hemorrhagic diathesis (abnormal bleeding). Needed by the liver to manufacture clotting factors II, VII, IX, and X and proteins C and S. | None known | Manufactured by bacteria in the colon and is present in green vegetables. Given to infants as an injection soon after birth to prevent hemorrhagic disease of the newborn. |

## VITAMIN DEFICIENCIES AND EXCESSES—WATER-SOLUBLE VITAMINS

☞ To remember which vitamin is $B_1$, $B_2$, or $B_3$, use the word TRaiN. The letters correspond to thiamine ($B_1$), riboflavin ($B_2$), and niacin ($B_3$). All B vitamins function as coenzymes.

| Vitamin | Symptoms of Vitamin Deficiency | Symptoms of Vitamin Excess | Notes and Findings |
|---|---|---|---|
| **Vitamin $B_1$ (Thiamine)** | Wet beriberi—cardiac failure and edema (this is why it is wet). | None known | Endemic beriberi is found in areas where white or polished rice is the predominant food staple (e.g., Japan, Philippines, and India). |
| | Dry beriberi—flaccid paralysis, muscular atrophy, and lack of reflexes. | | |
| | Cerebral beriberi or Wernicke syndrome—triad of confusion, ataxia, and ophthalmoplegia. This can progress to Korsakoff syndrome—confabulation and memory loss in addition to the triad. See Pathology of Smoking, Alcoholism, and Lead Intoxication—Alcohol-Related Disorders above. | | Korsakoff syndrome is due to periventricular demyelination. |
| **Vitamin $B_2$ (Riboflavin)** | Glossitis (inflammation of the tongue) and dermatitis (skin inflammation). | None known | Vitamin $B_2$ is needed for cellular respiration. |
| **Vitamin $B_3$ (Niacin)** | Pellagra manifests with dementia, dermatitis, and diarrhea. | None known | ☞ All symptoms start with "D". |
| **Vitamin $B_6$ (Pyridoxine)** | Glossitis, anemia, convulsions, and central nervous system dysfunction. | None known | Vitamin $B_6$ is found in most foods. |
| **Vitamin $B_{12}$ (Cobalamin)** | Pernicious anemia, an autoimmune disorder in which antibodies against intrinsic factor prevent $B_{12}$ absorption. Results in megaloblastic anemia and can cause peripheral neuropathy and degeneration of posterolateral spinal cord tracts. See Chapter 4, Macrocytic Anemias; Chapter 13, Other Degenerative Diseases – Subacute Combined Degeneration of the Spinal Cord. | None known | Vitamin $B_{12}$ is needed for nucleic acid synthesis. Need intrinsic factor from parietal cells in the stomach to deliver vitamin $B_{12}$ to the distal ileum, where it is absorbed. |
| **Folic Acid** | Megaloblastic anemia. Neural tube defects (spina bifida) can result in infants of mothers who are folate deficient during pregnancy. See Chapter 4, Macrocytic Anemias; Chapter 15, Congenital Neurologic Diseases. | None known | Folic acid is needed for nucleic acid synthesis. Amounts needed are doubled during pregnancy. |
| **Vitamin C** | Scurvy; defective wound healing. Bleeding is due to fragile blood vessels. | None known | Vitamin C is needed for collagen synthesis. |

## DIET-RELATED DISORDERS

| Disease or Condition | Foods That Should Be Avoided | Substance That Accumulates | Symptoms if Untreated |
|---|---|---|---|
| Galactosemia | Lactose in cow milk, breast milk, and dairy products | Galactose in the blood | Failure to thrive, mental retardation, steatosis, hepatomegaly, and cataracts |
| Phenylketonuria | Those that contain phenylalanine | Phenylalanine in the blood | Mental retardation. See Chapter 15, Congenital Neurologic Diseases. |
| Lactose Intolerance | Dairy products | Lactose is broken down by colonic bacteria instead of by lactase in the small intestine. | Cramping, abdominal pain, bloating, and diarrhea. Also see Chapter 9 for diarrhea. |
| Dermatitis Herpetiformis | Wheat and rye | Gluten hypersensitivity | Vesicular skin rash |
| Celiac Sprue | Wheat and rye | Intestinal hypersensitivity to gluten | Stunted growth; atrophy of the intestinal villi with resulting malabsorption. Also see Chapter 9, Malabsorption Syndromes. |

# CHAPTER 15
# DISEASES OF INFANCY TO CHILDHOOD

I. CONGENITAL DISEASES

Transmission of Congenital Infections

Perinatal AIDS Infection

Teratogens

Congenital Infections

Congenital Heart Diseases

Congenital Jaundice

Congenital Neurologic Diseases

II. NEONATAL AND POSTNATAL DISEASES

Neonatal Infections

Respiratory Diseases

Rashes and Skin Lesions

Skin Infections

Gastrointestinal Diseases

Neonatal Jaundice

Urogenital Diseases

Chromosome Abnormality Diseases

Sex Chromosome Diseases

Childhood Tumor Epidemiology

**ABBREVIATIONS**

**HIV** = human immunodeficiency virus

**Ig** = immunoglobulin

**IUGR** = intrauterine growth retardation

**ToRCHS** = toxoplasmosis, other infections, rubella, cytomegalovirus, herpes simplex virus, and syphilis

## MOST COMMON Causes and Types

| Disorder | Common Cause |
| --- | --- |
| Congenital jaundice | Gilbert disease |
| Skin infection | Impetigo |
| Malignant tumor of infancy | Acute lymphoblastic leukemia |
| Benign tumor of infancy | Hemangioma |
| Chromosomal disorder | Down syndrome (trisomy 21) |
| Intrauterine infection | Cytomegalovirus |

| Disorder | Common Type |
| --- | --- |
| Teratogen | Alcohol (ethanol) |

| | |
|---|---|
| Congenital | Any condition present at the time of birth, genetic or not |
| Neonatal | Time period between birth and the first 4 weeks of life |
| Nonspecific Signs of a Neonatal Infection | Constellation of signs not localizing to the specific infection (e.g., meningitis, urinary tract infection, pneumonia); these include fever, poor feeding, diarrhea, vomiting, irritability, lethargy, jaundice, and hepatosplenomegaly |
| Perinatal | Time period from 3 months before birth to 1 month after |
| Postpartum | Time period of the immediate few days after birth |
| Prenatal | The time before birth |
| Teratogen | Any substance that induces the formation of fetal abnormalities |

# I. Congenital Diseases

## TRANSMISSION OF CONGENITAL INFECTIONS

| Type of Transmission | Type of Congenital Infection |
|---|---|
| Intrauterine or Transplacental | *Toxoplasma, Listeria,* rubella, cytomegalovirus, syphilis, parvovirus B19, and HIV |
| During Delivery | *Streptococcus agalactiae* (group B), *Neisseria gonorrhoeae,* hepatitis B, herpes simplex virus type 2, varicella zoster virus, *Escherichia coli,* *Chlamydia trachomatis,* cytomegalovirus, HIV, and *Candida* |
| During Breast-Feeding | HIV |

## PERINATAL AIDS INFECTION

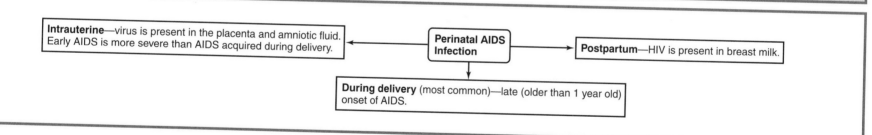

## TERATOGENS

| Teratogen | Crucial Time for Exposure | Signs and Symptoms |
| --- | --- | --- |
| Alcohol (ethanol) | Anytime | Most common teratogen. Fetal alcohol syndrome manifests as facial and developmental abnormalities. Level of defects is proportional to the amount of alcohol used. Infants present with microcephaly, cardiac and renal abnormalities, and mental and growth retardation. |
| Angiotensin-Converting Enzyme Inhibitors | Second or third trimester | Fetal renal damage, lack of cranial ossification, and IUGR. |
| Chloramphenicol | Third trimester | Gray baby syndrome affects premature neonates. Consists of cyanosis, hypotension, and death (from inability to metabolize the drug). |
| Diethylstilbestrol[1] | First trimester | Clear cell adenocarcinoma and vaginal adenosis in daughters of mothers who used it during pregnancy. |
| Isotretinoin (Accutane)[1] | First trimester | Central nervous system defects, thymic agenesis, cardiovascular defects, craniofacial dysmorphism (cleft lip and palate), and mental retardation. |
| Lithium | Third trimester | Congenital heart disease, particularly Ebstein anomaly. Also toxic to kidneys, thyroid, and neuromuscular system. |
| Methyl Mercury | Third trimester | Cerebral atrophy, mental retardation, seizures, blindness, and cerebral palsy. |
| Phenytoin (Dilantin) | Chronic use throughout pregnancy | IUGR, mental retardation, dysmorphic craniofacial features, and hypoplastic nails. |
| Streptomycin | Chronic use throughout pregnancy | Hearing loss. |
| Tetracycline | Second or third trimester | Hypoplastic tooth enamel, permanent discoloration of deciduous teeth. |
| Thalidomide[1] | First trimester | Bilateral limb deficiencies, cardiac and gastrointestinal anomalies. |
| Valproic Acid[1] | First trimester | Neural tube defects in the fetus. |
| Warfarin[1] | First trimester | Nasal hypoplasia, CNS abnormalities. |

[1]Period of organogenesis (day 18–60) during gestation is the period of greatest sensitivity and vulnerability to teratogens.

## CONGENITAL INFECTIONS

| ☞ | Organism | Symptoms | Notes on Transmission |
|---|---|---|---|
| T | Toxoplasmosis | Most infants are asymptomatic at birth. Microcephaly, mental retardation, intracranial calcifications, jaundice, hepatosplenomegaly, and a purpuric maculopapular rash occur later. Chorioretinitis can occur at birth or later. | *Toxoplasma gondii* is a protozoan parasite carried by members of the cat family. Transmission occurs via ingestion of oocytes. Only primary infection of the mother (often asymptomatic) causes the congenital infection. |
| O | Varicella Zoster Virus | Congenital chickenpox causes cutaneous scars, defects in the eye, central nervous system anomalies, and low birth weight. | Most pregnant women are already immune. The rest have a 25% risk of causing disease if infected. |
| R | Rubella Virus | Congenital rubella produces heart defects, cataracts, glaucoma, chorioretinitis, deafness, microcephaly, and mental retardation. Chronic infection presents with growth retardation, hepatosplenomegaly, jaundice, and blueberry muffin spots (purple skin lesions). | Greatest risk is in the first trimester. Vaccine given just before or during pregnancy poses a theoretical risk for congenital rubella. |
| C | Cytomegalovirus | The most common congenital infection. Most infants are asymptomatic. Encephalitis, IUGR, purpura, jaundice, chorioretinitis, microcephaly, hepatosplenomegaly, and pneumonia may occur. | Results from primary or reactivation of maternal infection. Infected cells have a characteristic "owl eye" appearance (halo around the nucleus). |
| H | Herpes Simplex Virus Type 2 | Vesicular ulcerations and scars on the body, microcephaly, intracranial calcifications, bone abnormalities, and hepatosplenomegaly. If untreated, infection leads to herpes encephalitis or chorioretinitis. | Mother may be asymptomatically infected. |
|  | Hepatitis B | Asymptomatic. | > 90% of infants become asymptomatic chronic carriers and become at risk for cirrhosis and hepatocellular carcinoma later in life. |
|  | Human Immunodeficiency Virus | Asymptomatic at birth. Later, recurrent thrush, lymphadenopathy, hepatosplenomegaly, intractable diarrhea, and failure to thrive. | Rate of transmission from mother to infant is 30% without azidothymidine and 8% with azidothymidine. |
| S | Syphilis | The most common cause of stillbirth. Survivors have congenital syphilis. Intermittent fevers; bone inflammation; hepatosplenomegaly; lymphadenopathy; rash involving the palms, soles, and trunk; persistent rhinitis (sniffles); jaundice; and failure to thrive. Late manifestations are Hutchinson teeth, mulberry molars, saddle nose, frontal bossing, interstitial keratitis, and nerve deafness. | Due to *Treponema pallidum*, transmitted from an untreated infected woman before or during pregnancy. Mother may be asymptomatic. |

## CONGENITAL HEART DISEASES

| Condition | Description and Symptoms | Notes |
|---|---|---|
| Coarctation of the Aorta | Postductal type is asymptomatic until adult life (collateral flow develops by dilated intercostal arteries). Causes intercostal rib notching. Preductal type is fatal without surgery. | Hypertension is similar to that in bilateral renal artery stenosis (blood flow reduced to both kidneys, leading to kidney failure). Renin independent (renin levels are normal). See Chapter 2, Types of Hypertension. |
| **Noncyanotic Diseases** | **No shunt or left-to-right shunt. Oxygenated blood is diverted back to the lungs.** | |
| Patent Ductus Arteriosus | Asymptomatic unless there is left ventricular heart failure or pulmonary hypertension. Infants are at risk for infective endocarditis. Eisenmenger syndrome can occur in a small number of patients. (See Chapter 2.) | Usually closes at birth when prostaglandin levels decline. Can be closed by administering prostaglandin antagonists (nonsteroidal anti-inflammatory drugs). |
| Atrial Septal Defect | Patent foramen ovale (small shunt) is asymptomatic. Larger shunts (septum secundum defect) cause Eisenmenger syndrome later in life. Lesions in the septum primum (lower septum) are associated with Down syndrome. | Risk for paradoxic embolus. Later in life, emboli originating in the venous system (entering the right side of the heart) can traverse the atrial septal defect into the arterial side (into the left side of the heart and aorta). |
| Ventricular Septal Defect | Most common congenital cardiac anomaly. Presents with a holosystolic regurgitant murmur. Most are in the membranous septum. Large holes may lead to Eisenmenger syndrome and right-sided heart failure. | At risk for infective endocarditis. Some defects close spontaneously late in childhood, and many small shunts do not need surgical repair. |
| Rubella Infection | Congenital rubella syndrome produces cardiovascular defects: patent ductus arteriosus, aortic stenosis, ventricular septal defect, pulmonary valve stenosis, and others. | See Congenital Infections—ToRCHS above. |
| **Cyanotic Diseases** | **Right-to-left shunt whereby deoxygenated blood is diverted back to the body instead of to the lungs.** | |
| Tetralogy of Fallot | • Pulmonary valve stenosis    • Right ventricular hypertrophy<br>• Ventricular septal defect    • Overriding aorta | Children tend to squat. Squatting increases afterload and flow through the defect and improves the cyanotic condition. Pulmonary valve stenosis can occur by itself (not part of this syndrome). |
| Transposition of the Great Vessels | Aorta originates from the right ventricle and pulmonary artery originates from the left ventricle. Patent ductus arteriosus or atrial or ventricular septal defect is needed to survive. | More common in children of mothers with diabetes mellitus. |
| Truncus Arteriosus | Failure of aorta and pulmonary trunk separation, resulting in mixing of right ventricular and left ventricular blood. | Poor prognosis unless surgically corrected at an early age. |

## CONGENITAL JAUNDICE

| Disease | Description | Pathology |
| --- | --- | --- |
| Gilbert Syndrome | Most common type of jaundice. Infant is born with mild unconjugated hyperbilirubinemia (liver function is normal). Jaundice is exacerbated with stress or starvation. | Reduced liver uptake of bilirubin. Reduced glucuronosyltransferase levels. |
| Crigler-Najjar Syndrome | Severe unconjugated hyperbilirubinemia that can cause kernicterus. Type I is severe and fatal; type II is mild. | Absence of glucuronosyltransferase. |
| Dubin-Johnson Syndrome | Rare, autosomal recessive disease. Presents with a mild conjugated hyperbilirubinemia. Normal life expectancy. | Defective transport of conjugated bilirubin out of the liver. Brown or black liver from bile deposition. |
| Rotor Syndrome | Presentation is similar to that of Dubin-Johnson syndrome. | No black liver. |
| Biliary Atresia | Presents with jaundice and pale, gray stools by the third week of life. By 8 weeks, there is hepatosplenomegaly. Syndrome is associated with trisomy 13 and 18. Must be surgically corrected or death occurs from liver cirrhosis by 2 years. | Unknown etiology. Obstructive jaundice from obstructed extrahepatic bile ducts. |

See also Neonatal Jaundice.

# CONGENITAL NEUROLOGIC DISEASES

| Disease | Description | Pathologic Findings |
|---------|-------------|---------------------|
| Neural Tube Defects | Neural tube defects occur from failure of neural tube closure at 3–4 weeks of gestation. They accompany spina bifida, in which several posterior vertebral arches fail to fuse.<br>• Spina bifida occulta—1–2 vertebrae are affected. Asymptomatic.<br>• Spina bifida meningocele—Meninges herniate through the defect in the arches.<br>• Meningomyelocele—Spinal cord herniates with the meninges. Most severe type. Occurs often in the lumbosacral area.<br>• Anencephaly—Absence of cerebral hemispheres, cerebellum, and overlying skull. Most infants die within a few days of birth. | Elevated maternal $\alpha$-fetoprotein in the serum is diagnostic. $\alpha$-Fetoprotein, present in cerebrospinal fluid, leaks from the defect in the spinal cord. |
| Hydrocephalus | Production of cerebrospinal fluid is greater than absorption. Obstruction from stenosis of the cerebral aqueduct produces a noncommunicating hydrocephalus (ventricle immediately before the block becomes enlarged). In a communicating hydrocephalus, the subarachnoid villi are nonfunctional (all ventricles enlarge). Presents with increased head circumference, a bulging fontanelle, poor feeding, and irritability or lethargy. | Communicating hydrocephalus is caused by bacterial meningitis, intra-uterine infections, or intraventricular bleeding.<br>Noncommunicating hydrocephalus is caused by intracranial brain tumors. |
| Arnold-Chiari Malformation | Malformation of the fourth ventricle causes its foramina to open below the foramen magnum. Reabsorption of the cerebrospinal fluid draining from these foramina is blocked, creating a communicating hydrocephalus. Cerebellar tonsils herniate through the foramen magnum, and there is pressure atrophy of the brain. | Presence of thoracolumbar meningomyelocele (spina bifida). |
| Tuberous Sclerosis | Progressive autosomal dominant disorder with ash-leaf spots (hypopigmented areas) on the skin and shagreen patches. Local knob tumorlike swellings or hamartomas (tubers) compress local structures and can cause hydrocephalus. Mental retardation and seizures result. | Benign tumor masses are composed of giant astrocytes and other hamartomatous neural tissue. |
| Neurofibromatosis | Autosomal dominant disorder known as von Recklinghausen disease (type 1) is associated with *NF-1* (on chromosome 17) or *NF-2* (on chromosome 22) gene. Multiple neural tumors in the skin and internal organs, café au lait spots (large brown macules over the trunk), and Lisch nodules (pigmented iris; only in type 1). Type 2 presents with bilateral acoustic neuromas instead of Lisch nodules. | Proliferation of axons and fibroblasts in loose myxoid stroma. Lesions contain entangled nerves. |
| Phenylketonuria | Autosomal recessive disorder involving a deficiency of phenylalanine hydroxylase (normally converts phenylalanine into tyrosine). Mental retardation, hypertonicity, tremors, and behavioral problems occur. Hypopigmentation from lack of melanin (tyrosine is a precursor). Can prevent by changing the diet to eliminate phenylalanine. | Toxic metabolites form without a functional enzyme and cause neurologic manifestations later in childhood. |

# II. Neonatal and Postnatal Diseases

## NEONATAL INFECTIONS

| Infection | Organisms Involved | Description and Symptoms |
|---|---|---|
| Thrush | *Candida albicans*. | Most common neonatal infection. Under the curdlike white plaques, there is an erythematous base. Also see Chapter 9, Oral Cavity Lesions. |
| Meningitis | < 1 month: *E. coli*, group B streptococci, *Listeria*, viruses. 1–3 months: viruses, *Streptococcus pneumoniae*, *Haemophilus influenzae*, *N. meningitidis*. | High fever, vomiting, irritability, lethargy, photophobia, bulging fontanelles, and nuchal rigidity. Patients younger than 1 month with fever must have a workup for sepsis. Must be treated immediately with antibiotics if cause is bacterial. |
| Pneumonia | 2 weeks: group B streptococci and gram-negative bacteria. 2 weeks to 2 months: *Chlamydia*, viruses, *S. pneumoniae*, *Staphylococcus aureus*, *H. influenzae*. | Fever, dyspnea, retractions, nasal flaring, and possible apnea. Patients younger than 1 month with fever must have a workup for sepsis. |
| Neonatal Sepsis | Early onset (first week): group B streptococci (most common), *E. coli* (second most common), *Klebsiella*, and *Listeria*. Late onset (7 days to 1 month): group B streptococci (most common), *S. aureus*, *N. gonorrhoeae*, gram-negative bacteria, *H. influenzae*, and *S. pneumoniae*. | Early: multiorgan system failure, respiratory failure, meningitis, and shock. Risk factors include maternal colonization with group B streptococci, prolonged rupture of membranes (> 24 hours), chorioamnionitis, and preterm birth. Late: bacteremia, meningitis, osteomyelitis, septic arthritis, or urinary tract infection. |
| Urinary Tract Infections | ≤ 1 month: see Neonatal Sepsis above. > 1 month: *E. coli*, *S. enterococci*, *Enterobacter*, *S. saprophyticus*, *Klebsiella*. | Low-grade fever, vomiting, diarrhea, irritability, jaundice, and failure to gain weight. Patients younger than 1 month with fever must have a workup for sepsis. Also see Urogenital Diseases below. |
| Botulism | *Clostridium botulinum* neurotoxin. | Transmitted by spores in home-canned foods or honey. Ingested spores germinate and release a toxin that prevents presynaptic acetylcholine release. Sudden onset of ileus, constipation, pupillary dilatation, bilateral ptosis, and apneic spells. Progressive weakness and hypotonia may lead to respiratory failure. |

| Disease | Cause | Description and Symptoms |
|---|---|---|
| Meconium Aspiration | Hypoxia | Postterm infants (42 weeks and older) are especially at risk for fetal hypoxia, which may trigger the release of meconium into the amniotic fluid. Meconium can be swallowed by the infant and aspirated at delivery. May result in meconium pneumonitis. Risk of developing persistent pulmonary hypertension. |
| Neonatal Respiratory Distress Syndrome | Unknown | Also known as hyaline membrane disease. See Chapter 5. |
| Cystic Fibrosis | Defective chloride channel | Autosomal recessive disorder. Patients are prone to pneumonias (*S. aureus, H. influenzae,* and *Pseudomonas*), bronchiectasis, and lung fibrosis. Decreased pancreatic enzyme secretion leads to fat malabsorption and pale gray stools. Meconium ileus (thickened meconium) can cause a small-bowel obstruction (pathognomonic in neonates with cystic fibrosis). |
| Pharyngitis | Viruses (most common) | Mild fever, cough, runny nose, sneezing, and sore throat (pharyngitis). |
| | "Strep throat"—group A streptococci | Occurs in children > 2 years with fever, exudative pharyngitis (oropharyngeal mucous membrane is covered by an exudate), and tonsillar enlargement. Complications include glomerulonephritis and rheumatic fever. |
| | Pertussis—*Bordetella pertussis* | Uncommon infection because of vaccination. Whooping cough (lasts for months) starts after 1–2 days of fever, coryza, and cough. |
| | Diphtheria—*Corynebacterium diphtheriae* | Fever, exudative pharyngitis, and airway edema (possible loss of upper airway). Toxin-mediated damage to the nerves and heart. |
| Mononucleosis | Epstein-Barr virus (most common)—heterophile positive Cytomegalovirus—heterophile negative | Mild infection with pharyngitis, fatigue, hepatosplenomegaly, and generalized lymphadenopathy. Atypical lymphocytes are found on a peripheral blood smear. |
| Mumps | Mumps virus | Presents with swollen salivary and parotid glands. |
| Measles | Measles virus | High fever, cough, coryza, conjunctivitis, Koplik spots (white and blue spots in the mouth), and a maculopapular red rash that starts on the head and face and progresses downward. Rash lasts a week. |

## RASHES AND SKIN LESIONS[1]

| Disease | Cause | Description and Symptoms | Findings and Complications |
|---|---|---|---|
| Atopic Dermatitis | Autoimmune mechanism | Affects 5% of children by age 5. Itchy erythematous papules cause a characteristic itch-scratch cycle. In the first 2 years, rash appears on the face, neck, scalp, trunk, and extensor surfaces. In older children, rash predominates on the flexor surfaces. | Associated with allergic disorders such as allergic rhinitis and atopic asthma. |
| Café au Lait Spots | Neurofibromatosis, Turner syndrome | Light brown pigmented macules. | |
| Erythema Toxicum Neonatorum | Unknown | Affects > 50% of all newborns. Red papules or macules resembling flea bites may disappear within a day. Large areas of erythema surround each lesion. | Scraping the lesion and staining it with Wright stain will show eosinophils. |
| Birthmarks | Hemangioma | Flammeus nevus—light pink to red macule or patch (also known as a salmon patch) that usually regresses with age. Flammeus nevus can also occur as a dark red-purple patch. | |
| | | Port-wine stain occurs on the face and grows with the child. | |
| | | Strawberry hemangioma grows with the child, then regresses by 3 years of age. | |
| | Nevi | Nevocellular nevus (common mole) is a black or brown macule or papule. May be junctional (in the epidermis), compound (epidermis and dermis), or intradermal (dermis). | |
| | | Spitz nevus is composed of spindle and epithelioid nevus cells and can be junctional, compound, or dermal. | |
| | | Blue nevus is a black-blue mole composed of dendritic nevus cells. | |
| | | Congenital nevus is present at birth but is not inherited. Ranges from brown macules to patches with hair. | It is a compound nevus. May predispose to malignancy. |
| | | Dysplastic nevus may be inherited. | Potentially premalignant. |
| Seborrheic Dermatitis | Unknown | On the scalp, appears as a yellowish greasy scale. May also involve the nose, ears, and eyebrows. Often clears on its own. | |

| Urticaria | Autoimmune mechanism | Also known as hives. Affects up to 20% of children. Caused by a hypersensitivity reaction (IgE mediated) to foods such as eggs, peanuts, and chocolate; by medications such as penicillin; and by various infections. Raised itchy wheals with pale centers. Is limited to 1 or 2 days. | May be complicated by anaphylactic shock. |

[1]See Chapter 11 before reading this section.

## SKIN INFECTIONS

| Disease | Cause | Description and Symptoms | Findings and Complications |
|---|---|---|---|
| Chickenpox | Varicella zoster virus | Primary infection presents with fever and malaise followed by successive crops of itchy vesicles on the skin and mucous membranes. Starts on the trunk and spreads peripherally. Reactivation occurs in adults. See Chapter 11, Viral Skin Infections. | In immunocompromised children, may see disseminated disease (meningoencephalitis or hepatitis) or death |
| Erythema Infectiosum (Fifth Disease) | Parvovirus B19 | Self-limited illness. Facial "slapped cheek" rash progresses to an erythematous, itchy maculopapular rash on the arms, trunk, and legs. | Complications include arthritis, hemolytic anemia, and encephalopathy |
| Hand-Foot-Mouth Disease | Coxsackie A virus | Summer illness. Fever, anorexia, and oral pain are followed by ulcers over the posterior third of the mouth and hands and feet. | Bacterial superinfection of the ulcers |
| Impetigo | S. aureus or Streptococcus pyogenes | Most common skin infection. Painless red macules on the face and hands progress to pustules with eventual erosion and yellow crusting. Lesions are epidermal and do not cause scarring. Spreads by scratching. | May lead to acute poststreptococcal glomerulonephritis if the agent is streptococcal |
| Roseola Virus (Roseola Infantum) | Herpes simplex virus type 6 | Abrupt, high fever (up to 106°F) in a well-looking child. On the fourth day, a maculopapular rash appears on the trunk and spreads peripherally. | None |
| Rubella | Rubella virus | Mild fever, generalized lymphadenopathy, and a self-limited maculopapular rash on the face and neck. Rash lasts 5 days. | Transient arthralgias and arthritis may be seen in adolescents |

Also see Chapter 11 for adult skin infections.

## GASTROINTESTINAL DISEASES

| Disease | Description and Symptoms | Causes and Pathologic Findings |
| --- | --- | --- |
| Infectious Diarrhea | Viruses cause low-grade fever, runny stools, vomiting, and upper respiratory complaints. Bacterial diarrhea presents with high fever, abdominal cramping, malaise, and tenesmus. Stools contain blood and white blood cells. Also see Chapter 9 for diarrhea. | • Viral (most common)—rotavirus, enteroviruses, adenovirus, and Norwalk virus<br><br>• Bacterial—*Salmonella, Shigella, Campylobacter, Yersinia,* and *E. coli*<br><br>• Parasitic—*Giardia* (e.g., at day care centers) |
| Meckel Diverticulum | Most common congenital anomaly of the small intestine. Usually asymptomatic. If symptomatic, presents with gastrointestinal bleeding and abdominal pain. Complications include bowel obstruction or volvulus. | Diverticulum can contain ectopic gastric, duodenal, colonic, or pancreatic tissue. |
| Hirschsprung Disease | Also called congenital megacolon. No peristalsis in the affected segment. Colon remains tonically contracted, preventing the flow of feces. Section in front of the affected segment dilates. Death occurs from dehydration and electrolyte imbalance unless the condition is surgically corrected. More common in boys. | Absence of ganglion cells in plexuses. ☞ Think of a "sprung colon." |

## NEONATAL JAUNDICE

| Disease | Description | Cause |
|---|---|---|
| Neonatal jaundice leads to kernicterus (staining and damage to the basal ganglia). Indirect (unconjugated) bilirubin is toxic to the central nervous system. | | |
| Physiologic Jaundice | Transient unconjugated hyperbilirubinemia that begins after the first 24 hours of life | Secondary to minor red blood cell lysis, inadequate bilirubin conjugation, and increased circulation to the liver |
| Hemolytic Disease of the Newborn | Unconjugated hyperbilirubinemia in the first 24 hours of life | Secondary to Rh or ABO incompatibility |
| Breast Milk Jaundice | Common; occurs with breast-feeding. Self-limited. | Cause is not known |
| Other Important Causes | ToRCHS congenital infections, congenital jaundice (see above), and neonatal sepsis. Also see Chapter 10, Jaundice. | |

## UROGENITAL DISEASES

| Disease | Causes | Description and Symptoms |
|---|---|---|
| Cryptorchidism | Low serum level of human chorionic gonadotropin or testosterone. Associated with trisomy 13 or 18 and Klinefelter syndrome. | Testes that have not fully descended into the scrotum. Increased risk of testicular cancer later in life if not corrected surgically. If both testes are affected, patient is infertile. Hyalinized basement membrane is found around the tubules. Parenchymal atrophy sparing the Leydig cells. |
| Vesicoureteral Reflux | Primary (most common type in children)—defect in the attachment of the ureters to the bladder. Secondary—increased bladder pressure. | Retrograde urine flow from the bladder into the kidneys. Most common presenting complaint is recurrent urinary tract infections. Low-grade reflux may resolve spontaneously. May lead to renal scarring and hypertension if severe and not repaired. Also see Chapter 6. |
| Urinary Tract Infections | E. coli, Klebsiella, Proteus, S. enterococci, Enterobacter S. saprophyticus. | Cystitis (bladder infection) presents with fever, incontinence, urgency, bed-wetting, dysuria, frequency, abdominal pain, or foul-smelling urine. Girls predominate over boys except in the newborn period. Pyelonephritis (kidney infection) presents with high fever, chills, and flank pain. A serious complication is renal parenchymal damage. |

## CHROMOSOME ABNORMALITY DISEASES

| Disease | Description and Symptoms | Chromosomal Abnormality |
|---|---|---|
| Down Syndrome (Trisomy 21) | Most common chromosomal inherited disorder (incidence of 1 in 1000 live births). Patients present with mental retardation and dysmorphic facial features including a flat face and nasal bridge, oblique palpebral fissures with epicanthal folds, small mouth, and short ears. The eyes may have Brushfield spots (white spots) on the periphery of the iris. The hands may have a simian crease (single palmar crease instead of two). May also have congenital heart disease such as septal defects, duodenal atresia and Hirschsprung disease, increased risk of acute leukemia, and premature Alzheimer disease occurring around the 30s to 40s. | Risk of extra chromosome 21 increases with maternal age, peaking after 35 years. Most cases occur de novo from nondisjunction. The rest may occur from a balanced translocation in which two chromosomes 21 are stuck together. |
| Edwards Syndrome (Trisomy 18) | Incidence is 1 in 4000–5000 live births. Presents with micrognathia (small jaw), rocker-bottom feet, cleft lip and palate, congenital heart disease (septal), and growth retardation. Most infants die by 1 year of age. | Most are the result of nondisjunction. Increased risk with increasing maternal age, but not as great as with Down syndrome. |
| Patau Syndrome (Trisomy 13) | Incidence is 1 in 10,000 live births. Presents with midline malformations including cleft lip and palate, polydactyly, congenital heart disease (septal), microphthalmia, growth retardation, and scalp defects. Most infants die by 1 year of age. | Most occur from nondisjunction, with an increased risk with increasing maternal age. Some may have mosaicism. |
| Cri du Chat Syndrome (5p-) | Incidence is 1 in 50,000 live births. Presents with severe mental retardation, a catlike cry (hence its name), wide-set eyes (hypertelorism) with cataracts and optic atrophy, growth retardation, and congenital heart disease (septal). Many infants survive into adulthood. | Deletion of the short arm of chromosome 5 or inherited balanced translocation. |

## SEX CHROMOSOME DISEASES

| Disease | Karyotype | Cause | Description |
|---|---|---|---|
| Klinefelter Syndrome | 47,XXY | Unknown | Incidence is 1 in 1000 live male births. Often not recognized until puberty. Males are incompletely masculinized and have decreased body hair, gynecomastia, small penis, and small, soft, atrophic testes. Patients are infertile and tall. May have mild retardation. Follicle-stimulating hormone is elevated and testosterone is decreased. |
| Turner Syndrome | 45,X | Defective embryonic division after fertilization | Incidence is 1 in 5000 live births. Female phenotype with neck webbing, short stature, broad chest with wide-spaced nipples, renal anomalies, Hashimoto thyroiditis, no breast or genitalia development, primary amenorrhea (atrophic ovaries), and congenital heart disease including coarctation of the aorta, aortic stenosis, and bicuspid aortic valve. |
| Fragile X Syndrome | 46,XY (it is X-linked recessive) | Amplification of a trinucleotide repeat (CGG) | Occurs in 1 out of 1000 males. Long face, prominent jaw, large ears, and macro-orchidism (large testicles). Female carriers may have lower than average IQ. |

## CHILDHOOD TUMOR EPIDEMIOLOGY

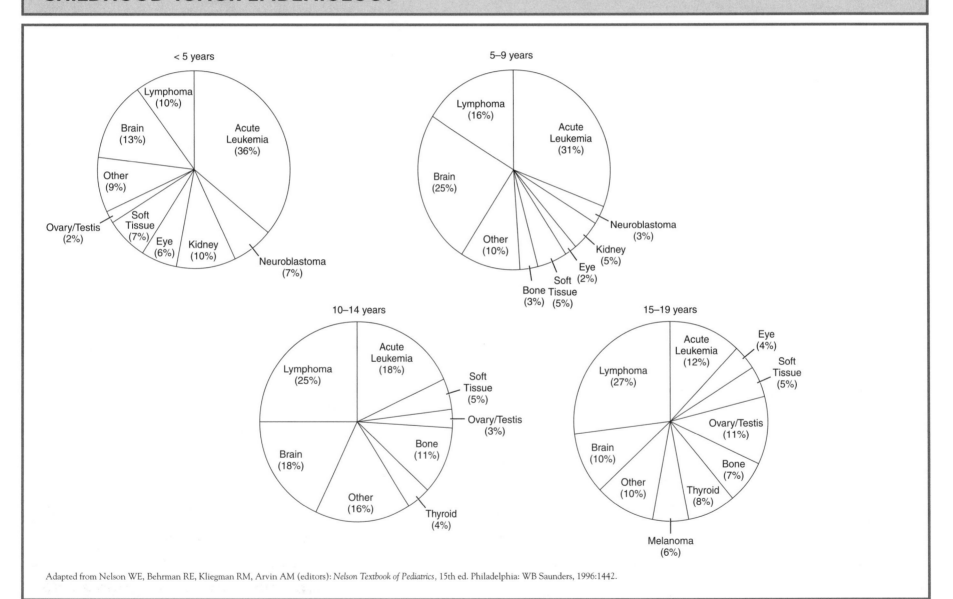

Adapted from Nelson WE, Behrman RE, Kliegman RM, Arvin AM (editors): *Nelson Textbook of Pediatrics*, 15th ed. Philadelphia: WB Saunders, 1996:1442.

# APPENDIX A
# GENETIC CAUSES OF DISEASE

I. SUMMARY OF GENETIC CAUSES
OF DISEASE

Autosomal Dominant Diseases

Autosomal Recessive Diseases

X-Linked Recessive Diseases

# I. Summary of Genetic Causes of Disease

| Autosomal Dominant Diseases | Autosomal Recessive Diseases | X-Linked Recessive Diseases |
| --- | --- | --- |
| Adult polycystic kidney disease (see Chapter 6) | **Lysosomal storage diseases (see Chapter 1)** | Hunter syndrome (see Chapter 1) |
| Familial hypercholesterolemia (see Chapter 2) | Pompe disease (type II) | Fabry disease (see Chapter 1) |
| von Hippel-Lindau disease (see Chapter 15) | Tay-Sachs disease | Hemophilia A and B (see Chapter 4) |
| Hereditary hemorrhagic telangiectasia (Rendu-Osler-Weber syndrome) | Gaucher disease | Lesch-Nyhan syndrome (see Chapter 4) |
| Hereditary spherocytosis (see Chapter 4) | Sandhoff disease | Duchenne muscular dystrophy (see Chapter 12) |
| Huntington disease (see Chapter 13) | Niemann-Pick disease | Glucose-6-phosphate dehydrogenase (G6PD) deficiency (see Chapter 4) |
| Tuberous sclerosis | Hurler disease | |
| Osteogenesis imperfecta (see Chapter 12) | **Glycogen storage diseases (see Chapter 1)** | |
| Marfan syndrome (see Chapter 1) | von Gierke disease (type I) | |
| McArdle disease (type V) | McArdle disease (type V) | |
| | Pompe disease (type II) | |
| | **Other diseases** | |
| | Galactosemia (see Chapter 14) | |
| | Cystic fibrosis (see Chapter 15) | |
| | Phenylketonuria (see Chapters 14 and 15) | |
| | Sickle cell anemia (see Chapter 4) | |
| | Alkaptonuria | |

# APPENDIX B
# INFECTIOUS PATHOGENS

## I. SUMMARY OF IMPORTANT INFECTIOUS PATHOGENS

Gram-Positive Organisms

Gram-Negative Organisms

Intracellular Parasites

Acid-Fast Organisms

Other Organisms

Fungi

Helminths

DNA Viruses and RNA Viruses

**ABBREVIATIONS**

**HIV** = human immunodeficiency virus
**HSV** = herpes simplex virus
**HTLV** = human T-lymphotropic virus

**PID** = pelvic inflammatory disease
**TB** = tuberculosis

# Summary of Important Infectious Pathogens

## GRAM-POSITIVE ORGANISMS

| Bacteria | Species | Representative Diseases |
|---|---|---|
| Staphylococcus | aureus | Acute endocarditis (most common cause), enterotoxin food poisoning, toxic shock syndrome, scalded skin syndrome, skin infections, osteomyelitis (most common cause) |
| | saprophyticus | Cystitis (urinary tract infection) |
| | epidermidis | Subacute endocarditis |
| Streptococcus | pyogenes (group A) β-hemolytic | Pharyngitis, scarlet fever, rheumatic fever (if not treated), acute poststreptococcal glomerulonephritis, impetigo, necrotizing fasciitis, and myositis |
| | agalactiae (group B) α-hemolytic | Common infection in neonates as pneumonia or meningitis |
| | pneumoniae | Lobar pneumonia and meningitis |
| | bovis (group D) | Urinary tract infections and subacute bacterial endocarditis |
| | viridans | Subacute bacterial endocarditis (most common cause) |
| Enterococcus | | Subacute bacterial endocarditis |
| Listeria (intracellular) | monocytogenes | Meningitis in neonates |
| Corynebacterium | | Diphtheria |

| Clostridium | perfringens | Toxinogenic enterocolitis and gas gangrene |
|---|---|---|
| | botulinum | Botulism |
| | tetani | Tetanus |
| | difficile | Pseudomembranous colitis |
| Bacillus | cereus | Toxinogenic enterocolitis |
| Actinomyces | | PID in women with an intrauterine device (most common cause) |
| Nocardia | | Pulmonary infection in immunocompromised patients |

## GRAM-NEGATIVE ORGANISMS

| Bacteria | Genus or Species | Representative Diseases |
| --- | --- | --- |
| *Neisseria* (diplococci) | *meningitidis* (meningococcus) | Meningitis and Waterhouse-Friderichsen syndrome (results from bacteremia) |
| | *gonorrhoeae* (gonococcus) | Gonococcal gonorrhea, PID as initial infection in females, urethritis and proctitis in males, pharyngitis, septic arthritis, and neonatal conjunctivitis (ophthalmia neonatorum) |
| Enterobacteriaceae (rods) | *Escherichia coli* | Urinary tract infection including cystitis and pyelonephritis (most common cause), toxinogenic enterocolitis, invasive enterocolitis (dysentery), meningitis and sepsis in neonates |
| | *Salmonella typhi* | Typhoid fever |
| | *Proteus* | Urinary tract infection |
| | *Klebsiella* | Bronchial pneumonia |
| *Campylobacter* and *Helicobacter* | *Helicobacter pylori* | Duodenal ulcers, chronic gastric ulcers, and increased incidence of gastric lymphomas and carcinomas |
| *Pseudomonas* | | Burn infections, nosocomial pneumonia, and osteomyelitis in children with sickle cell disease |
| *Vibrio* | *cholerae* | Cholera, a toxinogenic enterocolitis |
| | *parahaemolyticus* | Invasive enterocolitis caused by eating raw shellfish |
| Respiratory pathogens | *Haemophilus influenzae* type b | Meningitis in neonates and epiglottitis in children |
| | *Haemophilus ducreyi* | Painful chancroid lesion on the external genitalia |
| | *Legionella* | Legionnaires' disease, an atypical pneumonia |
| | *Bordetella* | Whooping cough |
| Anaerobes | *Bacteroides, Fusobacterium* | Common in abscesses; may see in aspiration pneumonia; infections are prevalent in patients with diabetes or immunocompromise |

## INTRACELLULAR PARASITES

| Bacteria | Species | Representative Diseases |
| --- | --- | --- |
| Chlamydia | psittaci | Atypical pneumonia. See Chapter 5. |
| | trachomatis | Acute conjunctival infection; PID in women and urethritis in men. Also causes lymphogranuloma venereum. It is the most common sexually transmitted disease. |
| Rickettsia (all-cause vasculitis) | rickettsii | Rocky Mountain spotted fever, transmitted by Dermacentor (dog tick). |
| | typhi | Typhus fever, transmitted by a flea. Do not confuse with typhoid fever, caused by Salmonella. |
| Coxiella | burnetii | Q fever and an atypical pneumonia. See Chapter 5. |

## ACID-FAST ORGANISMS

| Bacteria | Species | Representative Diseases |
| --- | --- | --- |
| Mycobacterium (must be cultured in a special medium, Lowenstein-Jensen) | | |
| | tuberculosis | TB of the lungs. See Chapter 5. |
| | leprae | Leprosy, which manifests itself as a peripheral neuropathy. See Chapters 11 and 13. |
| | avium-intracellulare | Chronic diarrhea in patients with AIDS. |

## OTHER ORGANISMS

| Organism or Category | Genus or Species | Representative Diseases |
| --- | --- | --- |
| *Mycoplasma* (no cell wall) | | Atypical pneumonia (most common cause) |
| *Ureaplasma* | | Urinary tract infections |
| Spirochetes (all need a special medium to culture) | | |
| | *Borrelia burgdorferi* | Lyme disease; see Chapters 11 and 13 |
| | *Leptospira* | Leptospirosis, which can cause hepatitis or meningitis; see Chapters 10 and 13, respectively |
| | *Treponema pallidum* | Congenital and sexually acquired syphilis; see Chapters 15 and 7, respectively |
| Protozoans | *Entamoeba* | Most patients are asymptomatic; can cause amebiasis, evident as a "teardrop ulcer," and dysentery (a low-volume, bloody, purulent diarrhea) |
| Flagellates | *Giardia* | Giardiasis |
| | *Trichomonas* | Sexually transmitted disease |
| Hemoflagellates | *Leishmania donovani* | Kala azar (visceral leishmaniasis), transmitted by a sand fly, causes damage to the mononuclear-reticulo-endothelial system in the skin, liver, spleen, and in bone |
| | *Trypanosoma cruzi* | Chagas disease, transmitted by the reduviid bug, causes a chancre at the site of the bite followed by dissemination of the organism into the brain, heart, and skeletal and smooth muscle |
| | *Trypanosoma brucei* | African sleeping sickness, transmitted by the tsetse fly, causes meningoencephalitis and is fatal unless treated |
| Sporozoa | *Cryptosporidium* | Noninvasive enterocolitis (watery diarrhea) in immunocompromised individuals |
| | *Plasmodium* | Malaria |
| | *Toxoplasma* | Toxoplasmosis |

## FUNGI

| Type of Fungus | Genus | Representative Diseases |
|---|---|---|
| Systemic fungi | *Coccidioides* | Coccidiomycosis, transmitted by inhaling contaminated soil and dust, is a serious infection in AIDS and immunocompromised patients, disseminating to the lungs (TB-like) and the brain (meningitis) |
| | *Paracoccidioides* | Paracoccidiomycosis causes ulcerations in the mucosa of the mouth and infects the lymph nodes, forming sinus tracts to the skin |
| | *Blastomyces* | Blastomycosis looks like TB and can disseminate into bone and skin |
| | *Histoplasma* | Histoplasmosis looks like TB and forms caseous granulomas; can reactivate |
| | *Pneumocystis* | Interstitial pneumonia in patients with AIDS |
| Opportunistic fungi | *Candida* | Candidiasis can occur orally, vaginally, in the esophagus, and systemically |
| | *Cryptococcus* | Cryptococcosis, transmitted by inhalation of soil contaminated with bird droppings, occurs in AIDS and other immunocompromised conditions as meningitis |
| | *Aspergillus* | Allergic aspergillosis (eosinophilia) |
| | *Zygomycetes (Mucor)* | Pneumonia in immunocompromised patients, especially diabetic patients with ketoacidosis |
| Superficial fungi | Dermatophytes | Tinea (ringworm) in various places |
| | *Malassezia* | Tinea versicolor |
| | *Cladosporium* | Tinea nigra |
| | *Sporothrix* | Subcutaneous infection, usually as a result of being pricked by a thorn (common in gardeners) |

## HELMINTHS

| Parasite Category | Genus or Species | Representative Diseases |
|---|---|---|
| Intestinal Roundworms (Nematodes) | Ascaris | Pulmonary eosinophilia and interstitial disease |
| | Enterobius | Also known as pinworm; causes anal itching, especially at night; commonly infects children |
| | Trichuris | Mostly asymptomatic; infests the small intestine |
| | Ancylostoma and Necator | Asthmalike reaction and iron-deficiency anemia (the worm eats blood) |
| | Strongyloides | Watery, chronic diarrhea in patients with AIDS; can cause pulmonary eosinophilia |
| Zoonotic Roundworms (humans are dead-end hosts) | Toxocara | Fever, muscle aches, malnutrition, meningitis, and encephalitis |
| | Anisakis | Causes eosinophilic granulomas in stomach; found in raw seafood |
| | Trichinella spiralis | Trichinosis causes gastrointestinal manifestations, then becomes disseminated |
| Cestodes (Tapeworms) | Diphyllobothrium latum | Vague abdominal complaints and vitamin $B_{12}$ deficiency anemia (worm consumes vitamin $B_{12}$) |
| | Taenia saginata | Vague abdominal complaints |
| | Taenia solium | Cysticercosis—cysts in muscle or brain |
| | Echinococcus granulosus | Slow granulomalike growth in lungs and liver |
| Trematodes (Flukes) | Schistosoma | Involves the liver and the bladder |
| | Clonorchis | Mostly asymptomatic; infests the biliary ducts |
| | Paragonimus | Infests the lung parenchyma with bloody sputum, dyspnea, pleuritic chest pain, and recurrent bacterial pneumonias |

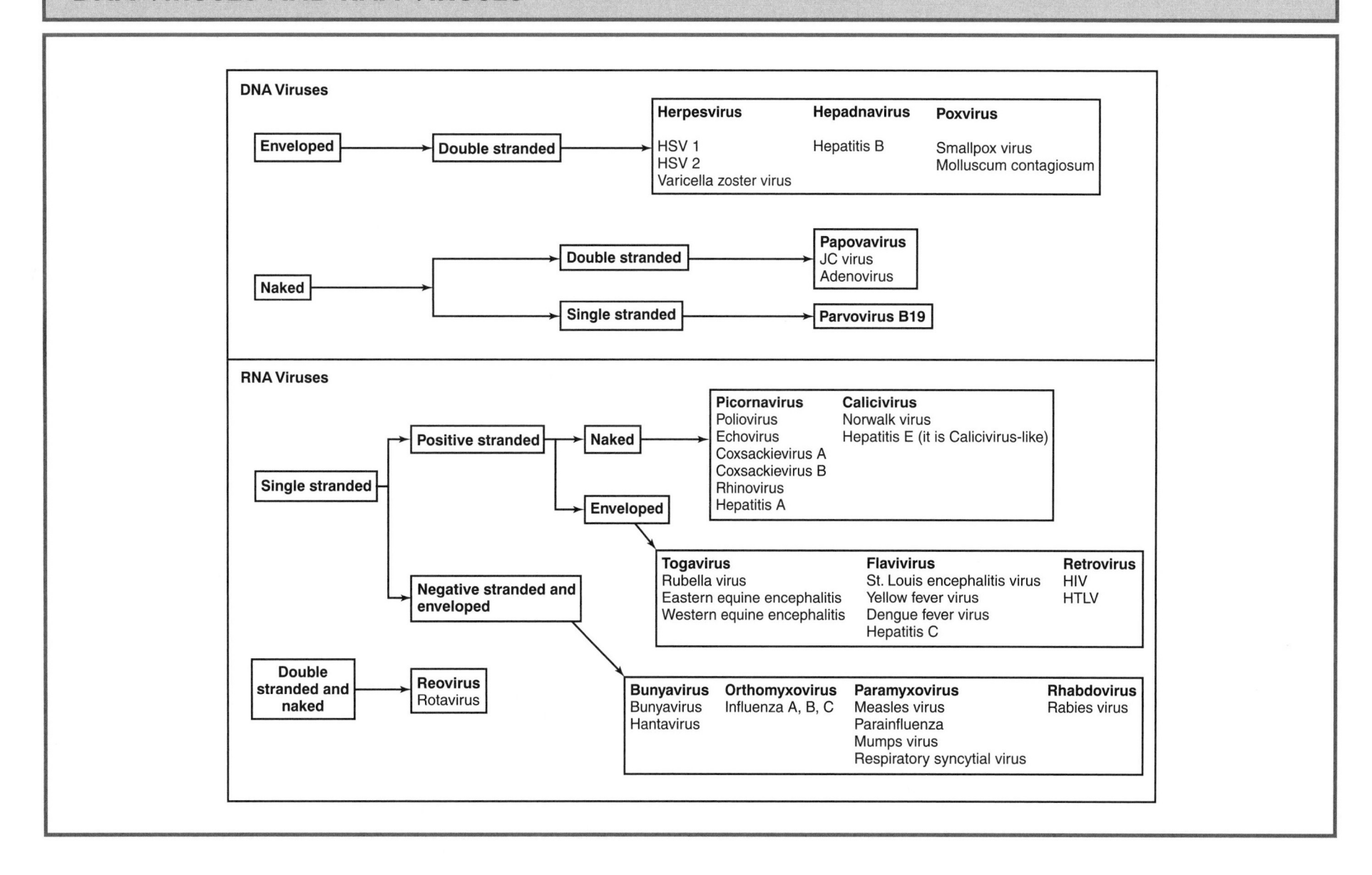

**DNA Viruses**

Enveloped → Double stranded →

| **Herpesvirus** | **Hepadnavirus** | **Poxvirus** |
|---|---|---|
| HSV 1 | Hepatitis B | Smallpox virus |
| HSV 2 | | Molluscum contagiosum |
| Varicella zoster virus | | |

Naked → Double stranded →

**Papovavirus**
JC virus
Adenovirus

Naked → Single stranded →

**Parvovirus B19**

**RNA Viruses**

Single stranded → Positive stranded → Naked →

| **Picornavirus** | **Calicivirus** |
|---|---|
| Poliovirus | Norwalk virus |
| Echovirus | Hepatitis E (it is Calicivirus-like) |
| Coxsackievirus A | |
| Coxsackievirus B | |
| Rhinovirus | |
| Hepatitis A | |

Positive stranded → Enveloped →

| **Togavirus** | **Flavivirus** | **Retrovirus** |
|---|---|---|
| Rubella virus | St. Louis encephalitis virus | HIV |
| Eastern equine encephalitis | Yellow fever virus | HTLV |
| Western equine encephalitis | Dengue fever virus | |
| | Hepatitis C | |

Negative stranded and enveloped →

| **Bunyavirus** | **Orthomyxovirus** | **Paramyxovirus** | **Rhabdovirus** |
|---|---|---|---|
| Bunyavirus | Influenza A, B, C | Measles virus | Rabies virus |
| Hantavirus | | Parainfluenza | |
| | | Mumps virus | |
| | | Respiratory syncytial virus | |

Double stranded and naked → **Reovirus** Rotavirus

# INDEX

## A

α-cell tumor (glucagonoma), 186
abciximab, 90
abrasion, 14, 27
abruptio placentae, 159
abscess
  cerebral, 277, 279
  lung, 95
acanthocytosis, 59
acanthosis nigricans, 247
Accutane, 303
acetaminophen toxicity, 292
achalasia, 195
acid-fast organisms, 323
acne vulgaris, 241
acoustic schwannoma, 286
acquired Immunodeficiency syndrome (AIDS). *See*
    AIDS
acquired inflammatory myopathies, 253
acrochordon, 245
acromegaly, 168
ACTH (adrenocorticotropic hormone), 163, 166,
    167, 179, 180
  deficiency, 169
actinic keratosis, 247
*Actinomyces*, 321
acute diseases
  allergic contact dermatitis, 238

appendicitis, 212
cholecystitis, 232
cystitis, 128
disseminated encephalomyelitis, 282
endometritis, 144
erosive gastropathy, 197
hemorrhagic anemia, 71
infectious thyroiditis, 173
infective endocarditis, 38
inflammatory demyelinating polyradiculoneurop-
    athy, 274
inflammatory response, 74
leukemias, 81
liver failure, 228
mastitis, 153
necrotizing ulcerative gingivitis, 191
osteomyelitis, 259
pancreatitis, 234
pelvic inflammatory disease, 143
proliferative poststreptococcal glomerulonephri-
    tis, 116
prostatitis, 141
rashes, 238
renal failure, 17, 110
salpingitis, 143
subdural hematoma, 275
tubular necrosis, 118
tubulointerstitial nephritis, 119
viral hepatitis, 222

acyclovir toxicity, 291
Addison disease, 164, 184
  antibodies involved, 52
addisonian crisis (adrenal insufficiency), 179
adenocarcinomas, 107, 194
  adrenal, 180
  clear cell, 148
  colorectal, 205
  of extrahepatic biliary ducts, 233
  follicular, 175
  of gallbladder, 233
  gastric, 198
  pancreatic, 234
  papillary, 175
  of prostate, 141, 142
  small intestine, 205
adenoid cystic carcinoma, 194
adenomas
  adrenal cortical, 180, 183
  colon, 204
  cortical, 127
  corticotropic, 167
  corticotropic pituitary, 180
  follicular, 175
  hepatic, 231
  islet cell, 186
  nonfunctional, 167
  parathyroid, 176, 177
  pituitary, 167, 286

adenomas (*continued*)
  pleomorphic, 194
  somatotropic, 167
  tubular, 204
  villous, 204
adenomatous polyps, 204
adenomyosis. *See* endometriosis interna
adenosine diphosphate (ADP), 45
adenosine triphosphate (ATP), 1
ADH (antidiuretic hormone), 163, 166
  deficiency, 169
  inappropriate secretion, 167
ADP (adenosine diphosphate), 45
adrenal adenocarcinoma, 180
adrenal cortical adenoma, 180, 183
adrenal gland disorders, 178–83
  Cushing syndrome, 182
  tumors, 183
  types of, 179–81
adrenal glands
  structure, 178
  tumors, 180, 183
adrenal hypercorticoidism, 184
adrenal hypocorticoidism, 184
adrenal insufficiency (addisonian crisis), 179
adrenal pheochromocytoma, 187
adrenocorticotropic hormone. *See* ACTH (adrenocorticotropic hormone)
adult renal malignancy, 110
adult respiratory distress syndrome (ARDS), 93,
  100
African sleeping sickness, 324
agenesis, 2
AIDS (acquired Immunodeficiency syndrome), 25,
  55
  diarrhea and, 209
  perinatal infection, 302
air and gas embolus, 13
alanine aminotransferase (ALT), 1, 215

albinism, 240
alcohol
  congenital diseases and, 303
  disorders related to, 293
  macrocytic anemias and, 69
  steatosis (fatty change) and, 303
alcoholic cirrhosis, 229
alcoholic hepatic steatosis, 227
alcoholic hepatitis, 224
alcoholic liver disease, 215
alcoholic polyneuropathy, 273
aldolase, 251
aldosterone, 181
alkaline phosphatase (ALP), 213, 256
alkaptonuria, 318
Allbright syndrome, 262
allergic contact dermatitis
  acute, 238
  chronic, 238
ALP (alkaline phosphatase), 213, 256
Alport syndrome, 116
ALT (alanine aminotransferase), 1, 215
alveolitis, 95
Alzheimer disease, 283, 284
amebiasis, hepatic, 224
amine precursor uptake and decarboxylation
  (APUD), 93
aminotransferases, 215
amniotic embolus, 13
amphotericin B toxicity, 291
amyloidosis, 6
  renal, 114
  secondary, 6
amyotrophic lateral sclerosis, 285
anaerobes, 322
anaerobic pneumonias, 105
anaphylactic shock, 16
anaplasia, 2
anaplastic carcinoma, 175

*Ancylostoma*, 326
androgens, 255
anemias
  abnormal blood indices in, 64
  acute hemorrhagic, 71
  aplastic, 59, 71
  autoimmune hemolytic, 69
  of chronic disease, 66
  defined, 59
  hemoglobin types, 67
  hemolytic, 71, 72
  hereditary spherocytosis, 66, 318
  hypoproliferative, 71
  iron-carrying proteins, 62
  iron-deficiency, 66
  lead poisoning, 66
  macrocytic, 58, 68–69
  macrocytic hyperchromic, 64
  megaloblastic, 297
  microcytic, 58, 65, 66
  microcytic hypochromic, 64
  myelophthisic, 60, 71
  normochromic, 71
  normocytic normochromic, 64
  pernicious, 297
  red blood cell morphology in, 63
  refractory, 80
  Schilling test, 70
  sickle cell, 318
  sideroblastic, 66
  spur cell, 69
  thalassemias, 66, 68
anencephaly, 307
aneurysms
  atherosclerotic, 29
  berry, 29
  defined, 27
  dissecting, 29
  syphilitic, 29

angina
  pectoris, 35
  Prinzmetal, 35
  stable, 35
  unstable, 35
  Vincent (trench mouth), 191
angiosarcoma (hemangiosarcoma), 32, 231, 267
angiotensin-converting enzyme inhibitors, 303
aniline dyes, 290
animal bites, 280
Anisakis, 326
anisocytosis, 59
ankylosing spondylitis, 264
ankylosis, 264
anterior pituitary hormones, 166
anthracosis, 101
anticoagulation medications, 90
anticoagulators (clotting system), 90
antidiuretic hormone (ADH). See ADH (antidi-
    uretic hormone)
antiepileptic medication toxicity, 291
antifungal agent toxicity, 291
antihypertensive agent toxicity, 292
antilipidemic drug toxicity, 292
antimetabolite drugs, 69
antimicrobial agent toxicity, 291
antiplatelet medications, 90
antiseizure medication toxicity, 291
antithrombin III, 90
α₁-antitrypsin deficiency, 229
antiviral agent toxicity, 291
anuria, 111
aorta, coarctation of, 305
aortic valve regurgitation, 41
aortic valve stenosis, 41
aphthous stomatitis, 191
aplasia, 2
aplastic anemias, 59, 71
apoptosis, 2
appendicitis, acute, 212

appendix tumor, 190
APUD (amine precursor uptake and decarboxyla-
    tion), 93
ARDS. See adult respiratory distress syndrome
    (ARDS)
Arnold-Chiari malformation, 307
arsenic, 290
arterial septal defect, 305
arterial thrombosis, 12
arteriosclerosis, 27, 28
arteriosclerotic disorders, 28
arthralgia, 251
arthritis, 250
  chronic, 265
  defined, 251
  gonococcal, 265, 266
  gouty, 264
  infectious, 265
  nongonococcal, 265, 266
  osteoarthritis, 263
  reactive, 264
  rheumatoid, 263
  viral, 265
arthropathy, enteropathic, 264
arthropod-borne viral encephalitis, 280
arthropod-caused skin infections, 243
arthrosis (arthropathy), 251
Arthus reaction, 46
asbestos, 290
asbestosis, 101
Ascaris, 326
ascending cholangitis, 232
aseptic necrosis, 262
ash-leaf spots, 307
aspartate aminotransferase (AST), 1, 215
Aspergillus, 325
aspiration pneumonias, 105
aspirin, 90
  toxicity, 292

asplenia, 53
AST (aspartate aminotransferase), 1, 215
asthma
  bronchial, 98
  cardiac, 98
  status, 98
astrocytoma, 286, 287
atelectasis, 100
atherosclerosis, 7, 28, 30
atherosclerotic aneurysm, 29
athlete's foot. See tinea pedis
atopic dermatitis, 238, 310
ATP (adenosine triphosphate), 1
atrophic gastritis, 197
atrophy, 2
atypical pneumonias, 94, 105
Auer bodies, 74
autoimmune adrenalitis, 179
autoimmune chronic viral hepatitis, 229
autoimmune disorders
  hypersensitivity diseases, 50
  summary, 52
  systemic autoimmune disorders, 51
  type I (immediate), 50
  type II (cytotoxic or antibody mediated), 50
  type III (immune complex), 50
  type IV (cell mediated), 50
autoimmune hemolytic anemia, 69
autoimmune hepatitis, 225
autosomal dominant diseases, 318
autosomal recessive diseases, 318
avascular necrosis. See aseptic necrosis
avulsion, 14

# B

β-cell tumor (insulinoma), 186
Bacillus cereus, 321
bacterial arthritis, 265

bacterial diarrhea, 210
bacterial endocarditis, 38
bacterial meningitis, 277, 278
bacterial skin infections, 241
*Bacteroides*, 322
basal cell carcinoma, 247
basement membrane deposits, 113
B cells, 54
Becker muscular dystrophy, 252
benign nephrosclerosis, 122
benign prostatic hyperplasia, 141, 142
benign tumors
    bone, 250, 260–61
    breast, 132
    central nervous system, 287
    hepatic, 231
    of infancy, 300
    liver, 214
    nomenclature, 19
    oral epithelial, 190
    ovarian, 132
    primary vascular, 32
    renal, 127
    skin, 245–46
    soft tissue, 250, 267
benzene, 290
Berger disease. *See* IgA nephropathy
beriberi
    cerebral, 285, 297
    dry, 297
    wet, 297
berry aneurysm, 29
berylliosis, 3, 101
bilateral hydronephrosis, 125
"bile lakes," 221
biliary atresia, 306
biliary cirrhosis, 229
    primary, 221
    secondary, 221

biliary colic, 232
biliary tree cancers, 233
bilirubin
    conjugated, 219
    unconjugated, 219
birthmarks, 310
blackheads, 241
blast crisis, 81
*Blastomyces*, 325
blastomycosis, 325
bleeding disorders, 86
bleomycin toxicity, 291
blood disorders, 293
blood urea nitrogen (BUN), 109, 112
blue bloaters, 98
blue nevus, 310
boils, 241
bone
    architecture, 254
    atrophy, 257
    metabolism, 255
    mineralization, 256
    softening, 257
bone diseases, 254–62
    differential diagnosis of, 256
    metabolic, 257–58
    primary bone tumors, 260–61
    pyogenic osteomyelitis, 259–60
bone marrow transplant complications, 49
*Bordetella*, 322
*Borrelia burgdorferi*, 324
botryoid sarcoma, 148
botulism, 253, 308
Bouchard's nodes, 263
bowel obstruction, 201
Bowen disease. *See* squamous carcinoma in situ
bradykinin, 48
brain
    primary malignant lymphoma of, 287

breast cancers
    common features of, 156
    distribution pattern, 156
    incidence of, 157
    prognostic indicators of, 156
    risk factors, incidence and mortality, 146
    types of, 157–58
breast diseases, 132, 153–58
    cancers, 156–58
    fibrocystic disease, 155
    inflammatory conditions, 153
    lesions, 154
    terminology, 153
    tumors, 157–58
breast-feeding
    congenital infection and, 302
breast milk jaundice, 313
breast tumors
    benign, 157
    malignant, 157–58
Brenner tumor, 138
bronchial adenoma, 108
bronchial asthma, 98
bronchial obstruction, 107
bronchiectasis, 99
bronchogenic tumors, 95
    carcinomas, 94, 107
bronchopneumonias, 105
Brushfield spots, 314
Buerger disease (thromboangiitis obliterans), 30, 31
"buffalo hump," 180
bullous pemphigoid, 239
BUN (blood urea nitrogen), 109, 112
BUN-creatinine ratio, 112
Bunyavirus, 327
burns, 294
bursitis, 251

# C

café au lait spots, 310
calcitriol, 255
calcium
    bone diseases and, 256
    bone metabolism and, 255
calcium pyrophosphate deposition disease. *See*
        pseudogout
calcium stones, 124
calicivirus, 327
*Campylobacter*, 322
cancers. *See also* specific cancers
    characteristics of, 19
    epidemiology, 21
    in women, risk factors, incidence and mortality,
        146–47
*Candida*, 133, 325
    *esophagitis*, 196
candidiasis, 325
canker sores. *See* aphthous stomatitis
capillary hemangioma, 32
capillary permeability, 12
carbamazepine toxicity, 291
carbon monoxide, 290
carbon tetrachloride, 290
carcinogenesis, 18
carcinoid syndrome, endocarditis of, 40
carcinoid tumors
    defined, 19
    intestinal, 206
    lung, 108
    small intestine, 206
carcinomas
    adenoid cystic, 194
    anaplastic, 175
    basal cell, 247
    bronchogenic tumors, 94, 107
    characteristics of, 19

clear cell, 137
ductal carcinoma in situ, 157
embryonal, 136
endometrial, 146, 149
esophageal squamous cell, 196
hepatocellular, 231
inflammatory, 158
invasive colloid, 158
invasive ductal, 158
invasive lobular, 158
invasive medullary, 158
invasive mucinous, 158
invasive squamous cell, 135
large cell, 107
lobular carcinoma in situ, 157
medullary, 175
medullary thyroid, 187
mucoepidermoid, 194
parathyroid, 176
renal cell, 110, 127
small cell (oat cell), 107
squamous cell, 107, 129, 148, 192, 196, 247
transitional cell, lower urinary tract, 129
verrucous, 135
yolk sac, 136
cardiac asthma, 98
cardiac diseases, 33–42
    cardiomyopathies, 37
    congenital, 305
    infective endocarditis, 38–39
    ischemic, 35
    myocardial infarction timetable, 36
    noninfective endocarditis, 40
    pericarditis, 42
    primary heart tumors, 42
    terminology, 33–34
    valvular diseases, 41
cardiogenic shock, 16
cardiomyopathies

dilated, 37
    hypertrophic obstructive, 37
    restrictive, 37
cardiovascular system, 25–43
    cardiac diseases, 33–42
    hypertension, 43
    injury, 293
    most common disorders, 26
    uncontrolled diabetes mellitus and, 186
    vascular diseases, 27–32
carpal tunnel syndrome, 274
caseous, 9
cavernous hemangioma, 32
celiac disease, 208
celiac sprue, 298
cell blebs, 5
cell death, 5
cellular and tissue changes, 2–7
    cellular necrosis, 5
    granuloma, 3
    hypoxic cellular injury, 5
    steatosis (fatty change), 4
    storage diseases, 6–7
    terminology, 2
cellulitis, 241
    necrotizing, 241
central nervous system (CNS), 25
central nervous system (CNS) diseases, 275–81
    cerebral trauma, 275
    cerebrospinal fluid analysis and, 277
    cerebrovascular diseases, 276
    hydrocephalus, 277
    infections, 278–79
    slow viral encephalitis/encephalopathies, 281
    viral encephalitis, 280
centrilobular emphysema, 97, 99
cerebral abscess, 279
    cerebrospinal fluid analysis, 277
cerebral beriberi, 285, 297

cerebral contusion, 275
cerebral edema, 10
cerebral infarction, 276
cerebral trauma, 275
cerebrospinal fluid (CSF), 269
    cytologic analysis of, 277
cerebrovascular diseases, 276
cervical intraepithelial neoplasia (CIN), 131
cervical tumors, 132
    cancer risk factors, incidence and mortality, 147
    Papanicolaou smear classification and, 150
    types of, 148
cervicitis, 133
Cestodes, 326
Chagas disease, 324
chancroid, 134
Chédiak-Higashi anomaly, 74
Chédiak-Higashi syndrome, 53
chemical injuries, 290
chemotherapeutic agent toxicity, 291
chemotherapy toxicity, 55
CHF (congestive heart failure), 1
chickenpox, 311
    congenital, 304
childhood diseases, 299–316
    common disorders and causes, 300
    congenital diseases, 302–8
    neonatal and postnatal, 308–16
    terminology, 301
childhood leukemia, 58
childhood renal malignancy, 110
childhood thrombocytopenia, 58
Chlamydia
    psittaci, 323
    trachomatis, 133, 323
chloramphenicol, 303
chloroquine toxicity, 291
cholangiocarcinoma, 231
cholangitis, ascending, 232

cholecystitis
    acute, 232
    chronic, 233
cholelithiasis (gallstones), 214, 232
cholestasis markers, 215
cholestasis of pregnancy, 221
cholesterolosis, 233
chondroblastoma, 261
chondrocalcinosis. See pseudogout
chondroma, 260
chondrosarcoma, 261
chorioamnionitis, 160
choriocarcinoma, 149
    gestational, 161
    testicular, 136
choristoma, 18
Christmas disease, 87
chromium, 290
chromosomal disorder, 300
chromosome abnormality diseases, 314–15
chronic diseases
    allergic contact dermatitis, 238
    arthritis, 265
    autoimmune viral hepatitis, 229
    bronchitis (COPD), 98
    cholecystitis, 233
    chronic obstructive pulmonary disease (COPD),
      93, 98, 99
    constrictive pericarditis, 42
    diarrhea, 209
    endometritis, 144
    gastritis, 197
    glomerulonephritis, 117
    granulomatous disease, 53
    hepatitis, 214, 225, 226, 229
    inflammatory response, 74
    leukemias, 81
    mastitis, 153
    meningitis, 277, 278

myelomonocytic leukemia, 80
    osteomyelitis, 259
    pelvic inflammatory disease (PID), 143
    prostatitis, 141
    pyelonephritis, 120
    rashes, 238–39
    relapsing pancreatitis, 234
    renal failure, 110, 177
    subdural hematoma, 275
    tissue transplant rejection, 49
    tubulointerstitial nephritis, 119
    viral hepatitis, 225, 229
chylocele, 139
CIN (cervical intraepithelial neoplasia), 131
cirrhosis
    liver, 229
    macronodular, 214, 229
    micronodular, 214, 229
    primary biliary, 221
    secondary biliary, 221
CK. See creatine kinase (CK)
CK-MB (creatine kinase MB fraction). See creatine
      kinase MB fraction (CK-MB)
Cladosporium, 325
clear cell adenocarcinoma, 148
clear cell carcinoma, 137
Clonorchis, 326
clopidogrel, 90
Clostridium
    botulinum, 321
    difficile, 321
    perfringens, 321
    tetani, 321
clotting cascade, 84, 89
clotting factor deficiencies, 86
clotting system (anticoagulators), 90
CMV. See cytomegalovirus (CMV)
CNS. See central nervous system (CNS)
coagulative, 9

coal worker's pneumoconiosis, 101
coarctation of the aorta, 305
cobalamin (vitamin B$_{12}$) deficiency, 68, 70, 285, 297
   neuropathy, 273
*Coccidioides*, 325
coccidioidomycosis, 325
colic, biliary, 232
colitis
   ischemic, 200
   ulcerative, 202, 203
collagen vascular disease, 103
colon adenoma, 204
colonic diverticula, 200
colon inflammatory diseases, 200
colorectal adenocarcinoma, 205
communicating hydrocephalus, 277, 307
community-acquired pneumonias, 105
compensated (nonprogressive) shock, 17
complement, 54
concussion, 275
congenital conditions, 46, 301
congenital diseases, 302–7
   anomaly of small intestine, 190
   heart diseases, 305
   infections, 304
   jaundice, 300, 306
   megacolon, 312
   neurologic, 307
   neurologic diseases, 307
   nevus, 310
   nipple inversion, 153
   perinatal AIDS, 302
   teratogens and, 303
   transmission of, 302
congestive heart failure (CHF), 1
conjugated bilirubin, 219
conjugated hyperbilirubinemia, 219

Conn syndrome (primary hyperaldosteronism), 43, 164
consolidation, 95
constrictive pericarditis, chronic, 42
contact dermatitis, acute allergic, 238
contusion
   cerebral, 275
   defined, 14
Coombs' test, 46
COPD (chronic obstructive pulmonary disease), 93, 98, 99
cor pulmonale, 33
corpus luteum cysts, 145
cortical tumors, 183
   adenoma, 127
corticosteroid toxicity, 292
corticotrophs, 166
corticotropic adenoma, 167
corticotropic pituitary adenoma, 180
*Corynebacterium*, 320
*Coxiella burnetii*, 323
craniopharyngioma, 286
craniotabes, 257
creatine kinase (CK), 25
   defined, 33
      myocyte damage and, 251
creatine kinase MB fraction (CK-MB), 1, 25, 33
creatinine, 112
crepitus, 263
crescentic glomerulonephritis, 116
Creutzfeldt-Jakob disease, 281, 283
cri du chat syndrome, 314
Crigler-Najjar syndrome, 306
Crohn disease, 202, 203
cryptococcosis, 325
*Cryptococcus*, 325
cryptogenic fibrosing alveolitis, 103
cryptorchidism, 313

cryptorchism, 140
*Cryptosporidium*, 324
CSF (cerebrospinal fluid), 269
Cushing disease. *See* primary hypercorticoidism (Cushing disease)
Cushing syndrome. *See* secondary hypercorticoidism (Cushing syndrome)
cyanide, 290
cyanotic diseases, 305
cyclophosphamide toxicity, 291
cyclosporine toxicity, 291
cystadenocarcinoma
   mucinous, 137
   serous, 137
cystic disease
   dialysis, 126
   uremic medullary, 126
cystic fibrosis, 309, 318
cystine stones, 124
cystitis
   acute, 128
   in children, 313
cysts
   epidermal inclusion, 245
   simple, 126
   skin, 245
   trichilemmal, 245
cytokines, 48
cytomegalovirus (CMV), 45, 280
   congenital, 304

# D

decompensated (progressive) shock, 17
degenerative diseases, 282–87
   brain areas affected, 283
   central nervous system tumors, 287
   demyelinating diseases, 282

degenerative diseases (*continued*)
    incurable dementias, 284
    intracranial tumors, 286
    treatable/curable dementias, 285
delivery
    infection transmission during, 302
dementia, 270
    brain areas affected, 283
    infectious causes of, 285
    multiple infarct, 283, 284
    pellagra-associated, 285
demyelinating diseases, 270, 282
demyelinating polyradiculoneuropathy, acute
    inflammatory, 274
de Quervain thyroiditis. *See* subacute thyroiditis
dermal tumors, 246
dermatitis, 297
    acute allergic contact, 238
    atopic, 238, 310
    chronic allergic contact, 238
dermatitis herpetiformis, 239, 298
dermatofibroma, 246
dermatofibrosarcoma protuberans, 248
dermatomyositis, 253
Dermatophytes, 325
desmoplasia, 18
desquamation syndromes, 243
diabetes mellitus, 53
    antibodies involved, 52
    primary, type 1, 185
    primary, type 2, 185
    secondary, 185
    uncontrolled, 186
diabetic ketoacidosis, 185
diabetic nephropathy, 114
diabetic neuropathy, 273
dialysis cystic disease, 126
diarrhea
    AIDS and, 209

bacterial, 210
chronic, 209
infectious, 209, 312
mechanisms of, 207
diethylstilbestrol, 303
diet-related disorders, 295, 298
diffuse alveolar damage. *See* adult respiratory distress
    syndrome (ARDS)
DiGeorge syndrome, 55
Dilantin, 303
dilated cardiomyopathy, 37
DIP (distal interphalangeal), 249
diphtheric neuropathy, 273
*Diphyllobothrium latum*, 211, 326
dissecting aneurysm, 29
disseminated encephalomyelitis, acute, 282
disseminated intravascular coagulation, 91
distal interphalangeal (DIP), 249
diverticula
    colonic, 200
    esophageal, 195
diverticulitis, 200
diverticulosis, 200
DNA viruses, 327
Döhle bodies, 74
Down syndrome, 314
doxorubicin toxicity, 291
dry beriberi, 297
Dubin-Johnson syndrome, 306
Duchenne muscular dystrophy, 252, 318
ductal carcinoma in situ, 157
ductal hyperplasia, 155
ductal papilloma, 157
duodenal ulcers, 199
dysgerminoma, 136
    pinealoma, 286
dysphagia, 190
dysplasia, 2
dysplastic nevus, 310

dyspnea, 17
dystrophic calcification, 7

## E

EBV (Epstein-Barr virus), 45
ecchymosis, 84
ECG (electrocardiogram), 25
*Echinococcus granulosus*, 224, 326
eclampsia, 159, 228
ectopic ACTH production, 180
ectopic pregnancy, 160
edema
    causes of, 10–11
    defined, 8
    mechanisms of, 12
    pulmonary, 106
    types of, 10–11
Edwards syndrome, 314
Eisenmenger syndrome, 33
electrocardiogram (ECG), 25
ELISA, 46
embolism, 8, 13
embryonal carcinoma, 136
emphysema, 99
    centrilobular, 97, 99
    irregular, 99
    lung morphology and, 97
    panacinar, 97, 99
    paraseptal, 99
empyema, 95
encephalitis, 270, 278
    cerebrospinal fluid analysis, 277
    defined, 271
    slow viral, 280
    viral, 280
encephalomyelitis, acute disseminated, 282
encephalopathy
    hypertensive, 276

Wernicke, 285
endocarditis
  acute infective, 38
  bacterial, 38
  of carcinoid syndrome, 40
  defined, 33
  infective, 38–39
  Libman-Sacks, 40
  nonbacterial thrombotic, 40
  noninfective, 40
  rheumatic fever, 40
  subacute infective, 39
endocrine system
  adrenal disorders, 178–83
  common disorders and causes, 164
  diabetes mellitus, 185, 186
  disease summary, 184
  pancreatic diseases, 185–87
  parathyroid disorders, 176–77
  pituitary disorders, 166–69
  terminology, 165
  thyroid disorders, 170–75
endometrial carcinoma, 146, 149
endometriosis externa, 143, 144
endometriosis interna, 143, 144
endometritis, 143, 144
  acute, 144
  chronic, 144
*Entamoeba*, 324
  *histolytica*, 224
Enterobacteriaceae, 322
*Enterobius*, 326
*Enterococcus*, 320
  *faecalis*, 320
enterocolitis
  invasive, 210
  noninvasive, 324
enteropathic arthropathy, 264
enterotoxin (toxinogenic gastroenteritis)

noninvasive, 210
environmental disorders, 294
enzyme-linked immunosorbent assay (ELISA), 46
enzyme markers, tumors associated with, 20
eosinophilia, 74
eosinophilic granuloma, 83, 248
ependymoma, 286
ephelis, 240
epidermal inclusion cysts, 245
epidermal tumors, 245
epididymitis, 132, 139
epididymo-orchitis, 139
epidural hematoma, 275
epistaxis, 84
epithelial hyperplasia, 155
epithelial tumors, 137
Epstein-Barr virus (EBV), 45
eptifibatide, 90
erosive gastropathy, acute, 197
erysipelas, 241
erythema infectiosum (fifth disease), 311
erythema multiforme, 239
erythema nodosum, 239
erythema toxicum neonatorum, 310
Erythroplasia of Queyrat. *See* squamous carcinoma
  in situ
erythropoiesis, 61
  defined, 59
  extramedullary, 59
  ineffective, 59
  reactive, 60
*Escherichia coli*, 322
esophageal disorders, 195–96
esophageal diverticulum, 195
esophageal squamous cell carcinoma, 196
esophageal varices, 195
esophagitis
  Candida, 196
  reflux, 196

viral, 196
essential hypertension, 33, 43
essential polycythemia, 76
essential thrombocytosis, 76
estrogen, 255
ethanol, 303
ethylene glycol, 290
Ewing sarcoma, 261
exogenous estrogen toxicity, 292
exogenous progestin toxicity, 292
external genital tumors, 135
extradural hematoma. *See* epidural hematoma
extrahepatic biliary ducts, adenocarcinoma of, 233
extramammary Paget disease, 135
extramedullary erythropoiesis, 59
extrinsic allergic alveolitis. *See* pulmonary eosinophilia
exudative generalized edema, 11
exudative localized edema, 10–11
eyes, diabetes mellitus and, 186

# F

Fabry disease, 318
Fallot, tetralogy of, 305
familial adenomatous polyposis, 205
fasciitis, necrotizing, 241
fat, 9
  embolus, 13
  necrosis, 153
fat-soluable vitamin deficiencies, 296
fatty change (steatosis), 4, 215
fatty liver, 227
femoral hernias, 201
FEP (free erythrocyte protoporphyrin), 65
ferritin, 62
fetal alcohol syndrome, 303
fibrinoid, 9
fibrinoid necrosis, 9

fibrinolysis, 84, 90
fibrinous pericarditis, 42
fibroadenoma, 157
fibrocystic breast changes, 132
    defined, 153
    simple, 155
fibroepithelial polyps, 245
fibroma, 267
fibroma-thecoma tumor, 138
fibrosarcoma, 267
fibrous dysplasia, 262
fibrous histiocytoma
    benign, 267
    malignant, 267
fifth disease, 311
first-intention healing, 14
flagellates, 324
flammeus nevus, 310
Flavivirus, 327
fluke, 326
focal segmental glomerulosclerosis, 115
folic acid deficiency, 69, 297
follicle-stimulating hormone (FSH), 131, 169
follicular adenocarcinoma, 175
follicular adenoma, 175
follicular cysts, 145
folliculitis, 241
food poisoning (preformed exotoxin), 210
foreign-body giant cell, 3
fragile blood vessels, 86
fragile X syndrome, 315
freckles, 240
free erythrocyte protoporphyrin (FEP), 65
frostbite, 294
FSH (follicle-stimulating hormone), 131
    deficiency, 169
fungal skin infections, superficial, 243
fungi, 39, 325

furuncles, 241
*Fusobacterium*, 322

## G

GABA (gamma-aminobutyric acid), 269
galactosemia, 229, 298, 318
gallbladder disorders, 232–33
    adenocarcinoma, 233
    cancers, 233
    obstructive diseases, 232
    stones, 214, 232
    tumors, 214, 233
gamma-aminobutyric acid (GABA), 269
gamma-glutamyl transpeptidase (GGTP), 213
gammopathy, monoclonal, 82
ganglion and synovial cyst, 251
ganglioneuromas of oral cavity, 187
gangrene, infectious, 241
gangrenous, 9
Gardner syndrome, 205, 261
Garner duct cyst, 143
gastric adenocarcinoma, 198
gastric lymphoma, 198
gastric ulcers, 197
gastrinoma, 186
gastritis, chronic, 197
gastroenteritis (stomach flu), 209
gastroesophageal reflux (heartburn), 196
gastrointestinal tract, 189–212
    alcohol and, 293
    appendicitis, 212
    common disorders and causes, 190
    diarrhea, 207, 209–10
    diseases in children, 312
    esophageal disorders, 195–96
    intestinal disorders, 199–206
    intestinal infections, 211

malabsorption, 208
    oral cavity disorders, 191–94
    peritoneum disorders, 212
    stomach disorders, 197–98
    terminology, 190
gastropathy, acute erosive, 197
Gaucher disease, 6, 318
genetic causes of disease, 318
genital herpes, 242
genital tumors, external, 135
germ cell tumors, 136
gestational choriocarcinoma, 161
gestational disorders, 159–61
    tumors, 161
GGTP (gamma-glutamyl transpeptidase), 213
GH. *See* growth hormone (GH)
giant cell arteritides, 31
giant cell bone tumor, 258, 261
giant cells
    foreign-body, 3
    Langhans-type, 3
*Giardia*, 324
Gilbert syndrome, 306
gingivitis, acute necrotizing ulcerative, 191
gliomas, 286
    pontine, 286
globin-chain genes, 68
glomangioma (glomus tumor), 32
glomerular deposits, 113
glomerular diseases, 113–17, 121
glomerular nephritis. *See* glomerulonephritis
glomerulonephritis, 110
    acute proliferative poststreptococcal, 116
    chronic, 117
    defined, 111
    membranous, 114
    rapidly progressing, 116
glomus tumor, 32

glossitis, 190, 297
glucagonoma (α-cell tumor), 186
glucose-6-phosphate dehydrogenase (G6PD), 57, 318
glycogen storage diseases, 6, 318
goiters
  nontoxic, 174
  thyroid, 174
  toxic, 174
gonadal tumors, 136–38
gonadotrophs, 166
gonococcal arthritis, 265, 266
gonorrhea, 133
Goodpasture syndrome, 52, 116
gout, 7
gouty arthritis, 264
G6PD (glucose-6-phosphate dehydrogenase), 57, 318
gram-negative organisms, 39, 322
granulation tissue, 14
granuloma
  caseous, 3
  defined, 2
  eosinophilic, 83
  giant cells in, 3
  noncaseating, 3
  pyogenic, 192
granulomatosis, Wegener, 117
granulomatous disease
  chronic, 53
granulomatous mastitis, 153
granulomatous thyroiditis, 173
granulosa cell tumor, 138
granulosa-theca cell tumor, 138
Graves disease, 52, 171
gray baby syndrome, 303
great vessels, transposition of, 305
growth hormone (GH), 163, 166, 167
  deficiency, 169

Guillain-Barré syndrome, 274
gynecologic diseases, 143–52
  abnormal uterine bleeding, 152
  cancer risk factors, incidence, and mortality, 146–47
  cervical carcinoma and Papanicolaou smear classification, 150
  cervical tumors, 148
  menstrual cycle, 151
  ovarian cysts, 145
  terminology, 143
  uterine conditions, 144
  uterine tumors, 149
  vaginal tumors, 148
gynecomastia, 153

# H

Haemophilus
  *ducreyi*, 322
  *influenzae*, 322
hairy leukoplakia, 192
hamartoma, 18. *See also* lipoma
hamartomatous polyps, 204
hand-foot-mouth disease, 311
Hand-Shüller-Christian disease, 83, 248
haptoglobin, 62
Hashimoto thyroiditis, 52, 170, 173
HBcAb (antibody to hepatitis B core antigen), 213, 223
HBeAb (antibody to hepatitis B early antigen), 213, 223
HBeAg (hepatitis B early antigen), 213, 223
HBsAb (antibody to hepatitis B surface antigen), 213, 223
HBsAg (hepatitis B surface antigen), 213, 223
HBV (hepatitis B virus), 213, 222, 223, 304
hCG (human chorionic gonadotropin), 131
Hct (hematocrit), 57, 59

HCV (hepatitis C virus), 213, 222
HDL (high-density lipoprotein), 25, 27
HDV (hepatitis D virus), 213, 222
healing, 14
heartburn (gastroesophageal reflux), 196
heart cells (myocytes), 5
heart diseases. *See* cardiac diseases
heart failure, 33
heatstroke, 294
heavy-chain disease, 82
Heberden's nodes, 263
Heinz body, 59
*Helicobacter pylori*, 322
HELLP, 213
Helminths, 326
hemangioblastoma, 286, 287
hemangioma, 32, 267, 310
  capillary, 32
  cavernous, 32
  hepatic, 231
  strawberry, 310
hemangiosarcoma, 32, 231, 267
hemarthrosis, 84
hematemesis, 84, 195
hematocele, 139
hematochezia, 84
hematocrit (Hct), 57, 59
hematology
  hematopoiesis, 61
  terminology, 59–60
hematoma, 275
  chronic subdural, 275
  defined, 84
  epidural, 275
  subdural, 275
hematopoiesis, 59, 61
hematopoietic disorders, 57, 58
hematuria, 84, 111
hemochromatosis, 7, 229

hemoflagellates, 324
hemoglobin (Hgb), 57
  function, 62
  types of, 67
hemolytic anemias, 71, 72
hemolytic disease of the newborn, 313
hemolytic (iron overload) jaundice, 220
hemolytic-uremic syndrome, 88
hemophilia, 87, 318
  A, 87
  B (Christmas disease), 87
hemoptysis, 84
hemorrhage, subarachnoid, 276
hemorrhagic anemia, acute, 71
hemorrhagic pericarditis, 42
hemorrhagic stroke, 276
hemorrhoids, 200
hemosiderin, 62
hemosiderosis, 7
hemostasis, 84, 90
hemostatic disorders, 84–91
  bleeding disorders, 86
  clotting cascade, 89
  disseminated intravascular coagulation, 91
  hemophilia, 87
  hemostasis system modifiers, 90
  terminology, 84–85
  thrombocytopenia, 88
  Von Willebrand disease, 87
Henoch-Schönlein purpura, 114
hepadnavirus, 327
heparin, 90
hepatic adenoma, 231
hepatic amebiasis, 224
hepatic hemangioma, 231
hepatic steatosis, alcoholic, 227
hepatic tumors, 231
hepatitis
  acute hepatitis B serology, 223

acute viral, 222
alcoholic, 224
anicteric, 222
autoimmune, 225
autoimmune chronic viral, 229
chronic, 214, 225–26
chronic viral, 225, 229
defined, 215
fatty liver, 227
viral, 224
hepatitis A, 222
hepatitis B, 213, 222, 223
  congenital, 304
  recovery from, 223
  serology, 223
hepatitis C, 213, 222
hepatitis D, 213, 222
hepatitis E, 222
hepatobiliary system, 213–33
  common disorders and causes, 214
  fatty liver, 227
  gallbladder disorders, 232–33
  hepatic tumors, 231
  hepatitis, 222–26
  jaundice, 218–21
  liver architecture and necrosis, 216–17
  liver cirrhosis, 229
  liver failure, 228
  liver infections, 224
  pancreatic disorders, 234
  portal hypertension, 230
  terminology, 215
hepatocellular carcinoma, 231
hepatocellular jaundice, 220
hepatoma. See hepatocellular carcinoma
hepatomegaly, 215
hereditary G6PD deficiency, 69
hereditary hemorrhagic telangiectasia, 32, 318

hereditary nephritis. See Alport syndrome
hereditary spherocytosis, 66, 318
hernias, 201
  esophageal, 195
  femoral, 201
  inguinal, 201
  umbilical, 201
herpes genitalis, 133, 242
herpes labialis, 242
herpes simplex virus (HSV), 189, 319
  type 1, 224, 280
  type 2, 224, 280
  type 2 congenital, 304
herpes stomatitis, 191
herpesvirus, 327
herpes zoster (shingles), 242
Hgb. See hemoglobin (Hgb)
high-density lipoprotein (HDL), 25, 27
high grade non-Hodgkin lymphoma, 78
high-pressure hydrocephalus, 277
Hirschsprung disease, 312
histiocytoma, fibrous, 267
Histoplasma, 325
histoplasmosis, 3, 325
HIV. See human immunodeficiency virus (HIV)
hives, 238, 311
HLA (human leukocyte antigen), 45
HMG-CoA (3-hydroxy-3-methylglutaryl coenzyme A), 289
H₂O₂ (hydrogen peroxide), 45
Hodgkin lymphomas, 58, 74, 77
hookworm, 211
hordeolum, 241
Horner syndrome, 107
hospital-acquired pneumonias, 105
Howell-Jolly body, 59
HPV (human papillomavirus), 131, 134
HSV. See herpes simplex virus (HSV)
human chorionic gonadotropin (hCG), 131

human immunodeficiency virus (HIV), 45, 280
  congenital, 304
human leukocyte antigen (HLA), 45
human papillomavirus (HPV), 131, 134
Hunter syndrome, 6, 318
Huntington disease, 284, 318
Hurler syndrome, 6, 318
Hutchinson freckle, 247
hyaline membrane disease, 100, 309
hydatidiform mole, 161
hydrocele, 139
hydrocephalus, 307
  communicating, 277, 307
  high-pressure, 277
  noncommunicating, 277
  normal-pressure, 277, 284
hydrogen peroxide ($H_2O_2$), 45
hydronephrosis, 125
hydrostatic pressure, 12
3-hydroxy-3-methylglutaryl coenzyme A
      (HMG-CoA), 289
hyperacute tissue transplant rejection, 49
hyperaldosteronism, 43
  primary, 181
  secondary, 181
hypercalcemia, 176, 177
hypercholesterolemia, 28, 318
hypercorticoidism
  adrenal, 184
  primary (Cushing disease), 164, 180
  primary adrenal (Addison disease), 164 (*See also*
      Addison disease)
  secondary (Cushing syndrome), 164, 180, 182,
      184
hyperemia (congestion), 8
hyperosmolar nonketonic coma, 185
hyperparathyroidism, 184, 258
  primary, 164, 176, 256
  secondary, 164, 177, 256

hyperplasia, 2
hypersensitivity pneumonitis, 103
hypersensitivity vasculitis, 30, 31
hypertelorism, 314
hypertension
  defined, 33
  essential, 43
  malignant, 43
  portal, 230
  secondary, 43
hypertensive encephalopathy, 276
hyperthyroidism, 174, 184
  clinical signs of, 172
  primary, 164, 171
  secondary, 171
hypertrophic obstructive cardiomyopathy, 37
hypertrophy, 2
hypoalbuminemia, 12
hypocorticoidism
  adrenal, 184
  primary, 179
  secondary, 179
hypoparathyroidism, 176, 184
hypopituitarism, 167, 169, 170
hypoplasia, 2
hypoproliferative anemia, 71
hypoproteinemia, 12
hypothalamic nuclei, 166
hypothyroidism, 170, 174, 184
  clinical signs of, 172
  primary, 164, 170
  secondary, 170
hypovolemic shock, 16
hypoxic cellular injury, 5

I

idiopathic hypertrophic subaortic stenosis, 37
idiopathic pulmonary fibrosis, 103

idiopathic pulmonary hemosiderosis, 103
idiopathic thrombocytopenic purpura, 88
Ig (immunoglobulin), 45
IgA deficiency, 55
IgA nephropathy, 114
immature teratoma, 19
immune complement cascade system, 47
immune components, 54
immune-mediated rashes, 238–39
immunodeficiencies, 53–56
  conditions, 55–56
  by immune component, 54
  inflammatory response failure, 53
  types of, 55–56
immunoglobulin (Ig), 45
immunology
  cytokines, 48
  immune complement cascade system, 47
  MHC antigen type and associated diseases, 48
  terminology, 46
  tissue transplant complications, 49
impetigo, 311
inappropriate ADH secretion, 167
incision, 14
inclusion body myositis, 253
ineffective erythropoiesis, 59
infancy, tumors of, 300. *See also* neonatal diseases
infantile polycystic kidney disease, 126
infarct, 8
infarction
  cerebral, 276
  intestinal, 199
  lacunar, 276
infectious arthritis, 265
infectious diarrhea, 209, 312
infectious gangrene, 241
infectious pathogens, 319–27
  acid-fast organisms, 323
  DNA viruses, 327

infectious pathogens (*continued*)
    fungi, 325
    gram-negative organisms, 322
    gram-positive organisms, 320–21
    Helminths, 326
    intracellular parasites, 323
    RNA viruses, 327
infectious thyroiditis, acute, 173
infective endocarditis
    acute, 38
    bacterial, 38
    subacute, 39
infiltrative diseases, 103
inflammation, 8
inflammatory bowel disease
    Crohn disease, 202, 203
    ulcerative colitis, 202, 203
inflammatory breast conditions, 153
inflammatory carcinoma, 158
inflammatory demyelinating polyradiculoneuropathy, acute, 274
inflammatory esophageal conditions, 196
inflammatory mediators, 10
inflammatory myopathies
    acquired, 253
    inherited, 252
inflammatory response
    acute, 74
    chronic, 74
inguinal hernias, 201
inherited inflammatory myopathies, 252
inherited kidney disease, 110
inherited myopathies, 250
    inflammatory, 252
initiation, 18
insect bits, 243
insulinoma (β-cell tumor), 186
interleukin-1, 48
interleukin-2, 48

interleukin-3, 48
intermediate grade non-Hodgkin lymphoma, 78
interstitial disease, 121
interstitial lung edema, 12
interstitial tumors, 138
intestinal disorders, 199–206
    bowel obstruction, 201
    colon inflammatory diseases, 200
    inflammatory bowel diseases, 202–3
    peptic ulcers, 200
    polyps, 204
    small intestine, 199
    tumors, 205–6
intestinal infarction, 199
intestinal metaplasia, 129
intestinal polyps, 204
intestinal roundworm, 326
intestinal tumors, 205–6
intracellular parasites, 323
intracerebral hemorrhage. *See* hemorrhagic stroke
intracranial tumors, 270
    defined, 271
    distribution of, 286
    primary, 270
intrauterine growth retardation (IUGR), 299
intrauterine infection, 300
intrauterine transmission of congenital infections, 302
intravenous (IV), 213
intussusception, 201
invasive carcinoma
    colloid, 158
    ductal, 158
    lobular, 158
    medullary, 158
    mucinous, 158
    squamous cell, 135
invasive enterocolitis, 210
invasive mole, 161

iodine deficiency, 170
iron-carrying proteins, 62
iron-deficiency anemia, 66
irregular emphysema, 99
irreversible shock, 17
ischemic acute tubular necrosis, 118
ischemic colitis, 200
ischemic heart diseases
    angina pectoris, 35
    defined, 34
    myocardial infarction, 35
islet cell adenoma, 186
Islet cell tumor, 164
isoimmune thrombocytopenia (post-transfusion purpura), 88
isotretinoin, 303
IUGR (intrauterine growth retardation), 299
IV (intravenous), 213

## J

jaundice, 7, 218–21
    categories of, 220
    congenital, 306
    defined, 215
    hemolytic, 220
    hepatocellular, 220
    mechanisms of, 219
    neonatal, 313
    obstructive, 220, 221
    physiologic, 313
jock itch. *See* tinea cruris
joint diseases, 263–65
joint effusion, 10
joint fluid analysis, 266

## K

kala azar, 324

Kaposi sarcoma, 32
Kawasaki disease, 30, 31, 244
Kayser-Fleischer ring, 229
Kearns-Sayre syndrome, 252
keloid, 246
keratoacanthoma, 246
keratosis, seborrheic, 245
kernicterus, 313
kidney disease
    infantile polycystic, 126
    inherited, 110
    medullary sponge, 126
    polycystic adult, 110, 126, 318
kidneys
    lead toxicity and, 293
    size patterns in disease states, 123
    uncontrolled diabetes mellitus and, 186
kidney stones, 124–25
kidney tubular cells, 5
*Klebsiella*, 322
Klinefelter syndrome, 315
Koplik spots, 309
Korsakoff syndrome, 297
Krukenberg tumor, 143
kuru, 281
kwashiorkor, 295

# L

laceration, 14
lactate dehydrogenase (LDH), 1, 25
    defined, 34
    myocyte damage and, 251
lactose intolerance, 298
lactotrophs, 166
lacunar infarction, 276
Lamber-Eaton syndrome, 253
Langerhans cell histiocytosis, 83, 248
Langhans-type giant cell, 3

large cell carcinoma, 107
LDH. *See* lactate dehydrogenase (LDH)
LDL (low-density lipoprotein), 25, 27
lead neuropathy, 274
lead poisoning, 66
lead toxicity, 293
leg edema, 12
*Legionella*, 322
leiomyoma, 149, 267
leiomyosarcoma, 149, 267
*Leishmania donovani*, 324
leishmaniasis, visceral, 324
lentigo, 240
lentigo maligna melanoma, 247
lepromatous leprosy, 241
lepromatous neuropathy, 273
leprosy, 241, 273, 323
*Leptospira*, 224, 324
Leptospirosis, 324
lesions
    breast, 154
    lytic bone, 256
    oral, 190, 191
    pigmented, 240
    sunlight-caused, 240
Letterer-Siwe disease, 83, 248
leukemias
    acute, 81
    childhood, 58
    chronic, 81
    chronic myelomonocytic, 80
    defined, 74
    lymphocytic, 81
    myelocytic, 81
leukemoid reaction, 74
leukocytic disorders, 74–83
    Hodgkin lymphomas, 77
    Langerhans cell histiocytosis, 83
    leukemias, 58, 74, 80, 81

myelodysplastic syndromes, 80
myeloproliferative syndromes, 76
non-Hodgkin lymphomas, 78–79
plasma cell dyscrasias, 82
terminology, 74–75
leukocytosis, 74
leukoencephalopathy, progressive multifocal, 281
leukoplakia, 192
    hairy, 192
    oral, 190, 192
leukopoiesis, 60
Lewy bodies, 284
LH. *See* luteinizing hormone (LH)
Libman-Sacks endocarditis, 40
lice, 243
lines of Zahn, 12
lipid storage diseases, 6
lipoid nephrosis. *See* minimal-charge disease
lipoma, 42, 267
liposarcoma, 267
liquefactive, 9
*Listeria monocytogenes*, 320
lithium, 303
liver
    architecture and necrosis patterns, 216–17
    cells (hepatocytes), 5
    cirrhosis, 215, 227, 229
    disease, 214
    function tests, 215
    infections, 224
    malignancy, 214
    necrosis, 216–17
    primary malignancy, 214
liver failure, 229
    acute, 228
    defined, 215
    of pregnancy, 228
lobar hyperplasia, 155
lobar pneumonias, 94, 105

lobular carcinoma in situ, 157
Löffler syndrome, 103
Lou Gerhrig's disease, 285
lovastatin toxicity, 292
low-density lipoprotein (LDL), 25, 27
lower urinary tract
  diseases, 128
  tumors, 129
low grade non-Hodgkin lymphoma, 78
lung diseases
  abscess, 95
  cancers, 107–8
  distribution, 102
  morphology, 97
  primary cancers, 107–8
  tobacco and, 293
  vascular, 106
lupoid autoimmune cirrhosis, 52
lupus, 238
lupus nephropathy, 115
luteinized follicular cysts, 145
luteinizing hormone (LH), 131, 166
  deficiency, 169
Lyme disease, 265, 273, 278
lymphatic obstruction, 12
lymphocyte depletion Hodgkin lymphoma, 77
lymphocyte predominant Hodgkin lymphoma, 77
lymphocytic leukemias, 81
lymphocytic thyroiditis, subacute, 173
lymphogranuloma venereum, 323
lymphoma, 206
  brain, primary malignant, 287
  defined, 74
  gastric, 198
  Hodgkin, 58
lymphopenia, 54
lymphoreticular disorders, 57, 58
lysosomal storage diseases, 6, 318

Lytic bone lesions, 256

## M

macrocyte, 60
macrocytic anemias, 58
  causes of, 68–69
  hyperchromic, 64
macroglobulinemia, Waldenström, 82
macronodular cirrhosis, 214, 229
major histocompatibility complex (MHC), 45
  associated diseases, 48
  type I diseases, 48
  type II diseases, 48
malabsorption syndromes, 190, 208
malabsorptive diarrhea, 207
*Malassezia*, 325
malignancy, 18
malignancy-related neuropathy, 273
malignant fibrous histiocytoma, 267
malignant hypertension, 43
malignant lymphoma of the brain
  primary, 287
malignant melanoma, 248
malignant nephrosclerosis, 122
malignant tumors
  bone, 250, 261
  central nervous system, 287
  hepatic, 231
  of infancy, 300
  nomenclature, 19
  primary vascular, 32
  renal, 127
  sking, 247–48
  soft tissue, 267
Mallory-Weiss syndrome, 195
malnutrition, 295
marasmus, 295
Marfan syndrome, 318

mastitis
  acute, 153
  chronic, 153
  granulomatous, 153
May-Hegglin anomaly, 75
McArdle syndrome, 6, 318
MCH (mean corpuscular hemoglobin), 64
MCHC (mean corpuscular hemoglobin concentration), 64
MCP (metacarpophalangeal), 249
MCV (mean corpuscular volume), 57, 64
mean corpuscular hemoglobin (MCH), 64
mean corpuscular hemoglobin concentration (MCHC), 64
mean corpuscular volume (MCV), 57, 64
measles, 309
Meckel diverticulum, 312
meconium aspiration, 309
meconium ileus, 309
medial calcific sclerosis (Mönckeberg disease), 28, 30
medullary carcinoma, 175
medullary sponge kidney disease, 126
medullary thyroid carcinoma, 187
medullary tumors, 183
medulloblastoma, 286
megaloblastic anemia, 297
melanocyte-stimulating hormone (MSH), 163, 166, 167, 179
melanoma
  lentigo maligna, 247
  malignant, 248
  superficial spreading, in situ, 247
melasma, 240
melena, 84
membranoproliferative glomerulonephritis, 115
membranous glomerulonephritis, 114
MEN. *See* multiple endocrine neoplasia (MEN) syndromes

meningioma, 286, 287
meningitis, 278
   bacterial, 277, 278
   chronic, 277, 278
   defined, 271
   in infants, 308
   viral, 277, 278
meningomyelocele, 307
menorrhagia, 144
menstrual cycle, 151
mental retardation, 314
mercuric chloride, 290
mesothelioma, 108
metabolic acidosis, 17
metabolic bone disease, 257–58
metacarpophalangeal (MCP), 249
metaplasia, 2
   intestinal, 129
metastasis, 18
metastatic calcification, 7
metastatic tumors, 138
   bone, 261
   central nervous system, 287
   liver malignancy and, 231
metatarsophalangeal (MTP), 249
methanol, 290
methyldopa toxicity, 292
methyl mercury
   congenital diseases and, 303
MHC. *See* major histocompatibility complex
   (MHC)
MI. *See* myocardial infarction (MI)
microcyte, 60
microcytic anemias, 58, 65
   hypochromic, 64
   types of, 66
micrognathia, 314
micronodular cirrhosis, 214, 229
miliary tuberculosis, 105

minimal-charge disease, 114
mites, 243
mitral valve
   regurgitation, 41
   stenosis, 41
mixed cellularity Hodgkin lymphoma, 77
mixed cryoglobulinemia, 31
mixed germ cell neoplasms, 137
moles, 310
   hydatidiform, 161
   invasive, 161
molluscum contagiosum, 242
Mönckeberg disease (medial calcific sclerosis), 28, 30
monoclonal gammopathy of undetermined significance, 82
mononucleosis, 309
monostotic fibrous dysplasia, 262
mosquito bites, 280
MSH. *See* melanocyte-stimulating hormone (MSH)
MTP (metatarsophalangeal), 249
mucinous cystadenocarcinoma, 137
mucinous cystadenoma, 137
mucocele, 192
mucoepidermoid carcinoma, 194
mucosal edema, 11
mucosal erosion, 190
mucosal ulceration, 190
multiple endocrine neoplasia (MEN) syndromes, 163, 165, 187
multiple infarct dementia, 283, 284
multiple myeloma, 82
multiple polyposis syndromes, 205
multiple sclerosis, 282
mumps, 309
mural thrombus, 13
muscular diseases, 252–53
   myopathies, 250, 251, 252–53
   neuromuscular disorders, 253

muscular dystrophy
   Becker, 252
   Duchenne, 252, 318
   myotonic, 252
musculoskeletal system, 249–67
   bone diseases, 254–62
   common disorders and causes, 250
   joint diseases, 263–67
   muscular diseases, 252–53
   proteins and, 251
   terminology, 251
myasthenia gravis, 52, 253
myasthenic syndrome. *See* Lamber-Eaton syndrome
Mycobacterium
   *avium-intracellulare*, 323
   *leprae*, 323
   *tuberculosis*, 96, 323
*Mycoplasma*, 324
mycosis fungoides, 248
myelin figures, 5
myelitis, 279
myelocytic leukemias, 81
myelodysplastic syndromes, 75, 80
myelofibrosis, 76
myeloid cells, 60
myeloma, multiple, 82
myelomonocytic leukemia
   chronic, 80
myelophthisic anemia, 60, 71
myeloproliferative syndromes
   defined, 75
   types of, 76
myocardial infarction (MI), 25, 35
   timetable, 36
myocarditis, 34
myocyte damage, 251
myoglobin
   function, 62
   myocyte damage and, 251

myopathies, 252–53
    acquired inflammatory, 253
    defined, 251
    inherited, 250, 252
    inherited inflammatory, 252
    toxic, 253
myositis
    defined, 251
    inclusion body, 253
myotonic dystrophy, 252
myxoma, 42

# N

NADPH, 45
*Necator,* 326
    *americanus,* 211
necrosis
    acute tubular, 118
    aseptic, 262
    cellular, 5
    defined, 8
    fat, 153
    fibrinoid, 9
    ischemic acute tubular, 118
    liver, 216–17
    nephrotoxic acute tubular, 118
    renal papillary, 119
    tumor necrosis factor-$\alpha$, 48
necrotizing cellulitis, 241
necrotizing fasciitis, 241
necrotizing ulcerative gingivitis, acute, 191
Neisseria
    *gonorrhoeae,* 322
    *meningitidis,* 322
Nelson syndrome, 167
Nematodes, 326
neonatal, 301
neonatal diseases

childhood tumor epidemiology, 316
chromosome abnormalities, 314
gastrointestinal, 312
infections, 308
jaundice, 313
nonspecific signs of infection, 301
rashes and skin lesions, 310–11
respiratory, 309
sepsis, 308
sex chromosome, 315
skin infections, 311
urogenital, 313
neonatal respiratory distress syndrome, 100, 309
neoplasms
    alcohol and, 293
    mixed germ cell, 137
    parathyroid, 187
    pituitary, 187
    tobacco and, 293
neoplastic changes, 18–23
    cancer characteristics, 19
    cancer epidemiology, 21
    malignant and benign tumor nomenclature, 19
    oncogenes and defective tumor suppressor genes,
        20
    paraneoplastic syndromes, 23
    terminology, 18
    tumor and enzyme markers, 20
nephritic-nephrotic syndromes, 115
nephritic syndromes, 111, 116–17
nephritis, tubulointerstitial, 119
nephroblastoma. *See* Wilms tumor
nephrocalcinosis, 120
nephropathies
    defined, 111
    diabetic, 114
    IgA, 114
nephrosclerosis
    benign, 122

malignant, 122
nephrotic syndromes, 110
    defined, 111
    types of, 114
nephrotoxic acute tubular necrosis, 118
nerve tumors, peripheral, 272
nervous system, 269–87
    central nervous system diseases, 275–81
    common disorders and causes, 270
    degenerative diseases, 282–87
    peripheral nervous system diseases, 272–74
    terminology, 271
    uncontrolled diabetes mellitus and, 186
neural tube defects, 307
neuritis, 271
neuroblastoma, 183
neurofibroma, 272
neurofibromatosis, 307
neurogenic shock, 16
neurologic disorders
    alcohol and, 293
    congenital, 307
    lead toxicity and, 293
neuromas, 187
neuromuscular disorders, 253
neuropathies, 271
    peripheral, 273–74
neurosyphilis, 278
neutropenia, 54
neutrophils, 54, 61
nevi, 310
nevocellular nevus, 310
niacin (vitamin $B_3$) deficiency, 297
nickel, 290
nicotinamide adenine dinucleotide phosphate,
    reduced (NADPH), 45
Niemann-Pick disease, 6, 318
nipples, congenital inversion of, 153
*Nocardia,* 321

nodular sclerosis Hodgkin lymphoma, 77
nonbacterial thrombotic endocarditis, 40
noncommunicating hydrocephalus, 277
noncyanotic diseases, 305
non-elastic polyps, 204
nonfunctional adenoma, 167
nongonococcal arthritis, 266
   septic, 265
nongonococcal urethritis, 133
non-HIV-related chronic diarrhea, 209
non-Hodgkin lymphomas, 78–79
noninfective endocarditis, 40
noninvasive enterocolitis, 324
noninvasive enterotoxin (toxinogenic gastroenteritis), 210
nonspecific signs of neonatal infections, 301
nonsteroidal anti-inflammatory drugs (NSAIDs),
   57, 90, 197
   toxicity, 292
nontoxic goiters, 174
nontropical sprue. *See* celiac disease
normal-pressure hydrocephalus, 277, 284
normochromic anemias, 71
   normocytic, 64
nosocomial diarrhea, 209
NSAIDs. *See* nonsteroidal anti-inflammatory drugs
   (NSAIDs)
nutritional disorders, 295–97

# O

oat cell (small cell) carcinoma, 107
obesity, 295
obstructive jaundice, 220, 221
obstructive pulmonary diseases, 95–99
   defined, 95
   emphysema, 97
   terminology, 95–96
   types of, 98–99

$1,25(OH)_2$
   bone metabolism and, 255
oligodendroglioma, 287
oligohydramnios, 160
oliguria, 111
oncogenes, 20
oncotic pressure, 12
onion skinning, 9
opportunistic fungi, 325
opsonin, 46
oral cavity, 190, 191–94
   cancer, 190
   ganglioneuromas of, 187
   growths, 192
   lesions, 190, 191
   salivary gland diseases, 193
   salivary gland tumors, 194
   tumors, 190, 192
oral leukoplakia, 190
oral thrush, 191
orchitis, 132, 139
orthomyxovirus, 327
Osler-Weber-Rendu syndrome, 32
osteitis deformans. *See* Paget disease of bone
osteitis fibrosa cystica. *See* hyperparathyroidism
osteoarthritis, 263
osteoblastoma, 261
osteocartilaginous exostosis, 260
osteochondroma, 260
osteogenesis imperfecta, 257, 318
osteogenic sarcoma, 261
osteomalacia, 257
osteomalacia (rickets), 256
osteomas, 261
osteomyelitis
   acute, 259
   chronic, 259
   defined, 251
   mechanisms of, 260

   pyogenic, 259
osteonecrosis. *See* aseptic necrosis
osteopenia, 251
osteoporosis, 256, 257
osteosarcoma, 261
ovarian cancer, 147
ovarian cysts, 145
oxytocin, 166

# P

Paget disease of bone, 256, 258
Paget disease of breast, 158
panacinar emphysema, 97, 99
Pancoast syndrome, 107
pancreatic adenocarcinoma, 234
pancreatic cells (acinar cells), 5
pancreatic diseases, 185–87, 234
pancreatic islet cell tumors, 186, 187
pancreatitis
   acute, 234
   chronic relapsing, 234
pancytopenia, 54
panencephalitis, subacute sclerosing, 281
panniculitis, 239
pannus, 263
Papanicolaou smear classification, 150
papillary adenocarcinoma, 175
papovavirus, 327
Pappenheimer bodies, 60
*Paracoccidioides*, 325
paracoccidioidomycosis, 325
paradoxical embolus, 13
*Paragonimus*, 326
paramyxovirus, 327
paraneoplastic syndromes
   defined, 18
   types of, 22
paraseptal emphysema, 99

parathyroid adenoma, 176, 177
parathyroid carcinoma, 176
parathyroid gland disorders, 176–77
parathyroid hormone (PTH), 163, 176
    bone diseases and, 256
    bone metabolism and, 255
parathyroid hyperplasia, primary, 177
parathyroid neoplasm, 187
parenchymal storage diseases, 120
Parkinson disease, 284
parotiditis, 193
partial thromboplastin time (PTT), 57
parvovirus B19, 327
Patau syndrome, 314
patent ductus arteriosus, 305
patent foramen ovale, 305
peau d'orange, 158
pediculosis, 243
Pelger-Huët abnormality, 75
pellagra-associated dementia, 285, 297
pelvic inflammatory disease (PID), 131
    acute, 143
    chronic, 143
pemphigoid, bullous, 239
pemphigus vulgaris, 239
penetrating cerebral injuries, 275
penicillin toxicity, 291
penile tumors, 135
peptic ulcers, 199
    duodenal, 199, 200
    gastric, 200
pericardial effusion, 10
pericarditis
    chronic constrictive, 42
    defined, 34
    types of, 42
perinatal period, 46, 301
    AIDS infection, 302
peripheral nervous system diseases

neuropathies, 273–74
    tumors, 272
peritoneal effusion, 11
peritoneal infection, 212
peritoneal tumors, 212
peritoneum, 212
peritonitis, sterile, 212
pernicious anemia, 52, 297
petechia, 84
Peutz-Jeghers syndrome, 205
pharyngitis, 309
phenacetin toxicity, 292
phenylketonuria, 298, 307, 318
phenytoin
    congenital diseases and, 303
    toxicity, 291
pheochromocytoma, 43, 183
    adrenal, 187
phimosis, 139
phosphate
    bone diseases and, 256
    bone metabolism and, 255
Phyllodes tumor, 157
physiologic jaundice, 313
Pick disease, 283, 284
picornavirus, 327
PID. See pelvic inflammatory disease (PID)
pigmented lesions, 240
pigmented tumors, 247
pilar cysts, 245
pinealoma dysgerminoma, 286
pink puffers, 99
pinworm, 326
PIP (proximal interphalangeal), 249
pituitary cachexia, 164
pituitary disorders, 166–69
pituitary hormones, 166
pituitary tumors, 164
    adenomas, 167, 286

neoplasm, 187
    primary, 167
placentae accreta, 159
placental previa, 159
plasma cell dyscrasias, 58, 82
plasma cell mastitis, 153
plasmacytoma, solitary, 82
plasmacytosis, 75
plasminogen, 90
Plasmodium, 324
platelet down-regulators, 90
pleomorphic adenoma, 194
pleural effusion, 11
Plummer-Vinson syndrome, 195
PMN (polymorphonuclear leukocyte), 1, 25, 269
pneumoconioses, 94
    defined, 95
    types of, 101
Pneumocystis, 325
pneumonias
    anaerobic, 105
    aspiration, 105
    atypical, 105
    clinical classification, 105
    community-acquired, 105
    defined, 95
    hospital-acquired, 105
    in infants, 308
    lobar, 105
    pathologic classification, 104
pneumonitis, 95
poikilocytosis, 60
poliomyelitis, 279
polyarteritis nodosa, 30, 52, 117
polycystic kidney disease
    adult, 110, 126, 318
    infantile, 126
polycystic ovary syndrome, 145
polycythemia, 60, 73

polycythemia vera, 76
polyhydramnios, 160
polymorphonuclear leukocyte (PMN), 1, 25, 269
polymyositis, 253
polyostotic fibrous dysplasia, 262
polyps
    adenomatous, 204
    defined, 143
    fibroepithelial, 245
    intestinal, 204
    non-elastic, 204
polyradiculoneuropathy, acute inflammatory demyelinating, 274
polyuria, 111
polyvinyl chloride, 290
Pompe disease, 6, 318
pontine glioma, 286
pores of Kohn, 95
portal hypertension, 230
port-wine stains, 310
posterior pituitary
    hormones, 166
    hyperfunction, 167
postmenopausal osteoporosis. See osteoporosis
postpartum period, 301
poststreptococcal glomerulonephritis
    acute proliferative, 116
post-transfusion purpura (isoimmune thrombocytopenia), 88
Pott disease, 259
poxvirus, 327
preeclampsia, 159, 228
preformed exotoxin (food poisoning), 210
pregnancy
    cholestasis of, 221
    ectopic, 159
    liver failure of, 228
    toxemia of, 159
pregnancy tumor, 192

premalignant skin tumors, 247–48
prenatal period, 301
priapism, 139
primary adrenal hypercorticoidism, 164. See also Addison disease
primary benign tumors
    of bone, 250
    of soft tissue, 250
primary biliary cirrhosis, 52, 221
primary diabetes mellitus, 185
    type 1, 185
    type 2, 185
primary hyperaldosteronism (Conn syndrome), 43, 164, 181
primary hypercorticoidism (Cushing disease), 164, 180
primary hyperparathyroidism, 164, 176, 256
primary hyperthyroidism, 164, 171
primary hypocorticoidism, 179
primary hypoparathyroidism, 164
primary hypothyroidism, 164, 170
primary malignant lymphoma of the brain, 287
primary malignant tumors
    bone, 250
    breast, 132
    liver, 214
    ovarian, 132
primary parathyroid hyperplasia, 177
primary sclerosing cholangitis, 221
primary tuberculosis, 105
primary tumors
    benign uterine, 132
    bone, 260–61
    defined, 18
    heart, 42
    intracranial, 270
    pituitary, 167
    renal, 127
    thyroid, 175

Prinzmetal angina, 35
progressive multifocal leukoencephalopathy, 281
prolactin, 166
prolactinoma, 167
proliferative poststreptococcal glomerulonephritis, acute, 116
promotion, 18
prostacyclin, 90
prostate disorders, 132, 141
    adenocarcinoma, 141, 142
    distribution of, 142
prostatic hyperplasia, benign, 141, 142
prostatitis
    acute, 141
    chronic, 141
    defined, 139
prosthetic valves, 41
proteins
    associated with muscles, 251
    iron-carrying, 62
proteinuria, 111
Proteus, 322
prothrombin time (PT), 57
protozoans, 324
proximal interphalangeal (PIP), 249
pruritus, 215
pseudogout, 264
pseudohypertrophy, 252
Pseudomonas, 259, 322
psoriasis, 238
PT (prothrombin time), 57
PTH. See parathyroid hormone (PTH)
PTT (partial thromboplastin time), 57
pulmonary edema, 106
pulmonary embolism, 13, 106
pulmonary eosinophilia, 103
pulmonary fibrosis, idiopathic, 103
pulmonary hemorrhage, 94

pulmonary hypertension, 94, 106
pulmonary infections, 104–5
pure motor neuropathies, 274
purpura, 85
    Henoch-Schönlein, 114
purulent pericarditis, 42
pyelonephritis, 120, 313
    chronic, 120
pyknosis, 2
pyogenic granuloma, 192
pyogenic osteomyelitis, 259
pyridoxine (vitamin $B_6$) deficiency, 297
    neuropathy, 273
pyuria, 111

# Q

qualitative platelet disorders, 86

# R

rabies virus, 280
radiation exposure, 294
radioallergosorbent test (RIA), 46
rapidly progressing glomerulonephritis, 116
rashes, 238–40
    acute, 238
    in children, 310–11
    chronic, 238–39
Raynaud disease, 29
RBCs. See red blood cell (RBCs)
reactive arthritis (Reiter syndrome), 264
reactive erythropoiesis, 60
reactive thrombocytosis, 75
red blood cells (RBCs), 57
    morphology in anemias, 63
red cell aplasia, 71
reduced nicotinamide adenine dinucleotide phos-
        phate (NADPH), 45

reduced platelet count, 86
reduviid bug, 324
Reed-Sternberg cells, 78
reflux esophagitis, 196
refractory anemia, 80
    with excess blasts, 80
    with excess blasts in transformation, 80
    with ringed sideroblasts, 80
regurgitation
    aortic valve, 41
    mitral valve, 41
Reiter syndrome (reactive arthritis), 264
renal amyloidosis, 114, 120
renal artery stenosis, 122
renal cell carcinoma, 110, 127
renal cystic diseases, 126
renal failure
    acute, 17, 110
    chronic, 110, 177
    defined, 112
renal function tests, 112
renal infarct, 122
renal malignancy
    adult, 110
    childhood, 110
renal papillary necrosis, 119
renal tumors, primary, 127
Rendu-Osler-Weber syndrome, 318
reovirus, 327
reproductive system disorders
    abnormal uterine bleeding, 152
    breast diseases, 153–58
    breast lesions, 154
    breast tumors, 156–58
    cancers in women, 146–47
    cervical carcinoma and Papanicolaou smear clas-
        sification, 150
    cervical tumors, 148
    common types and causes, 132

    external genital tumors, 135
    fibrocystic disease, 155
    gestation diseases, 159–61
    gonadal tumors, 136–38
    gynecologic diseases, 143–52
    inflammatory breast conditions, 153
    menstrual cycle, 151
    ovarian cysts, 145
    prostate disorders, 141–42
    sexually transmitted infections, 133–34
    terminology, 139, 143, 153
    testicular diseases, 140
    urologic diseases, 139–42
    uterine conditions, 144
    uterine tumors, 149
    vaginal tumors, 148
respiratory system diseases, 93–108
    common types and causes, 94
    obstructive pulmonary diseases, 95–99
    pathogens, 322
    pulmonary infections, 104–5
    restrictive lung diseases, 100–103
    vascular disease and tumors, 106–8
restrictive cardiomyopathy, 37
restrictive pulmonary diseases, 100–103
    defined, 96
    distribution in lungs, 102
    infiltrative, 103
    pneumoconioses, 101
    types of, 100
reticulocytes, 61
retrovirus, 327
Reye syndrome, 4, 228
rhabdomyosarcoma, 267
rhabdovirus, 327
rheumatic fever, 34
rheumatic fever endocarditis, 40
rheumatoid arthritis, 51, 52, 263
rheumatoid factor, 263

RIA (radioallergosorbent test), 46
riboflavin (vitamin B$_2$) deficiency, 297
rickets, 256
Rickettsia
    *rickettsii*, 323
    *typhi*, 323
Riedel thyroiditis, 173
ringworm, 243
RNA viruses, 327
roseola virus (roseola infantum), 311
rotor syndrome, 306
Rouleaux formation, 60
roundworms
    intestinal, 326
    zoonotic, 326
rubella
    in children, 311
    congenital, 304, 305

# S

salivary gland diseases, 193
salivary gland tumors, 190, 194
Salmonella
    osteomyelitis, 259
    *typhi*, 211, 322
salpingitis, acute, 143
sand fly, 324
Sandhoff disease, 318
sarcoidosis, 3, 103
sarcoma, 19
scabies, 243
scalded skin syndrome, 244
scarlet fever, 244
scarring, 14
Schilling test, 70
schistocyte, 60
*Schistosoma*, 224, 326
schistosomiasis, 224

schwannoma, 272
    acoustic, 286
SCID (severe combined immunodeficiency disease),
    45, 55
scleroderma (systemic sclerosis), 51
sclerosing adenosis, 155
sclerosing cholangitis, primary, 221
sclerosing panencephalitis, subacute, 281
scurvy, 258
sebaceous cysts, 245
*Seborrheic dermatitis*, 310
seborrheic keratosis, 245
secondary adrenal hypocorticoidism, 164
secondary biliary cirrhosis, 221
secondary diabetes mellitus, 185
secondary hyperaldosteronism, 181
secondary hypercorticoidism (Cushing syndrome),
    164, 180, 184
    clinical signs of, 182
secondary hyperparathyroidism, 164, 177, 256
secondary hypertension, 33, 43
secondary hyperthyroidism, 171
secondary hypocorticoidism, 179
secondary hypothyroidism, 170
secondary (reactivated) tuberculosis, 105
secondary tumor, 18
second-intension healing, 14
seminoma, 136
sensory neuropathies, 273–74
sepsis, neonatal, 308
septal defect
    arterial, 305
    ventricular, 305
septic embolus, 13
septic shock, 16
septum secundum defect, 305
sequestered tissue, 46
serofibrinous pericarditis, 42
serology, 222

seronegative spondyloarthropathies, 264
serous cystadenocarcinoma, 137
serous cystadenoma, 137
serous pericarditis, 42
Sertoli-Leydig tumor, 138
Sertoli tumor, 138
severe combined immunodeficiency disease (SCID),
    45, 55
sex chromosome diseases, 315
sexually transmitted infections, 132, 133–34
SGOT (serum glutamicoxaloacetic transaminase).
    *See* AST (aspartate aminotransferase)
SGPT (serum glutamicpyruvic transaminase). *See*
    ALT (alanine aminotransferase)
shingles, 242
shock
    defined, 16
    stages of, 17
    types of, 16
sialolithiasis, 193
sickle cell, 60
sickle cell anemia, 318
sideroblastic anemias, 66
silicosis, 3, 101
simian crease, 314
Sipple syndrome, 187
Sjögren syndrome, 51, 193
skin, 235–48
    common disorders and causes, 236
    growths, 245–48
    infections, 241–44
    rashes, 238–40
    terminology, 236–37
    uncontrolled diabetes mellitus and, 186
skin cysts, 245
skin infections, 241–44
    arthropod-caused, 243
    bacterial, 241
    childhood, 300

skin infections (*continued*)
　in children, 311
　desquamation syndromes, 243
　superficial fungal, 243
　viral, 242
skin tags, 245
skin tumors
　benign, 245–46
　malignant, 247–48
　premalignant, 247–48
"slapped check" rash, 311
SLE (systemic lupus erythematosus), 25
slow viral encephalitis, 280
slow viruses, 271
small-bowel obstruction, 309
small cell (oat cell) carcinoma, 107
small intestine
　adenocarcinoma, 205
　diseases, 199
　tumors, 199
smoking-related disorders, 293
smudge cell, 75
sodium retention, 12
soft tissue, 251
　tumors, 267
solar keratosis. *See* actinic keratosis
solid tumors, 55
solitary plasmacytoma, 82
somatotrophs, 166
somatotropic adenoma, 167
spermatic cord, torsion of, 140
spermatocele, 139
spherocyte, 60
spherocytosis, hereditary, 66, 318
spider telangiectasia, 32
spina bifida meningocele, 307
spina bifida occulta, 307
spinal cord degeneration
　subacute combined, 285

Spirochetes, 324
Spitz nevus, 310
spondyloarthropathies, seronegative, 264
*Sporothrix*, 325
sporozoa, 324
sprue
　celiac, 298
　nontropical (*See* celiac disease)
　tropical, 208
spur cell anemia, 69
squamous carcinoma in situ, 135
squamous cell carcinoma, 107, 247
　cervical tumors, 148
　esophageal, 196
　lower urinary tract, 129
　oral cavity, 192
　vaginal tumors, 148
squamous papilloma, 245
stable angina, 35
Staphylococcus
　*aureus*, 259, 320
　*epidermidis*, 39, 320
　*saprophyticus*, 320
status asthma, 98
steatosis (fatty change), 4, 215
Stein-Leventhal syndrome. *See* polycystic ovary
　　syndrome
stem cells, 61
stenosis
　aortic valve, 41
　mitral valve, 41
sterile peritonitis, 212
steroid toxicity, 292
Stevens-Johnson syndrome, 239, 244
stillbirth, 304
Still disease, 263
stomach disorders, 197–98
　gastroenteritis (stomach flu), 209
stools, 84

storage diseases, 6–7
strawberry gallbladder, 233
strawberry hemangioma, 310
"strep throat," 309
Streptococcus
　*agalactiae*, 320
　*bovis*, 39, 320
　*pneumoniae*, 320
　*pyogenes*, 320
　*viridans*, 39, 320
streptokinase, 90
streptomycin
　congenital diseases and, 303
　toxicity, 291
stroke, 276
　hemorrhagic, 276
　thrombotic, 276
stromal tumors, 138
*Strongyloides*, 326
struma ovarii, 171
sty, 241
subacute diseases
　combined spinal cord degeneration, 285
　infective endocarditis, 39
　lymphocytic thyroiditis, 173
　sclerosing panencephalitis, 281
　thyroiditis, 173
subarachnoid hemorrhage, 276
subcutaneous edema, 11
subdural hematoma, 275
　acute, 275
　chronic, 275
subendothelial deposits, 113
subendothelial infarction, 35
subepithelial deposits, 113
sulfonamide toxicity, 291
sun exposure, 294
sunlight-caused lesions, 240
superficial fungal skin infections, 243

superficial fungi, 325
superficial spreading melanoma in situ, 247
superior vena cava syndrome, 107
symptomatic lung cancer, 107
synovial sarcoma, 267
synovitis, 251
syphilis, 134, 241
   congenital, 304
syphilitic aneurysm, 29
systemic autoimmune disorders, 51
systemic embolus, 13
systemic fungi, 325
systemic hypertension, 33
systemic lupus erythematosus (SLE), 25, 51
systemic sclerosis (scleroderma), 51

# T

$T_3$ (triiodothyronine), 163
$T_4$ (tryroxine), 163
Taenia
   *saginata*, 326
   *solium*, 326
Takayasu arteritis, 30
talc and silicone (silicosis), 3
tapeworms, 211, 326
target cell, 60
Tay-Sachs disease, 6, 318
TB. *See* tuberculosis
T-cell lymphoma, 79
T cells, 54
TdT (terminal deoxynucleotidyltransferase), 57
telangiectasia, 32
temporal arteritis, 30
teratogens, 300, 301, 303
teratoma, 136
terminal deoxynucleotidyltransferase (TdT), 57
testes, undescended, 140, 313
testicular atrophy, 132, 140

testicular choriocarcinoma, 136
testicular diseases, 140
testicular germ cell tumors, 132
tetanus, 279
tetracycline
   congenital diseases and, 303
   toxicity, 228, 291
tetralogy of Fallot, 305
thalassemias, 66, 68
thalidomide, 303
theca-lutein cysts, 145
therapeutic drug toxicity, 291–92
thiamine (vitamin $B_1$) deficiency, 297
   neuropathy, 273
thrombin time (TT), 57
thromboangiitis obliterans (Buerger disease), 30
thrombocytopenia, 58
   childhood, 58
   types of, 88
thrombocytosis, essential, 76
thrombolysis, 85
thrombolytic medications, 90
thrombomodulin, 90
thrombophlebitis, 12
thromboplastin, 91
thrombosis
   arterial, 12
   defined, 8
   venous, 12
thrombotic embolus, 13
thrombotic stroke, 276
thrombotic thrombocytopenic purpura, 88
thrush, 308
   oral, 191
thyroid disorders, 170–75
   hyperthyroidism (thyrotoxicosis), 171
   hypothyroidism, 170
thyroid goiters, 174
thyroiditis, 164, 173

   acute infectious, 173
   defined, 165
   Hashimoto, 173
   Riedel, 173
   subacute, 173
   subacute lymphocytic, 173
thyroid malignancy, 164
thyroid nodule, 165
thyroid-stimulating hormone (TSH), 163, 166
   deficiency, 169
thyrotoxicosis, 171
thyrotrophs, 166
tick bites, 280
ticlopidine, 90
tinea, 243
tinea capitis, 243
tinea corporis, 243
tinea cruris, 243
tinea pedis, 243
tinea versicolor, 243
tirofiban, 90
tissue and organ injury, 8–13
   edema, 10–12
   embolism, 12
   inflammatory mediators, 10
   terminology, 8–9
   thrombosis, 12
tissue factor, 91
tissue plasminogen activator, 90
tissue transplant rejection
   acute, 49
   chronic, 49
tissue transplants, 49
tobacco-related disorders, 293
togavirus, 327
ToRCHS, 299
torsion of the spermatic cord, 140
toxemia of pregnancy, 159
toxic epidermal necrolysis, 244

toxic goiters, 174
toxic granulation, 75
toxic myopathies, 253
toxic shock syndrome, 244
toxinogenic gastroenteritis (noninvasive enterotoxin), 210
*Toxocara*, 326
*Toxoplasma*, 324
  *gondii*, 304
toxoplasmosis, 279, 304
trabeculae, 256
transferrin, 62
transformation zone, 143
transfusion, 85
transient ischemic attack, 276
transitional cell carcinoma, lower urinary tract,
  129
transmural infarction, 35
transplacental transmission, of congenital infections, 302
transposition of great vessels, 305
transudative edema
  generalized, 11
  localized, 11
traveler's diarrhea, 209
Trematodes, 326
trench mouth (Vincent angina), 191
Treponema
  *pallidum*, 304, 324
trichilemmal cysts, 245
*Trichinella spiralis*, 211, 326
trichinosis, 211, 326
*Trichomonas*, 133, 324
*Trichuris*, 211, 326
triiodothyronine (T$_3$), 163
triple phosphate stones, 124
Trisomy 13, 314
Trisomy 18, 314
Trisomy 21, 314

tropical sprue, 208
truncus arteriosus, 305
Trypanosoma
  *brucei*, 324
  *cruzi*, 324
tryroxine (T$_4$), 163
tsetse fly, 324
TSH. *See* thyroid-stimulating hormone (TSH)
TT (thrombin time), 57
tuberculin reaction, 46
tuberculoid neuropathy, 273
tuberculosis (TB), 1, 3, 25
  of the bones, 259
  defined, 96
  miliary, 105
  primary, 105
  secondary (reactivated), 105
  types of, 105
tuberous sclerosis, 307, 318
tubular adenoma, 204
tubular disease, 121
tubular necrosis
  acute, 118
  ischemic acute, 118
  nephrotoxic acute, 118
tubulointerstitial diseases, 118–25
  kidney size patterns, 123
  kidney stones, 124–25
  types of, 118–20
  urinary tract obstruction, 124–25
  urine sediment assisting diagnosis, 121
  vascular kidney disorders, 122
tubulointerstitial nephritis, 119
  acute, 119
  chronic, 119
tumor embolus, 13
tumor grading, 18
tumor necrosis factor-α, 48
tumors

adrenal, 183
bone, 250, 260–61
central nervous system, 287
childhood, 316
defective tumor suppressor genes and, 20
enzyme markers, 20
external genital, 135
gallbladder, 214
gestational, 161
gonadal, 136–38
hepatic, 231
of infancy, 300
infectious causes of, 22
intestinal, 205–6
intracranial, 286
liver, 214
nomenclature, 19
oral cavity, 192
pancreatic islet, 186
peripheral nerve, 272
primary thyroid, 175
primary vascular, 32
salivary gland, 194
skin, 245–46
soft tissue, 250, 267
tumor staging, 18
tumor suppressor genes
  associated tumors, 20
  defined, 18
Turcot syndrome, 205
Turner syndrome, 315
typhoid fever, 211
typhus fever, 323
Tzanck preparation, 46

## U

ulcerative colitis, 202, 203
ulcerative gingivitis, acute necrotizing, 191

ulcers
    defined, 14
    duodenal, 199, 2000
    gastric, 197, 200
umbilical hernias, 201
unconjugated bilirubin, 219
unconjugated hyperbilirubinemia, 219
unilateral hydronephrosis, 125
unstable angina, 35
uranium, 290
urate nephropathy, 120
*Ureaplasma*, 324
uremia, 112
uremic medullary cystic disease, 126
uremic neuropathy, 273
urethritis
    defined, 112
    nongonococcal, 133
uric acid stones, 124
urinary system, 109–29
    common diseases and causes, 110
    glomerular diseases, 113–17
    lower urinary tract diseases, 128
    lower urinary tract tumors, 129
    renal cystic diseases, 126–27
    terminology, 111–12
    tubulointerstitial diseases, 118–25
urinary tract infections
    in children, 308, 313
    defined, 112
urinary tract obstruction, 124–25
urine sediment assisting diagnosis, 121
urogenital diseases, 313
urologic diseases
    prostate disorders, 141–42
    terminology, 139
    testicular diseases, 140
urticaria (hives), 238, 311
uterine bleeding, 152

uterine conditions, 144
uterine fibroids. *See* leiomyoma
uterine malignancy, 132
uterine tumors, 149

# V

vaginal adenosis, 143
vaginal infection, 132
vaginal tumors, 148
vaginitis, 133
valproic acid
    congenital diseases and, 303
    toxicity, 291
valvular diseases, 41
varicella zoster, congenital, 304
varicocele, 139
varicose veins, 29
vascular diseases, 27–32, 30–31
    aneurysms, 27, 29
    arteriosclerotic disorders, 28
    primary vascular tumors or tumorlike conditions, 32
    terminology, 27
    by vessel size, 30
vascular ectasia, 32
vascular kidney disorders, 122
vascular lung diseases, 106
vascular tumors, 246
vasculitides (vasculitis), 27, 30–31
vasopressin, 166
Venereal Disease Research Laboratory (VDRL), 45
venous stasis, 12
venous thrombosis, 12
ventricular hypertrophy, 34
ventricular septal defect, 305
verrucae vulgaris, 242
verrucous carcinoma, 135
very low-density lipoprotein (VLDL), 25

vesicoureteral reflux, 313
Vibrio
    *cholerae*, 322
    *parahaemolyticus*, 322
villous adenoma, 204
vipoma, 186
viral arthritis, 265
viral diarrhea, 209
viral encephalitis, 280
    arthropod-borne, 280
    slow, 280
viral esophagitis, 196
viral hepatitis, 224
    acute, 222
    autoimmune chronic, 229
    chronic, 225, 229
viral meningitis, 278
    cerebrospinal fluid analysis, 277
viral skin infections, 242
virilization, 165
viruses
    DNA, 327
    RNA, 327
    slow, 271, 280, 281
visceral leishmaniasis, 324
vitamin D
    bone diseases and, 256
    bone metabolism and, 255
    deficiency, 296
vitamin deficiencies, 296–97
    A, 296
    $B_1$, 297
    $B_2$, 297
    $B_3$, 297
    $B_6$, 297
    $B_{12}$, 68, 70, 285, 297
    C, 297
    D, 296
    E, 296

vitamin deficiencies (*continued*)
  fat-soluable vitamins, 296
    K, 296
vitamin deficiency neuropathies
  $B_1$, 273
  $B_6$, 273
  $B_{12}$, 273
vitiligo, 240
VLDL (very low-density lipoprotein), 25
volvulus, 201
Von Gierke disease, 6, 318
von Hippel-Lindau disease, 318
von Recklinghausen disease, 307
von Willebrand disease, 87
von Willebrand factor (vWF), 57
vulvar infection, 132
vulvar tumors, 132, 135

## W

Waldenström macroglobulinemia, 82
warfarin, 90, 303
Warthin tumor, 194

warts, 242
Waterhouse-Friderichsen syndrome, 179
WBCs (white blood cells), 57
Wegener granulomatosis, 30, 31, 117
weight disorders, 295
Wermer syndrome, 187
Wernicke encephalopathy, 285
Wernicke syndrome, 297
Western blot, 46
wet beriberi, 297
Whipple disease, 208
Whipple's triad, 186
whipworm, 211
white blood cells (WBCs), 57
whiteheads, 241
Wilms tumor, 110, 127
Wilson disease, 4, 7, 229
window period, 223
Wiskott-Aldrich syndrome, 55
wound healing
  terminology, 14
  timing of, 15

## X

xanthoma, 246
x-linked agammaglobulinemia, 55
x-linked recessive diseases, 318

## Y

yellow fever, 224
yolk sac carcinoma, 136

## Z

Zenker diverticulum, 195
Zollinger-Ellison syndrome, 186
zoonotic roundworms, 326
*Zygomycetes*, 325